THE FIFTEENTH CENTURY

VOLUME XII

The Fifteenth Century

ISSN 1479–9871

The series aims to provide a forum for the most recent research into the political, social, religious and cultural history of the fifteenth century in Britain and Europe. Contributions for future volumes are welcomed; prospective contributors should consult the guidelines at the end of this volume.

THE FIFTEENTH CENTURY
XII

SOCIETY IN AN AGE OF PLAGUE

Edited by
LINDA CLARK
and
CAROLE RAWCLIFFE

THE BOYDELL PRESS

First published 2013
The Boydell Press, Woodbridge

ISBN 978–1–84383–875–3

The Boydell Press is an imprint of Boydell & Brewer Ltd
PO Box 9, Woodbridge, Suffolk IP12 3DF, UK
and of Boydell & Brewer Inc.
668 Mt Hope Avenue, Rochester, NY 14620–2731, USA
website: www.boydellandbrewer.com

A catalogue record for this title is available
from the British Library

The publisher has no responsibility for the continued existence or accuracy of
URLs for external or third-party internet websites referred to in this book,
and does not guarantee that any content on such websites is,
or will remain, accurate or appropriate

Papers used by Boydell & Brewer Ltd are natural, recyclable products
made from wood grown in sustainable forests

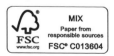

Printed from camera-ready copy supplied by the editor

Printed and bound in Great Britain by
CPI Group (UK) Ltd, Croydon, CR0 4YY

CONTENTS

LIST OF ILLUSTRATIONS

CONTRIBUTORS

J.L Bolton is a Professorial Research Fellow in the School of History at Queen Mary, University of London. His main research interests are in late-medieval international banking, credit and finance; his most recent book is *Money in the Medieval English Economy, 973–1489* (2012).

Elma Brenner is Specialist in Medieval and Early Modern Medicine at the Wellcome Library, London. Her research addresses medical history and religious culture in medieval France, particularly the history of leprosy in Normandy. She is co-editor of *Memory and Commemoration in Medieval Culture* (2013), and *Society and Culture in Medieval Rouen, 911–1300* (2013). She is completing a monograph, *Leprosy and Charity in Rouen, c.1100–c.1400*.

Samuel K. Cohn is Professor of Medieval History at Glasgow University. He has published books and articles on the labouring classes, women, art history, popular piety, political geography, popular protest, and disease, principally in late Medieval and Early Modern Europe. His most recent book is *Popular Protest in Late Medieval English Towns* (2013).

Jane Stevens Crawshaw is a Leverhulme Early Career Research Fellow in History at Oxford Brookes University. She has research interests in the social, medical and environmental history of early modern Italy; her first book, published in 2012, is entitled *Plague Hospitals: Public Health for the City in Early Modern Venice.*

John Henderson is Professor of Italian Renaissance History in the Department of History, Classics and Archaeology, Birkbeck, University of London. He has published a series of books and articles on the social, religious and medical history of medieval and renaissance Tuscany. His most recent book is *The Renaissance Hospital. Healing the Body and Healing the Soul* (1997) and he is at present completing a book on plague in early modern Florence.

Neil Murphy is a lecturer in early modern history at Northumbria University. He has published several articles on the urban history of later medieval and Renaissance France.

Carole Rawcliffe is Professor of Medieval History at the University of East Anglia. She has published several books and articles on medieval medical practice, hospitals and health, including *Leprosy in Medieval England* (2006) and *Urban Bodies: Communal Health in Late Medieval English Towns and Cities* (2013). She has also co-edited a two-volume *History of Norwich* (2004).

Elizabeth Rutledge is an honorary research fellow of the School of History, University of East Anglia. She has published a number of papers on social and economic aspects of medieval Norwich. Her most recent publication is 'The Medieval Jews of Norwich and their Legacy', in *Art, Faith and Place in East Anglia*, ed. T.A. Heslop, Elizabeth Mellings and Margit Thøfner (2012).

Samantha Sagui is a doctoral candidate at Fordham University. Her thesis is entitled 'Law, Order, and the Development of Urban Policing in Late Medieval England'. She is a Fulbright scholar and a recipient of the Schallek Award from the Medieval Academy of America, of the Dissertation Year Travel Grant from the North American Conference for British Studies, and of the Pollard Prize from the Institute of Historical Research.

Karen Smyth is Lecturer in Medieval Literature at the University of East Anglia. Her recent articles have focused on East Anglian authors. She has also published *Imaginings of Time in Lydgate and Hoccleve's Verse* (2011) and co-edited *Medieval Life-Cycles* (2013).

Sheila Sweetinburgh is a Research Fellow at the University of Huddersfield. She has published widely on different aspects of Kent's medieval history. Her most recent edited book is an essay collection entitled *Negotiating the Political in Northern European Urban Society, c.1400–c.1600* (2013).

PREFACE

'Society in an Age of Plague', the theme of the Fifteenth Century Conference of September 2011, and consequently of the present volume of *The Fifteenth Century*, emerged from Carole Rawcliffe's long-held fascination with the history of medicine, and her more recent interest in public health and the ways in which medieval societies responded to the threat of disease. Highlights of the conference, assembled under her expert direction at the University of East Anglia in Norwich, included tours of the Great Hospital (a venue entirely appropriate to the theme) and Dragon Hall, a reception in the Hostry of Norwich Cathedral and dinner in the Cathedral Refectory, all serving to enhance a thoroughly enjoyable and memorable occasion. We would like to express our warm appreciation to everyone involved in the organization of the conference, and extend particular thanks to the Master and staff of the Hospital for giving us a splendid welcome.

Ten of the nineteen papers presented at the conference are published in this present volume, while Samantha Harper's, which examined the fraught relations between Henry VII and the merchant companies of London, appeared in 2012 in volume XI of *The Fifteenth Century*, and Paul Cavill's on James Hobart and the clergy of Norwich diocese was published in the *Journal of Legal History*.

The following papers were also delivered at the conference:

Christopher Bonfield, *Surviving the Plague: Diet, Medical Advice and Regimens of Health, c.1348–1500.*
Philip Caudrey, *Death, War and Memory in Late Medieval East Anglia.*
Trevor Dean, *Plague and Crime in Italy in 1348.*
Hannes Kleineke, *Peasants and Ploughshares: Demonstrations at the Parliament of 1431.*
Christian Liddy, *The Politics of Enclosure in Fifteenth-Century English Towns.*
Edward Powell, *What the Foucault? Diseases and the Body Politic in the Fifteenth Century.*
Carole Rawcliffe, *Plague, Piety and the Provision of Institutional Care in Fifteenth-Century English Towns.*

Linda Clark

ABBREVIATIONS

AN	Archives Nationales, Paris
BIHR	*Bulletin of the Institute of Historical Research*
BJRL	*Bulletin of the John Rylands Library*
BL	British Library, London
BNF	Bibliothèque Nationale de France, Paris
Bodl.	Bodleian Library, Oxford
Cal. Inq. Misc.	*Calendar of Inquisitions Miscellaneous*
CChR	*Calendar of Charter Rolls*
CCR	*Calendar of Close Rolls*
CFR	*Calendar of Fine Rolls*
CIPM	*Calendar of Inquisitions Post Mortem*
CP	G.E. Cokayne, *The Complete Peerage of England, Scotland, Ireland, Great Britain and the United Kingdom*, ed. V. Gibbs *et al.* (12 vols., 1910–59)
CPL	*Calendar of Papal Registers. Papal Letters*
CPR	*Calendar of Patent Rolls*
EcHR	*Economic History Review*
EETS	Early English Text Society
EHR	*English Historical Review*
Foedera	Thomas Rymer, *Foedera, Conventiones, Literae, et Cujuscunque Generis Acta Publica* (20 vols., 1704–32)
HMC	Historical Manuscripts Commission
HR	*Historical Research*
Oxford DNB	*Oxford Dictionary of National Biography from the Earliest Times to the Year 2000*, ed. H.C.G. Matthew and Brian Harrison (61 vols., Oxford, 2004)
PCC	Prerogative Court of Canterbury
PPC	*Proceedings and Ordinances of the Privy Council of England*, ed. N.H. Nicolas (7 vols., 1834–7)
PROME	*Parliament Rolls of Medieval England, 1275–1504*, ed. Chris Given-Wilson *et al.* (16 vols., Woodbridge, 2005)
RO	Record Office
Rot. Parl.	*Rotuli Parliamentorum* (6 vols., 1767–77)
RS	Rolls Series
Statutes	*Statutes of the Realm* (11 vols., 1810–28)
TNA	The National Archives, Kew
TRHS	*Transactions of the Royal Historical Society*
VCH	*Victoria County History*

Unless stated otherwise, the place of publication of books cited is London.

INTRODUCTION

Carole Rawcliffe

> At first the sky weighed down upon the earth,
> Black and unbroken, and the clouds shut in
> Exhausting heat. Four times the crescent moon
> Filled her round orb, four times from her full orb
> She shrank and waned, and all that weary while
> The hot south wind blew furnace blasts of death.
> The vile infection spread, as all agree,
> Through springs and pools ...
> The doom weighed heavier as the plague attacked
> The wretched farmfolk and gained mastery
> Within the city walls.[1]

Ovid's description of the punishment inflicted upon the people of Aegina by Juno, in a fit of pique because they named their city after her rival for Jupiter's affections, ranks, along with Thucydides' celebrated account of the Athenian plague of 430–26 BC, as one of the great set-piece descriptions of pestilence. It has been regarded as a 'prototype' for an emerging genre that eventually gave rise to Defoe's *Journal of the Plague Year*,[2] and it clearly made a profound impression upon the monastic chronicler, Thomas Walsingham. He refers to the 'furnace blasts of death' borne on southerly winds when recording the devastating effects of the 1407 plague upon the people of London, 30,000 of whom reputedly died during what was to become a national epidemic.[3] Independent evidence suggests that this 'deadly plague' did, indeed, cause widespread mortality,[4] although, like many other fifteenth-century outbreaks, it has received considerably less attention than those of the late fourteenth century and early modern period. For many historians, visitations of pestilence seem by this point to have receded into the background as a familiar, but no longer newsworthy, part of late medieval life.

---

[1] Ovid, *Metamorphoses*, trans. A.D. Melville (Oxford, 1986), 160–1.

[2] *Ibid.*, 418.

[3] Thomas Walsingham, *Historia Anglicana*, ed. H.T. Riley (2 vols., Rolls Series, xxviii, 1863–4), ii. 276.

[4] In October the law courts at Westminster were adjourned because plague was spreading: *CCR, 1405–9*, p. 297. See also, Pamela Nightingale, 'Some New Evidence of Crises and Trends of Mortality in Late Medieval England', *Past and Present*, clxxxvii (2005), 33–68, on p. 48, for the suggestion that plague may have been endemic in 1406, too.

It is certainly true that from the 1400s onwards, plague became an increasingly localised phenomenon, striking more often at an urban or regional level, although this development rendered it no less disruptive or terrifying to the unfortunates caught in its path.[5] The wealth of documentary sources for the English capital (which inevitably attracted the attention of travellers from abroad, as well as the government at home) enables us to compile a particularly full, although still probably incomplete, list of epidemics in the London area, which numbered at least twenty-four between 1400 and 1530, in addition to around thirteen national, or at least very widespread, ones during which it was nearly always badly affected.[6] As several contributors to this volume point out, recurrent (and in the case of Venice almost annual) outbreaks of infectious disease had become the norm in the commercial centres of fifteenth-century Europe: pestilence struck on average once every decade in Canterbury, Florence, Ragusa (Dubrovnik), and Siena, and also in many northern French cities, such as Rouen.[7] Although, as we shall see, both personal and collective responses to these events were predicated upon certain common, and in many cases long-established, assumptions about the nature of physical and spiritual health, considerable variation occurred across the geographical spectrum, not simply between northern and southern Europe, but from one area or even town to another. By drawing together case studies from England, France and Italy it has been possible to highlight similarities and differences in approach, while also presenting the most recent research by medical, social and literary historians in an interdisciplinary context. Not surprisingly, the papers offered here challenge many preconceptions about strategies for coping with plague and the other infectious diseases that earned the long fifteenth century its unenviable sobriquet as 'the golden age of bacteria'.[8] The presumed conflict between medical professionals and urban magistrates over the aetiology and best means of combating epidemics is, for example, shown to have little, if any, basis in fact, while the involvement of lower status individuals in the business of municipal government testifies to the spread of administrative expertise and medical knowledge far beyond the ranks of the ruling elite. First of all, however, we address the contentious issue of what actually caused the Black Death and the successive waves of pestilence that persisted, in some parts of Europe, until the Napoleonic Wars, together constituting the second great plague pandemic of the Christian era.

---

[5]   Jim Bolton, '"The World Upside Down": Plague as an Agent of Economic and Social Change', in *The Black Death in England*, ed. W.M. Ormrod and P.G. Lindley (Stamford, 1996), 32; J.M.W. Bean, 'Plague, Population and Economic Decline in England during the Later Middle Ages', *EcHR*, 2nd series, xv (1963), 423–37, on p. 430; John Hatcher, 'Mortality in the Fifteenth Century: Some New Evidence', *ibid.*, xxxix (1986), 19–38, on p. 36.

[6]   Carole Rawcliffe, *Urban Bodies: Communal Health in Late Medieval English Towns and Cities* (Woodbridge, 2013), ch. 2 and Appendix.

[7]   In 1423 the Venetian senate noted that outbreaks were there occurring almost every year; and, indeed, 88 such 'pestilences' are recorded during the 15th century: R.J. Palmer, 'The Control of Plague in Venice and Northern Italy, 1348–1600' (Univ. of Kent Ph.D. thesis, 1978), 49–50. For Canterbury, see below, pp. 60–1; Florence, p. 179; Ragusa, p. 161; Siena, p. 204; Rouen, p. 126; and northern France in general, p. 158.

[8]   Sylvia Thrupp, 'The Problem of Replacement Rates in the Late Medieval English Population', *EconHR*, 2nd series, xviii (1965–6), 101–19, on p. 118.

Late medieval men and women generally ascribed these brutal onslaughts to divine wrath, discharged through the medium of malignant planetary forces, while at the same time blaming more immediate – and potentially more manageable – factors, such as poor diet, corrupt air and contact with infected persons.[9] Historians, by contrast, have found it far harder to reach a consensus framed in the language of modern bio-medicine, in some cases questioning the received orthodoxy that 'medieval' plague and the third major pandemic of the late nineteenth and early twentieth century were identical diseases.[10] Retrospective diagnosis can, of course, be fraught with difficulties, but several aspects of this lively, often acrimonious, exchange have recently been settled in the laboratory.[11] Thanks to the increasingly reliable and sophisticated techniques devised by molecular biologists and geneticists for testing samples derived from the teeth of medieval plague suspects, there can now be little doubt that *Yersinia pestis* was, indeed, the pathogen responsible for both pandemics. Yet it is also clear that the Black Death was spread by a different, previously unknown strain of the bacterium, which, given its remarkable speed of transmission, must have been carried by a different vector from the infamous black rat and its engorged fleas. Significantly, it also seems to have survived undisturbed for long periods in the soil and among a variety of wild and domesticated animals in both town and country.

These exciting developments are examined at the start of this volume by J.L. Bolton and at the end by Samuel Cohn, each of whom stress the important contribution that historians, as well as scientists, can make to on-going attempts to discover exactly how medieval plague may have been transmitted and why it proved so unusually lethal. Cohn's analysis of documentary sources from the later fourteenth and fifteenth centuries emphasises the many other factors, such as seasonality, patterns of recurrence, levels of immunity and recorded symptoms, that set 'the Black Death disease' apart from modern plague. The dependence between disciplines is, however, reciprocal, for, as Bolton observes, an awareness of advances in the field of microbiology is equally – if not more – valuable to students of history. It enables us, for instance, to explain the high mortality rates among young men, so often noted by contemporary chroniclers, and also to account for the existence of plague 'reservoirs', or specific places where the disease remained endemic for long periods. Whereas Bolton favours the suggestion that human fleas and more probably lice may have been the principal facilitators of rapid, person-to-person communication, Cohn queries the need for any insect vector, arguing instead that genetic changes in the ancestral strain of *Yersinia pestis* may have produced a pathogen that spread far more quickly and effectively through contaminated food and water.

Whatever the eventual outcome of this debate, it underscores the fact that the Black Death of 1346–53 was not only 'the greatest disaster in documented human

---

[9] From a copious literature on this topic, see Jon Arrizabalaga, 'Facing the Black Death: Perceptions and Reactions of University Medical Practitioners', in *Practical Medicine from Salerno to the Black Death,* ed. Luis García-Ballester *et al.* (Cambridge, 1994), 237–88; and *The Black Death*, ed. Rosemary Horrox (Manchester, 1995), chs. 3 and 4.

[10] See J.L. Bolton's paper, below, p. 16, for a summary of the various suggestions advanced.

[11] L.K. Little, 'Plague Historians in Lab Coats', *Past and Present*, ccxiii (2011), 267–90.

history',[12] but also the first in a long series of recurrent epidemics, the cumulative effects of which have yet to be fully evaluated and understood. Fear of *mors improvisa*, or sudden death, which might strike its victim at any moment without warning, was naturally widespread in a society so preoccupied with the frailty of the body and the need to prepare for the life to come. So too was a tendency to personify this unwelcome but irresistible visitor. The flourishing culture of the macabre (as reflected in the popularity of images of the Three Living and the Three Dead and of the Dance of Death) has often been regarded as an artistic expression of these anxieties; and although both the chronology and geographical distribution of examples defy any simple mono-causal explanation, there can be little doubt that the shadow of plague loomed over many of them.[13] Focusing upon verses composed in the 1420s by the Benedictine monk, John Lydgate, on the theme of the Dance, Karen Smyth detects a significant change in writing about mortality at this time, as the resigned acceptance of earlier periods gave way to a heightened consciousness of the unpredictable and arbitrary hand of fate. It is hardly coincidental that the Wheel of Fortune became such a common *topos* during the fifteenth century, or that Death's weapon of choice should be 'pestilence'. Significantly, too, these verses served as a vehicle for social criticism and subversion, developing themes familiar from contemporary estates satire, such as the perceived failings of newly appointed clergymen who lacked the moral and intellectual calibre to fill the many livings made vacant by plague.

Even so, beneath this superficial comedy of manners lies a powerful subtext on the theme of penance.[14] Clearly reflecting the psychological strain of 'living constantly in the face of random and indiscriminate death', the Dance offers a salutary lesson to the perceptive reader, who is urged to be prepared at all times for his or her summons.[15] Pilgrimage, which promised a dramatic improvement in spiritual, if not always physical, health, was an obvious step in the right direction, being officially recognised as a prophylactic against plague by Church and State alike.[16] Given the proliferation of holy images and miraculous relics in later medieval England, it might be assumed that the older and less currently fashionable shrines, such as that of St. Thomas Becket at Canterbury, would decline in popularity. Yet, as Sheila Sweetinburgh reveals, the martyr retained much of his earlier appeal, especially in times of crisis and during jubilees, when generous indulgences were available to speed the soul of the repentant pilgrim through purgatory. If the fears of an impending apocalypse that drew so many people to Canterbury in the decades following the Black Death had begun to recede, the Four Horsemen who heralded its arrival still remained behind to harass

---

[12] Mark Bailey, 'Introduction: England in the Age of the Black Death', in *Town and Countryside in the Age of the Black Death. Essays in Honour of John Hatcher*, ed. Mark Bailey and S.H. Rigby (Turnhout, 2012), p. xx.

[13] See Paul Binski, *Medieval Death* (1996), ch. 3. In John Aberth's words, the Dance of Death 'tapped into the mixed and complex responses to widespread mortality, becoming especially a pictorial and poetic summation of the plague': *From the Brink of the Apocalypse: Confronting Famine, War, Plague and Death in the Later Middle Ages* (London and New York, 2001), 206–7.

[14] Binski, *Medieval Death*, 155, 157.

[15] Below, p. 43.

[16] *The Black Death*, ed. Horrox, 26, 54, 82, 96, 97, 148–9. Pilgrimage was so popular, both for protection against plague and as an excuse for vagrancy, that additions to the Statute of Labourers made in 1388 insisted that working people should have written permission to go on one: *ibid.*, 323.

and intimidate anxious Christians. The chronicle of John Stone, a Benedictine monk from Christ Church priory, brings vividly to life the desperation with which members of his own community enlisted the support of healing saints during the plagues of 1457 and 1471.

There was, on the other hand, a hard-headed commercial element to the pilgrimage trade, which involved the active promotion of what might today be described as 'religious tourism' by the ecclesiastical authorities and townsfolk of Canterbury. It is worth stressing that their strategy hinged upon the provision of clean, well paved streets, wholesome food, a salubrious environment and attractive accommodation for visitors who were reluctant to risk their physical health in potentially lethal surroundings. While accepting that plague was ultimately an act of divine retribution, the rulers of late medieval towns and cities recognised that practical steps could be taken to deflect the arrows of pestilence. For this reason, they often adopted a dual approach that dealt simultaneously with sources of spiritual and physical infection. Orders promulgated in Leicester during the pestilence of 1467, for instance, targeted not only 'fylthe and swepynges' and other 'corrupcion in the strettes', but also the brothels, bawds and general misbehaviour that spread a moral miasma through the town.[17] Nevertheless, the assumption, so evident in the writing of Victorian sanitary reformers, that late medieval men and women remained supine in the face of epidemic disease, and that their only response lay in prayer and penitence, still lingers on today among academics, as well as writers for the popular market.[18] Ole Benedictow has, indeed, recently argued that the dramatic shift from a 'high pressure' to a 'low pressure' model of human population across northern Europe during the sixteenth century can best be explained in terms of the first stirrings of medical progress. In other words, numbers began to rise as pragmatism triumphed over superstition:

> It is evident that a key factor in this transition was the great change in the understanding of infectious diseases which began at the end of the fifteenth century (or perhaps slightly later). Now, instead of simply being fatalistically comprehended as a divine punishment for human sin, communicable disease began to be seen as a natural phenomenon, one that could be prevented, limited or halted by human counter measures, even though the transmission of diseases was still understood in terms of the classical notion of miasma.[19]

---

[17] *Records of the Borough of Leicester, II, 1327–1509*, ed. Mary Bateson (1901), 290–1. The closure of brothels performed a sanitary function, too, since sexual activity was discouraged in plague time. It was believed that, by raising the temperature, coitus would open the pores to noxious air, while also undermining the body's natural ability to combat infection: *The Liber de diversis medicinis*, ed. M.S. Ogden (EETS, original series, ccvii, 1938), 51 ('*Et super omnia alia nocet coitus & accelerat ad hunc morbum quod maxime aperit poros et destruit spiritus vitales*'); Christiane Nockels Fabbri, 'Continuity and Change in Late Medieval Plague Medicine' (Univ. of Yale Ph.D. thesis, 2006), 55–6.

[18] Rawcliffe, *Urban Bodies*, ch. 1.

[19] Ole Benedictow, 'New Perspectives in Medieval Demography: The Medieval Demographic System', in *Town and Countryside*, ed. Bailey and Rigby, 33. Significantly, in this context, when cholera reached Britain in 1831, the government's first response was to institute a 'Day of Fasting and Humiliation': Judith Flanders, *Victorian City: Everyday Life in Dickens' London* (2012), 213.

Research in the field of medieval environmental history demonstrates, by contrast, that however limited their technological and financial resources may have been, fifteenth-century magistrates adopted a proactive stance in matters of communal health.[20] Nor did they lack advice about the best means of preserving it. Bearing in mind that John Lydgate (like many other religious) was himself the author of a vernacular guide to the dietary and sanitary precautions necessary for avoiding plague, we should note the profusion of accessible self-help literature aimed at the educated laity throughout Europe.[21] As soon as the Black Death struck, members of the medical profession began to produce *consilia*, or advice manuals, for the benefit of heads of state and civic officials, as well as the general public.[22] One such was, indeed, sent by the 'masters and doctors of Oxford' to the mayor of London during the above-mentioned epidemic of 1407, perhaps at his request and evidently to widespread popular approval.[23] By this date, the Corporation had already mounted a systematic campaign for the removal of insanitary nuisances. The number of orders for cleansing the streets and water courses of noxious waste recorded in the official Letter Books increased fourfold from just sixteen between 1300 and 1349 to at least sixty-five during the second half of the century. Since the population fell by at least half during this period, and consequently generated far less refuse, these measures should have effected significant improvements. They were followed by several decades of sustained investment to the tune of at least £5,000 in the renewal and extension of the city's water pipes and conduits.[24] Lydgate, whose curiosity extended to hydraulics as well as medicine, paints an idealised picture of these costly public works in an encomium to the ancient city of Troy.[25] Elaborating, at considerable length, on the efficacy of the drainage system instituted by King Priam, he explains how river water was ingeniously diverted

> Thorugh condut pipis, large & wyde with-al,
> By certeyn meatis [channels] artificial,
> That it made a ful purgacioun
> Of al ordure & flythes in the toun,
> Waschyng the stretys as thei stod a rowe,
> And the goteris in the erthe lowe,
> That in the cite was no filthe sene ...
> So couertly euery thing was cured [hidden].

[20] For a survey of current literature, see R.J. Magnusson, 'Medieval Urban Environmental History', *History Compass*, xi (3) (2013), 189–200; and Guy Geltner, 'Public Health and the Pre-Modern City: A Research Agenda', *ibid.*, x (3) (2012), 231–45.

[21] *The Minor Poems of John Lydgate, Part II, Secular Poems*, ed. H.N. MacCracken and Merriam Sherwood (EETS, original series, cxlii, 1934, reprinted 1961), 702–7; and below, pp. 48–9.

[22] Arrizabalaga, 'Facing the Black Death', 237–88.

[23] BL, Sloane MS 3285, ff. 68–70. This Latin text was based on John of Burgundy's widely disseminated treatise of 1368: D.W. Singer and Annie Anderson, *Catalogue of Latin and Vernacular Plague Texts in Great Britain and Eire in Manuscripts Written before the Sixteenth Century* (1950), 27–8.

[24] Carole Rawcliffe, 'Sources for the Study of Public Health in the Medieval City', in *Understanding Medieval Primary Sources*, ed. J.T. Rosenthal (New York and London, 2012), 183; C.M. Barron, *London in the Later Middle Ages: Government and People, 1200–1500* (Oxford, 2004), ch. 10.

[25] According to Sylvia Federico, London was known as 'New Troy' at this time: *New Troy: Fantasies of Empire in the Late Middle Ages* (Minneapolis, Minn., 2003), ch. 1.

Wher-by the toun was outterly assured
From engenderyng of al corrupcioun,
From wikked eyr & from infeccioun,
That causyn ofte by her violence
Mortalite and gret pestilence.[26]

As this evidence reveals, throughout the later Middle Ages and beyond, assumptions about collective as well as individual health were profoundly influenced by Ancient Greek beliefs concerning the holistic relationship between man (the microcosm) and his surroundings (the macrocosm).[27] Through the proper management of a variety of external factors, of which air, food and water were the most important, it would be possible to protect both the human and urban body from disease. Conversely, however, such notorious hazards as 'wikked' or polluted air, contaminated meat and stagnant ponds and rivers could easily give rise to epidemics.[28] The 'central irony' of this concept has been neatly encapsulated by Charles Rosenberg, who observes that 'everything necessary to life was at the same time an occasion of vulnerability'.[29] In other words, magistrates were pitted in an unending battle to safeguard their communities against environmental threats that were difficult, if not sometimes impossible, to overcome. Their struggle can be documented particularly well in Norwich, whose remarkably full late medieval records, surviving infrastructure and archaeological resources offer an unusual insight into the challenge of bridging the gap between rhetoric and reality.

Not surprisingly, given its heavy losses during the Black Death and subsequent plagues, Norwich possessed at last one version of the Dance of Death, which was painted on glass in the parish church of St. Andrew at the start of the sixteenth century, thanks in part to a generous bequest by the former mayor, Robert Gardener.[30] The latter was posthumously celebrated as a champion of public works which served to beautify the city, but, as Elizabeth Rutledge demonstrates, the day to day experience of life within the massive flint walls did not always accord with official propaganda. (It is interesting to reflect that, in 1783, campaigners for sanitary reform described these very walls as 'a nuisance that smells rank in the nose of modern improvement' because they impeded the free flow of invigorating

---

[26] *Lydgate's Troy Book, Part I*, ed. Henry Bergen (EETS, extra series, xcvii, 1906), book ii. 166, lines 747–64. See also, Paul Strohm, 'Sovereignty and Sewage', in *Lydgate Matters: Poetry and Material Culture in the Fifteenth Century*, ed. L.H. Cooper and Andrea Denny-Brown (New York, 2007), 60–1. Lydgate's 'Dietary and Doctrine for Pestilence' also warned the reader to 'flee wikkyd heires [air]' and to 'eschew the presence off infect placys, causyng the violence': *The Minor Poems*, ed. MacCracken, 702.

[27] In other words, 'a human body is conceivable only in relation to its physical, social and moral surroundings': Luis García-Ballester, 'The Construction of a New Form of Learning and Practicing Medicine in Medieval Latin Europe', *Science in Context*, viii (no. 1) (1995), 75–102, on p. 88.

[28] For a more detailed discussion, see Rawcliffe, *Urban Bodies*, chs 3, 4 and 5; and for the tenacity of these ideas Andrew Wear, 'Making Sense of Health and the Environment in Early Modern England', in *Medicine and Society: Historical Essays*, ed. *idem* (Cambridge, 1992), 119–47.

[29] C.E. Rosenberg, 'Epilogue: Airs, Waters, Places. A Status Report', *Bulletin of the History of Medicine*, lxxxvi (4) (2012), 661–70, on p. 662.

[30] See the plate on p. 56, below; and Rawcliffe, *Urban Bodies*, Conclusion.

air from the countryside.)[31] Reinforcing Rosenberg's observation that, from a medieval perspective, 'geography was, in a sense, destiny',[32] she documents the struggle waged by members of the ruling elite to render a problematic urban landscape more salubrious and tractable. Notwithstanding their strenuous efforts to implement a wide range of health measures for the entire community, social status – or more accurately personal wealth – would often determine how far a resident might actually enjoy the benefits of fresh water, clean air, effective sanitation and green space. Ready access to these staples of the late medieval *regimen sanitatis* was not available to all, for even the greenest and most commodious of English cities could seem both claustrophobic and polluted to those who were obliged to live on the breadline in cramped lodgings.

Although by the fifteenth century plague was increasingly seen as a disease of the young and the poor, urban magistrates (or at least those who remained behind during epidemics) also suffered heavy losses. The replacement of seasoned office-holders by inexperienced newcomers with scant regard for authority could have serious political ramifications. At the most basic level, administrative continuity was hard to maintain in a society which still relied heavily upon collective memory for the transmission and implementation of civic custom. The *Liber Albus* (White Book) of London, which lists many 'ancient' regulations for the avoidance of environmental problems, was compiled in 1419 specifically because 'all the aged, most experienced and most discreet' aldermen had been 'carried off at the same instant, as it were, by pestilence'.[33] Being deprived of this repository of knowledge, the author notes, 'younger persons who have succeeded them in the government of the City, have on various occasions been often at a loss from the very want of written information; the result of which has repeatedly been disputes and perplexity among them as to the decisions which they should give'.[34] What began as wrangling over the interpretation of 'verbal traditions (*oracula*) not founded on the solid basis of clear conscience' could easily degenerate into conflict between surviving members of the old guard and ambitious parvenus of lower status, as happened in the plague-stricken cities of Shrewsbury in the 1360s and Lincoln in the 1390s.[35]

An effective way of containing such 'grievous debates and dissensions' was to allow lesser ranking citizens a modest share of political power through membership of consultative bodies and involvement in administration at ward or parochial level. As urban government grew more complex, not least with regard to

[31] *The Norwich Directory: Or Gentlemen and Tradesmen's Assistant* (Norwich, 1783, reprinted 1983), pp. iii–vi, presents a catalogue of 'Hints for Public Improvements' based on the Hippocratic concept of health.

[32] Rosenberg, 'Epilogue', 662.

[33] It is unclear which epidemic was responsible for culling the ranks of the elite, but in both 1417 and 1418 death rates among creditors whose loans were registered under the Statute Merchant rose to crisis level (Nightingale, 'Some New Evidence', 48), and we know that Canterbury was struck by 'acute plague' in 1418 (*John Stone's Chronicle, Christ Church Priory, Canterbury, 1417–1472*, selected, trans. and intro. Meriel Connor (Kalamazoo, Mich., 2010), 56).

[34] *Liber Albus: The White Book of the City of London*, ed. H.T. Riley (1861), 3.

[35] *CPR*, 1391–6, pp. 355–6; Stephen Rigby, 'Urban "Oligarchy" in Late Medieval England', in *Towns and Townspeople in the Fifteenth Century*, ed. J.A.F. Thomson (Gloucester, 1988), 65–6; *CPR*, 1358–62, p. 539; Hugh Owen and J.B. Blakeway, *A History of Shrewsbury* (2 vols., 1825), i. 167–72.

the enforcement of sanitary regulations, so the opportunities for participation increased. Beyond suggesting that service as a constable, searcher or some other 'mid-ranking' officer formed part of the conventional *cursus honorum* of civic life, historians have paid little attention to the occupants of these posts, rarely subjecting them to detailed prosopographical analysis in their own right. Samantha Sagui's study of the 651 individuals known to have held constableships and similar offices in Norwich between 1414 and 1473 demonstrates that, contrary to perceived wisdom, many of these men nursed few greater political ambitions, being either reluctant or unable to rise further in the hierarchy. Indeed, by according practitioners of less socially acceptable crafts and trades, such as leather-working, butchery and weaving (some of whom may not even have been freemen), a role in policing their communities, it was possible to engender a much-needed sense of cohesion between the aldermanic class and the 'middling' folk who carried much of the burden of routine civic business. Norwich may have been 'hevyly voysed for lak of good and vertuous governaunce' at various points between the 1370s and 1450s,[36] but below the fractious ranks of the mercantile elite a substantial body of artisans and retailers continued, undisturbed, to make certain that one of the country's largest and more prosperous cities functioned effectively on a day to day basis. It was, significantly, at this level that responsibility for implementing costly public works, such as cleansing the river and paving the streets, lay, as did the task of ensuring that thoroughfares remained clean and that food standards were observed by market traders. The dissemination of medical knowledge among the ordinary townsfolk of late medieval England, which Faye Getz has already traced in central legal records, clearly owed much to these activities.[37]

One of the many regulations enforced in Norwich's market concerned the sale of food to the servants employed in the city's extra mural *leprosaria*, who were prohibited from touching any items with their hands, lest they might infect the goods on display.[38] Introduced in the aftermath of the 1471 pestilence, which one local eyewitness described as 'the most vnyuersall dethe that euyre I wyst in Ingelonde',[39] this measure reveals that leprosy, a disease now chiefly associated with the twelfth and thirteenth centuries, continued to provoke extreme reactions long after it was in terminal decline. The paradox whereby anxiety about lepers increased as their numbers began dramatically to fall should hardly surprise us, since, as Elma Brenner explains, the spread of plague *consilia* and regimens of health made people nervous of such an obvious source of pollution. Her study of municipal responses in Rouen reveals a state of constant vigilance: fears that leprosy might be contracted from the consumption of rotten meat or proximity to the infected were compounded by the knowledge that an unwholesome diet would increase one's susceptibility to pestilential miasmas of the sort initially exhaled by

---

[36] Philippa Maddern, 'Order and Disorder', in *Medieval Norwich*, ed. Carole Rawcliffe and Richard Wilson (London and Rio Grande, 2004), 190.

[37] Faye Getz, *Medicine in the English Middle Ages* (Princeton, N.J., 1998), ch. 4.

[38] Norfolk RO, NCR, 16D/1, f. 95v.

[39] *Paston Letters and Papers of the Fifteenth Century*, ed. Norman Davis (2 vols., Oxford, 1971–6), i. 440.

the leprous. The need to provide hospital places for those few remaining lepers who posed such an apparent threat to their fellow citizens was clearly driven by sanitary considerations, although Brenner provides striking evidence of an attendant – if sometimes intermittent – sense of responsibility for their proper physical and spiritual care. Her article also presents another welcome reminder of the need to avoid anachronistic assumptions about the march of scientific progress. The widely held belief that 'conservative' ideas regarding the transmission of disease by miasmatic air were challenged at this time by more 'modern', and essentially incompatible, theories of contagion certainly finds little support in the surviving evidence.[40] As her account of a council meeting during the plague epidemic of 1499 reveals, the same individuals were keen to propose measures that would curb the generation of corrupt air and prevent contagion through proximity and touch, while simultaneously recommending the benefits of collective prayer.[41]

It was far easier to draft ordinances than to enforce them, especially during periods of endemic warfare, when financial resources were poured into defence, urban populations were swollen by hungry refugees from the countryside, and deprivation, along with cramped, unhygienic living conditions, encouraged the spread of epidemics.[42] Rouen was one of several northern French cities to suffer badly during the Hundred Years' War, and thus to introduce sanitary regulations and pest houses at a significantly later date than communities further south, which also fell more readily under Italian influence. Yet, although none of the northern cities examined by Neil Murphy established boards of health along the Milanese or Venetian model until the later sixteenth century, all had by then amassed decades of experience in dealing with plague. Murphy's analysis of the evidence to be found in municipal archives underscores the striking differences in response apparent from one region to another, and the ways in which particular networks for the exchange of information and ideas might develop. From the 1450s onwards, once most (but not all) of the fighting had ceased, magistrates were able to embark upon a more sustained programme for combating pestilence, with the result that a veritable 'industry' developed specifically for this purpose. In contrast to the situation in fifteenth-century England, physicians and surgeons were employed by the authorities both to treat the sick and to provide advice about public health. An initial focus upon the elimination of miasmas gave way to more stringent measures for the confinement of goods and people, including, predictably, lepers, whose freedom was increasingly curtailed. Once again, though, we can detect no signs of conflict between what might be termed the 'contagionist' and 'environmentalist' approaches to urban sanitation, or any significant divergence between professional or lay opinion.

The growth in institutional antagonism towards the feckless and vagrant poor documented by many historians during the later European Middle Ages was in part

---

[40] A.G. Carmichael, *Plague and the Poor in Renaissance Florence* (Cambridge, 1986), 125.
[41] Below, pp. 131–2.
[42] In an English context, the experience of Carlisle, which suffered repeatedly from arson attacks by the Scots, provides a striking example of the effects that warfare could have upon public health provision, or more properly the lack of it: Mark Brennand and K.J. Stringer, *The Making of Carlisle: From Romans to Railways* (Cumberland and Westmorland Antiquarian and Archaeological Society, extra series, xxxv, 2011), 125–6, 131–2.

fuelled by contemporary beliefs about the aetiology of plague.[43] On the one hand, moralists could point to the idle and sexually promiscuous behaviour of men and women whose conduct invited divine wrath, while on the other students of advice literature feared that indigents would be most likely to breed miasmatic air and spread infection among their betters.[44] The extent to which 'plague offered an opportunity for magistrates to discipline those whom they regarded as social parasites' seems, nonetheless, to have been determined, like so many other initiatives for communal health, by specifically local or regional factors.[45] Whereas Murphy observes a mood of 'undisguised intolerance' in the cities of northern France, Jane Stevens Crawshaw challenges the widespread assumption that Italian city states such as Florence adopted isolation procedures specifically in order to control undesirables. Her study of the early development of quarantine, which ranks as the best-known (but most frequently misunderstood) measure to be deployed against pre-modern plague, also questions the close connection so often made between leper houses and *lazaretti*, both of which have acquired an unfounded reputation for the enforced segregation and maltreatment of their inmates. Although they sought to protect the public from disease, the founders of plague hospitals in Milan, Ragusa and Venice were no less influenced by renaissance concepts of good governance and statehood. Some hoped to achieve political legitimacy through the very conscious projection of 'an image of solicitude and paternal care', while others were prompted by civic pride and a concern for the aesthetics of urban space. Here, as elsewhere in Europe, hospitals served as a mirror to society, reflecting its broader concerns and aspirations.

The conviction that charity towards the sick poor was itself a powerful prophylactic, guaranteed to safeguard the spiritual, and sometimes even the physical, health of benefactors, inspired many Italian hospital foundations both for victims of plague and the Great Pox, which spread rapidly across Europe from the 1490s onwards. Strategies for coping with the two diseases were, however, very different, as John Henderson reveals. This was largely due to the impact of medical ideas upon public policy, for whereas physicians and secular authorities agreed about the aetiology of plague and the sanitary measures to be deployed against it (he, too, is unconvinced by claims of tension between medical and urban authorities), there was less consensus regarding the causes of pox, which manifested itself as a chronically debilitating and disfiguring disease rather than one that killed within a matter of days or weeks. Indeed, since it appeared to be growing less aggressive with the passage of time, its victims were regarded not so much as a threat to the health of others as a growing social, economic and moral problem. In keeping with counter-reformation campaigns for piety, almsgiving and the rehabilitation of the undeserving poor, the *incurabili* hospital aimed to transform these ulcerated and wretched paupers into economically productive and

---

[43] M.K. McIntosh, *Poor Relief in England 1350–1600* (Cambridge, 2012), 43–5; Michel Mollat, *The Poor in the Middle Ages: An Essay in Social History*, trans Arthur Goldhammer (New Haven and London, 1986) part 4; Miri Rubin, *Charity and Community in Medieval Cambridge* (Cambridge, 1987), 296–9.

[44] Rawcliffe, *Urban Bodies*, ch. 2.

[45] See below, p. 157.

obedient citizens. Here, in Henderson's words, can be seen that striking combination of 'charity and disgust' so characteristic of renaissance attitudes to those who inspired compassion and distaste in equal measure, along increasingly with fear. Once again, we are made aware of the need to contextualise hospital foundations within a wider religious and political framework.

Medical historians have long since contested the Foucaultian view of pre-modern hospitals, and especially pest houses, as 'antechambers of death', where men and women were confined in squalor and abandoned to their fate.[46] Both Stevens Crawshaw and Murphy stress the effort expended on making these places appear clean and attractive, although it is easy to be seduced by the rhetoric of officials who placed such a high political premium on the trappings of philanthropy and the opinions of others. As Henderson points out, Florence's fifteenth-century *lazaretto* took thirty years to build (1464–94) and accommodated only twenty-six people, being more an exercise in republican propaganda than a major investment on behalf of the sick. A significant element of one-upmanship was also at play, since the commune was clearly afraid of seeming backward or less committed to the welfare of its people than was the case in Venice, which had boasted a *lazaretto* for decades.[47] The need to distinguish self-promotion of this kind from the mundane reality of care for the plague sick seems especially important in light of the reputation for innovation and excellence enjoyed by Italian renaissance cities. Henderson has noted elsewhere that fifteenth-century Florence was far less salubrious than humanists such as Leonardo Bruni would have us believe, although it is they who still influence the way in which we judge pre-modern public health provision (and against whose claims England invariably makes so poor a showing).[48]

On the other hand, the effort expended by magistrates from London to Dubrovnik to convince visitors of the healthfulness of their cities is indicative of rising expectations and grander ambitions, as articulated in Lydgate's paean to King Priam's public works and as documented in several of the papers presented in this volume.[49] Even if he or she was obliged to tolerate a raft of unpleasant and dangerous nuisances, the fifteenth-century citizen *aspired* to better things, not only as a defence against the miasmas of pestilence but also because clean streets and fresh water seemed desirable in their own right. Protests voiced in early Tudor Canterbury that, although the major thoroughfares were now well paved, lack of proper refuse collection rendered them 'foule and full of myre to the *grete dishonour* of the Cite and the *grete damage* of the inhabitaunts by the corrupte and

---

[46]   John Henderson, *The Renaissance Hospital: Healing the Body and Healing the Soul* (New Haven and London, 2006), pp. xxx–xxxi, 109, 261, 339.

[47]   See below, pp. 182–3; and Henderson, *The Renaissance Hospital*, 94. Since Florence did not suffer badly from plague during this period there was, admittedly, less incentive to complete the hospital quickly or accommodate more patients.

[48]   John Henderson, 'Public Health, Pollution and the Problem of Waste Disposal in Early Modern Tuscany', in *Le interazioni fra economia e ambiente biologico nell' Europa preindustriale, secc. XIII–XVIII*, ed. Simonetta Cavaciocchi (Florence, 2010), 373–82.

[49]   Echoing Lydgate, in 1452 the rulers of Salisbury expressed the hope that newly repaired drains and gutters would serve 'to the adornment of the city': *The First General Entry Book of the City of Salisbury, 1387–1452*, ed. D.R. Carr (Wiltshire Record Society, liv, 2001), no. 453.

infectuose heires', reflect these shared priorities. [50] Indeed, the association of hygiene with the wider '*bien commun de la chose publique*' occurs so often in the records of late medieval European towns as to appear almost platitudinous.[51] When considering the 'dyvers *good and godly* actes and ordynaunces' for environmental improvement passed by their predecessors, the rulers of sixteenth-century Norwich recognised that they had 'not only bene a great ease and heltheful commodyte to the inhabitauntes ... but also a goodly bewtefying and an occasyon that dyverse [people] havyng accesse to the same cittye from ffarre and strange places have moche comended and praysed'. [52] In short, the previous century had offered significant opportunities for the introduction of schemes for public health in towns that had been spared the blight of chronic overcrowding and widespread unemployment. If plague gave men and women a unique incentive for penitence and pilgrimage, it also prompted a range of strategies for survival that were anything but fatalistic.

---

[50] HMC, *Ninth Report Part I, Appendix* (1883), 174. The italics are mine. A carter was duly appointed to remove waste from the streets. See below, p. 73, for concerns that the poor state of the streets would deter visitors.

[51] See below, pp. 128, 168–9.

[52] *The Records of the City of Norwich*, ed. William Hudson and J.C. Tingey (2 vols., Norwich, 1906–10), ii. 109–10, 133–4.

LOOKING FOR *YERSINIA PESTIS*:
SCIENTISTS, HISTORIANS AND THE BLACK DEATH

J.L. Bolton

The fact that the plague in its bubonic, septicaemic and pneumonic forms is still with us in the twenty-first century often comes as a shock to the general public. Memories of school projects have made them vaguely aware of the great pandemic, which arrived in southern Italy in 1347 and then raged across Europe, reaching England and Norway in 1348, through Oslo in 1348 and then through Bergen in 1349, and European Russia in 1351, where the city state of Novgorod was first infected.[1] But then, surely, it went away? Not quite: outbreaks of plague in this second pandemic, first (allegedly) called the Black Death by Mrs Markham in 1823 in her *History of England*, from which the horrors of history and the complexities of party politics were removed as not suitable for young minds,[2] lasted in England until the early eighteenth century, whilst in Italy what is generally regarded as its final appearance came at Naja, near Bari, in 1815.[3] Even then the disease did not disappear. It merely became dormant until 1855, when a new pandemic began in China, spreading through the Pacific Rim and in 1899 to the United States where plague had previously been unknown. Indeed, as the well-known World Health Organisation map of plague *loci* and plague outbreaks 1970–1998 shows, the disease is enzootic or sylvatic (ever-present in certain animal populations and their fleas) in some fifty-eight different regions in the world and can still spread to more susceptible animals, including humans, in epizootic outbreaks.[4] The most important of these modern plague reservoirs are to be found in northern China and the adjacent states of the Former Soviet Union; sub-Saharan Africa and Madagascar; India; Iran and other areas of the Middle East; South America; and the Rocky Mountain states of the U.S.A.

Epizootic outbreaks are still, thankfully, rare, however, the most recent being in the Democratic Republic of the Congo in 2006, but individual cases of both bubonic and pneumonic plague are not uncommon. In 2012 a welder from Prineville, Oregon, was infected by a cat scratch and a young girl of seven by fleas

---

[1] The spread of the plague across Europe is described by Ole Benedictow, *The Black Death, 1346–1353: The Complete History* (Woodbridge, 2004), 57–215.

[2] Mrs. Markham [Elizabeth Penrose], *A History of England* (1829), 249–50.

[3] S.K. Cohn, Jr., 'Epidemiology of the Black Death and Successive Waves of Plague', in *Pestilential Complexities: Understanding Medieval Plague*, ed. Vivian Nutton, *Medical History*, supplement xxvii (2008), 74–5.

[4] For a version of the W.H.O. map see www.macroevolution.net/black-plague-map.html; this is updated to 2012 at www.cdc.gov/plague/maps/index.html; see below, n. 40 for further discussion of the terms enzootic and epizootic.

from a dead squirrel while on a camping site in south-west Colorado.[5] Both these cases were of bubonic plague, which is treatable with modern antibiotics. Pneumonic plague is not, and it was only prompt action by the highly effective health authorities in the People's Republic of China that prevented a major outbreak of that disease in Xinghai District, Qinghai Province, bordering Tibet. There, in July 2009, a shepherd and eleven of his human contacts contracted pneumonic plague from one of his dogs, which had probably been infected by eating a diseased marmoset. Three of them died, although the conclusion reached by those investigating the outbreak was that the transmissability of the disease was not as high as had been thought to be the case. Nevertheless, it highlights the importance of domestic animals in spreading the disease.[6]

Even today, when plague can be swiftly controlled by antibiotics, the mere mention of the word produces a highly emotive response. Amongst modern historians of medieval pandemics it seems to arouse even greater emotions. Much time and effort has been expended in recent years in trying to prove that the disease which swept through Europe from 1347 onwards could not possibly have been bubonic plague. Some have argued that it might have been Ebola fever, Marburg's disease or another form of haemorrhagic fever; anthrax or *Rinderpest* have also been suggested as the cause of the high death rates between 1347 and 1351. Perhaps the most eccentric explanation for the arrival of *Yersinia pestis*, the pathogen or bacterium that causes the plague, came from the distinguished mathematician and astronomer, the late Sir Fred Hoyle. He firmly believed that it and other pathogens arrived on Earth in the 'organic rain' from passing comets.[7] The debate between historians has reached new and perhaps unacceptable levels of ferocity in recent years, but alongside it, and sometimes completely separate from it, scientific research into the causes and vectors[8] of historic and modern plagues and why they have become 'persistent', that is, ever-present in some regions, has surged forward. New techniques, such as DNA sampling and genome sequencing, have been applied to evidence provided by archaeologists and have produced some very interesting answers. One of the main stimuli to research funding, however, has been the realization that bubonic and particularly pneumonic plague could be used as Class A bio-terrorist weapons. Consequently, in the last two decades, literally hundreds of articles on plague have appeared in print in scientific journals and, much more frequently, in the on-line versions of these or new journals that are freely available.

The problem for the historian is how to integrate these new scientific findings with received historical wisdom on the causes and consequences of the endemic plague that arrived in Europe in 1347. Experimental scientists are in most cases

---

[5] *The Guardian*, 18 July 2012; www.foxnews.com/health/2012/09/05/colorado-girl-recovering-from-bubonic-plague/; Hu Wang *et al.*, 'A Dog-Associated Primary Pneumonic Plague in Qinghai Province, China', *Clinical Infectious Diseases*, lii (2011), 185–9.

[6] Wang *et al.*, 'A Dog-Associated Primary Pneumonic Plague', 185–90.

[7] See, for example, the views expressed in J.D. Shrewsbury, *A History of Bubonic Plague in the British Isles* (Cambridge, 1970); Fred Hoyle and N.C. Wickramasinghe, *Diseases from Space* (1979); Graham Twigg, *The Black Death: a Biological Reappraisal* (1984); Susan Scott and C.J. Duncan, *Biology of Plagues: Evidence from Historical Populations* (Cambridge, 2001); and S.K. Cohn, Jr., *The Black Death Transformed: Disease and Culture in Early Renaissance Europe* (2002).

[8] A vector is an organism such as a flea or other ectoparasite that transfers disease-carrying micro-organisms from one host to another.

much more convinced that they, or rather their findings, are 'right'. Scientific proof is taken to be absolute: experiments properly conducted and repeatable cannot produce incorrect results. Medieval historians, on the other hand, have come to accept that they can only ever hope to uncover some of the 'truth', whatever that 'truth' might be. However, for one discipline to ignore the findings of another would be absurd, and the purpose of this paper is to review the most important of recent scientific experiments and to see how they can help historians better understand the cause of the second pandemic; how it spread so rapidly across Europe; and why it persisted in the following centuries, with serious long-term demographic, economic and social consequences.[9] Evaluating the methodology used and the evidence it produces is not easy for those without microbiological training, yet it is essential. Arguments are only as sound as the evidence on which they are based, provided that evidence itself is trustworthy. That has not always been the case, and some historical debates about the cause of the second great pandemic and the transmission of the disease have, frankly, been misinformed. However difficult it may be, assessing the microbiological evidence has to be, in this case, one of the historian's skills.

Looking for *Yersinia pestis* and trying to prove that the pathogen was the cause of three great pandemics has been a scientific quest since at least 1894, when Alexandre Yersin, the Franco-Swiss bacteriologist, finally identified the bacterium as the cause of plague shortly before his Japanese rival, Dr. Kitasato Shibasaburo, who deserves equal credit for the discovery. One significant stage in the quest was the division of the *Yersinia pestis* strain into three main biovars, *Antiqua*, *Mediaevalis* and *Orientalis*, by the French scientist René Devignat in 1951, which caused, respectively, the three great pandemics: Justinian's Plague, which began in Constantinople in A.D. 541–2 and then spread across Europe, lasting until c.750; the Black Death (1347–c.1815); and the nineteenth-century outbreak, which began in the Far East in the 1850s and whose consequences are still with us today.[10] Unfortunately, more recent research has shown that this neat division must be abandoned, since *Yersinia pestis* has many biovars, not all of which still exist today.[11] However, it was not until the 1990s that science began to catch up with archaeology, with the first major experiments trying to isolate the bacterium *Yersinia pestis* as the main cause of historic plague.

The skeletons of probable plague victims have long been excavated by European archaeologists. The difficulty was that such skeletons were usually precisely that, collections of bones and nothing else, with no material possessions or other surviving evidence that could be tested for the presence of *Yersinia pestis*. Ancient bones are not themselves good sources for the DNA of pathogens.[12] As

---

[9] I am indebted to Dr. R.E. Bolton of GlaxoSmithKline plc for his invaluable help in assessing the relative importance of the articles he read for me.

[10] René Devignat, 'Variétés de l'espèce Pasturella pestis. Nouvelle hypothèse', *Bulletin of the World Health Organisation*, iv (1951), 247–63; Cohn, 'Epidemiology of the Black Death', 74–5. A biovar is a group of bacterial strains that are distinguishable from other strains of the same species on the basis of their physiological characteristics.

[11] See below, pp. 23–4.

[12] Deoxyribonucleic acid is a nucleic acid that carries the genetic information in the cell and is a synthesis of RNA. DNA consists of two long chains on nucleotides twisted in a double helix. RNA is ribonucleic acid. It is present in all living cells and carries instructions from DNA to the protein-forming system of the cell.

long ago as 1937, however, Ruth Tunnicliff and Carolyn Hammond had discovered the presence of bacteria in the pulp of intact teeth, and it is dental pulp from ancient teeth that has provided the evidence for the growing body of palaeomicrobiologists who investigate ancient diseases.[13] Dental pulp is the soft tissue found in the central cavities of teeth, beneath the layers of enamel and dentine, the dense bony tissue that forms the bulk of the tooth. The pulp itself contains connective tissues, major nerves and blood vessels and it is they that provide the evidence needed. If an animal or a human being has died from septicaemia, or blood poisoning, the invasion of the bloodstream by a virulent pathogen, then it should be possible to identify the pathogen responsible from dental pulp. Since septicaemia is the final stage of bubonic plague, it follows that by analysing samples of dental pulp taken from the teeth of possible plague victims palaeomicrobiologists should be able to determine the presence of the DNA of *Yersinia pestis*. Such analyses should also be able to provide equally important negative evidence, that is, the absence of *Yersinia pestis* DNA and possibly the presence of other pathogens offered as alternative causes of the Black Death – anthrax, *Rinderpest* and haemorraghic fever – although no tests for cosmic dust seem to have been developed, as yet.[14]

Only the residue of dental pulp can be extracted from skeletal teeth, of course, usually in powder form. In 1998 Professor Michel Drancourt and his colleagues at what was then the University of Marseilles, and is now the University of the Mediterranean Aix-Marseilles II, decided to enter the fractious debate on the causes of ancient plague. Their intention was to test for the presence of *Yersinia pestis* in dental pulp taken from the teeth of skeletons found in two mass graves of supposed plague victims in Provence. One, at Lambesc, Bouches-du-Rhone, contained 133 skeletons buried between May and September 1590, the other, in Marseilles, approximately 200 skeletons buried in May 1722. Four un-erupted teeth were taken from two skeletons from Lambesc, eight from three skeletons from Marseilles, while seven teeth were used as negative controls since they came from skeletons from a cemetery in Toulon not associated with plague burials. The teeth were decontaminated and residue dental pulp extracted from them according to standard protocols. The specimens were then prepared for testing by a method known as Polymerase Chain Reaction, or PCR, a fast and inexpensive technique used to amplify or copy small segments of a specific and defined strand of DNA, in this case that of *Yersinia pestis*.[15]

What this experiment revealed was the presence of the *Yersinia pestis* DNA sequence in six of the twelve teeth taken from skeletons from the 'plague' cemeteries, but in none in the dental pulp of the seven teeth from the Toulon graveyard that had been used as controls. The authors proudly proclaimed that 'A nucleic acid-based confirmation of ancient plague was achieved from historically

---

[13] Ruth Tunnicliff and Carolyn Hammond, 'Presence of Bacteria in Pulps of Intact Teeth', *Journal of the American Dental Association and Dental Cosmos*, xxiv (1937), 1663–6.

[14] The use of ancient dental pulp as evidence is fully discussed by V.D. La *et al.*, 'Dental Pulp as a Tool for Retrospective Diagnoses of Infectious Diseases', in *Palaeomicrobiology: Past Human Infections*, ed. Didier Raoult and Michel Drancourt (Berlin and Heidelberg, 2008), 175–91.

[15] The history and specific workings of the PCR process are clearly described by J.M.S. Bartlett and David Sterling, 'A Short History of Polymerase Chain Reaction', in *PCR Protocols*, ed. Bartlett and Sterling, *Methods in Molecular Biology*, ccxxvi (Berlin and Heidelberg, 2003), 3–6.

identified victims', and that 'they had confirmed the presence of the disease at the end of the sixteenth century in France'.[16] Two years later much the same team, now led by Didier Raoult, carried out further tests, this time using a refinement of the earlier method known as 'Suicide' PCR. This was partly a response to mounting criticism of the original method, discussed further below, and partly to extend the chronological range of the evidence back to the fourteenth century and the beginnings of the second major plague pandemic. Standard PCR employs 'primers' made of oligonucleotides to create replicas of a specific strand of DNA, be it for *Yersinia pestis* or other diseases.[17] However, since they are used many times, there is a strong possibility of degradation and contamination, leading to false results. In 'Suicide' PCR the primer is used only once, with a negative result being followed by further tests using new primers, and a positive result by DNA sequencing, which reads the nucleotide bases in a DNA molecule. Nor are there any positive controls, that is, the testing of dental pulp taken from the teeth of people who could not have died of the plague, to show that the primers could produce negative as well as positive results. The experiment in 2000 used teeth taken from three skeletons found in a graveyard in Montpellier known to contain plague victims. One was of a man, whose skull provided ten teeth, the second of a woman (nine teeth) and the third a male child aged between eight to ten years (four teeth). The DNA of the *Yersinia pestis* bacterium was found in dental pulp residue from one of the child's teeth and in every single one of the nineteen teeth taken from the adults. Other tests, using templates and primers for the DNA of the bacteria causing anthrax and typhus, both suggested as alternative causes of the high death rates in 1347–51, proved negative. Then, in June 2005, the results of another study carried out in Munich on dental pulp from the teeth of two female skeletons found in an early medieval burial site at Aschheim in Upper Bavaria, dated to the second half of the sixth century, using both PCR and 'Suicide' PCR, were published. They showed the presence of *Yersinia pestis* DNA in the teeth, possibly as a result of Justinian's Plague.[18]

Although the results of the Bavarian study were not published until 2005, the paper had been submitted to *The American Journal of Physical Anthropology*, and had been accepted for publication in 2002. So, within the space of four years, it seemed as if the cause of two historical pandemics, Justinian's Plague and the Black Death, had been firmly and finally established. Alas, this was not the case. Already, in 2000, in a letter published in the journal *Science*, entitled 'Ancient DNA: do it right or not at all', Alan Cooper from Oxford and Hendrik N. Poinar from the Max Planck Institute, Leipzig, had severely criticised the methodology in these and other recent tests for ancient DNA. They argued that 'Ancient DNA

---

[16] Michel Drancourt *et al.*, 'Detection of 400-Year-Old *Yersinia pestis* DNA in Human Dental Pulp: an Approach to the Diagnosis of Ancient Septicemia', *Proceedings of the National Academy of Sciences of the USA*, xcv (1998), 12637–40.

[17] Oligoucleotides are short nucleic acid polymers. Nucleotides themselves form the basic structural unit of nucleic acids such as DNA.

[18] Didier Raoult *et al.*, 'Molecular Indentification by "Suicide PCR" of *Yersinia pestis* as the Agent of Medieval Black Death', *Proceedings of the National Academy of Sciences of the USA*, xcvii (2000), 12800–3; Ingrid Wiechmann and Gisela Grupe, 'Detection of *Yersinia pestis* DNA in Two Early Medieval Skeletal Finds from Aschheim (Upper Bavaria), 6th Century A.D.', *American Journal of Physical Anthropology*, cxxvi (2005), 48–55.

research presented extreme technical difficulties because of the minute amounts and degraded nature of surviving DNA and the exceptional risk of contamination.' They then gave a long list of standards to be adopted in PCR testing to avoid false or contaminated results, including the possibility of cross-contamination with target DNA and strict control of amplification procedures. Most importantly, all results should be repeatable from the same and different DNA extracts from the specimen, both in the same and in another independent laboratory.[19]

That experiments can be repeated and produce the same results is one of the key principles of scientific investigation. In their 2004 article in *Microbiology*, M.T.P. Gilbert and others, including Alan Cooper, took the Drancourt/Raoult school to task precisely on this issue. They attempted to amplify and sequence ancient *Yersinia pestis* DNA from the dental pulp of 108 human teeth taken from 61 skeletons from five archaeological sites in northern Europe known to contain plague victims: Copenhagen, Denmark; East Smithfield and Spitalfields, London; and Verdun and Angers, France. No traces of *Yersinia pestis* DNA could be amplified from the samples, and from these and other tests the team concluded that they could not confirm the identification of *Yersinia pestis* as the aetiological or main causative agent of the Black Death or other historical plagues. Additionally, because of the extreme dangers of contamination, the utility of the already published tooth-based ancient DNA techniques used to diagnose fatal bacteraemia in historical epidemics still awaited independent confirmation.[20] Such was the critical nature of their argument that the editors of the journal allowed Drancourt and Raoult instant right of reply, in the same issue. They defended their research vigorously, insisting that, as Gilbert and others had neither used their methods for extracting and analysing dental pulp, nor their PCR testing techniques, it was scarcely surprising that they had failed to reproduce the original results. In further correspondence, again in the same journal issue, Gilbert and his team agreed to disagree but admitted that 'further work [was needed] to involve independent processing in more than one laboratory of [dental pulp from] teeth taken directly from an archaeological site where *Yersinia pestis*-positive specimens [had] been obtained'. Drancourt's and Raoult's findings had been seriously challenged but the scientific debate as to the causes of the Black Death and other historic plagues was not likely to go away.

Nor has it, since between 2004 and 2012 old arguments have been rehearsed and re-rehearsed, while, much more fruitfully, the use of new techniques has amply confirmed the original findings of Drancourt, Raoult and others between 1998 and 2002. Here historians should be aware that the search for traces of *Yersinia pestis* in ancient DNA is only part of much wider investigations for the presence of bacteria in samples old and new. Some of the main targets are for the pathogens causing typhus (*Rickettsia typhi* or *prowazekii*), anthrax (*Bacillus anthracis*), leprosy (*mycobacterium leprae*) and tuberculosis (*mycobacterium tuberculosis*), and the parasites responsible for malaria (*Plasimodium falciparum*) and Leishman's disease (*Leishmaniasis*). The last is second only to malaria as a cause of death from parasitic diseases in the modern world and was, and still is,

---

[19] *Science*, cclxxxix, no. 5482 (2000), 1139.
[20] M.T.P. Gilbert *et al.*, 'Absence of *Yersinia pestis*-specific DNA in Human Teeth from Five European Excavations of Putative Plague Victims', *Microbiology*, cl (2004), 341–54.

widespread in southern Europe. Transmitted through the bite of the sand fly, it was certainly responsible for the death of Eleanor di Toledo (1522–62), wife of Cosimo de' Medici I, grand duke of Tuscany, and daughter of Don Alvarez di Toledo, Spanish viceroy of Naples, as research published in 2012 has shown. *Mycobacterium tuberculosis* has also been discovered in the 17,000-year-old skeleton of an extinct bison using gas chromatography mass spectrometry, whilst specimens from modern tuberculosis victims are still tested by PCR.[21] Looking for *Yersinia pestis* forms in ancient DNA constitutes only a very small part of modern microbiological research, but it uses the techniques developed in the search for the pathogens which cause widespread diseases in the modern world.

Consequently, when it became clear that the search for *Yersinia pestis* by looking for molecules of its DNA in dental pulp taken from the teeth of ancient skeletons was not the surest way forward,[22] other methods for identifying the presence of the pathogen were already to hand. The first to be exploited was testing for F1 antigens, again using dental pulp from the teeth of suspected plague victims as evidence. The *Yersinia pestis* pathogen carries on its surface three major proteins and the Fraction One or F1 capsular antigen is one of these. Its purpose is entirely defensive, since it offers the pathogen protection against phagocytosis, the process by which phagocytes, white blood cells in the human immune system, engulf and digest bacteria and other micro-organisms attacking it. Testing for F1 antigens specific or unique to *Yersinia pestis* provides evidence for the Yersinial proteome, that is, the full complement of proteins produced by a particular genome, the complete set of genetic material of an organism. Testing for proteins is considered more suitable for detecting plague in historical samples because proteins are more resistant to environmental degradation than DNA.[23]

The F1 antigen of *Yersinia pestis* had been isolated and characterised as long ago as 1952, as part of an on-going and so far largely unsuccessful attempt to develop a vaccine against plague.[24] Tests for the antigen were developed using a

---

[21] A.G. Nerlich *et al.*, 'Visceral Leishmaniasis during [the] Italian Renaissance, 1522–62', *Emerging Infectious Diseases*, xviii (2012), 184–6; O.Y. Lee *et al.*, 'Mycobacterium Tuberculosis Complex Lipid Virulence Factors in the 17,000 Year Old Skeleton of an Extinct Bison, Bison Antiquus', *Public Library of Science One*, vii (2012), e41923, Epublication 2012, July 30; V.J. Tavere *et al.*, 'Detection of Mycobacterium Tuberculosis by PCR Amplification with pan-Mycobacterium Primers and Hybridization to an M. Tuberculosis-Specific Probe', *Journal of Clinical Microbiology*, xxxiv (1996), 918–23.

[22] To their credit, the research team from the University of the Mediterranean/Aix-Marseilles II fully recognised the method's shortcomings in Thi-Nguyen-Tran *et al.*, 'Beyond Ancient Microbial DNA: Non-Nucleotidic Biomolecules for Palaeomicrobiology', *BioTechniques*, l (2011), 375; see also Daniel Antoine, 'The Archaeology of "Plague"', in *Pestilential Complexities*, ed. Nutton, 101–14, especially 110–11.

[23] For F1 antigens see S.D. Knight, 'Structure and Assembly of *Yersinia pestis* F1 Antigen', in *The Genus Yersinia. From Genome to Function*, ed. R.D. Perry and J.D. Fetherston (New York, 2007), 74–87.

[24] E.E. Barker *et al.*, 'The Isolation and Characterization of the Soluble Antigen of Pasturella Pestis', *Journal of Immunology*, lxviii (1952), 1331–45. For more recent research, see G.P. Andrews *et al.*, 'Fractional Capsular Antigen (F1) Purification for *Yersinia pestis* C092 and from an *Escherchia coli* Recombinant Strain and Efficacy Against a Lethal Plague Challenge', *Infection and Immunity*, lxiv, pt. 6 (1996), 2180–7; L.M. Runco *et al.*, 'Biogenisis of the Fraction 1 Capsule and Analysis of the Ultrastructure of *Yersinia pestis*', *Journal of Bacteriology*, cxc, pt. 9 (2008), 3381–5 and especially 3581; E.M. Galván *et al.*, 'Capsular Antigen Fraction 1 and Pla Modulate the Susceptibility for

process known as ELISA (Enzyme-Linked ImmunoSorbent Assay), which was introduced in the 1970s. This particular immunoassay uses an enzyme linked to an antibody or, in this case, an antigen as a marker for the detection of a specific protein, especially an antigen or antibody.[25] However, ELISA is both an expensive and destructive laboratory technique, in that the sample being tested is destroyed during the process, an obvious drawback for palaeomicrobiologists working with scarce dental pulp. It is also difficult to use ELISA in the field, outside the laboratory, when testing samples for plague or other diseases in modern society, and so an alternative was found in what is called the Rapid Dipstick Test or RDT. The RDT uses membranes of paper and nitrocellulose to which specific antibodies are attached. The latter then react when dipped in a solution containing the protein and detect the specific antigen, usually by a change in colour. They are less sensitive than ELISA tests, but provide, at much less cost, a straightforward way of indicating the presence of an antigen, which can then be tested further in the laboratory if necessary. As importantly, they can now be used to test for a variety of pathogens, not just for *Yersinia pestis*, and are widely deployed in the field by clinicians.

It was not until 2003, however, that a specific RDT for both bubonic and pneumonic plague was developed in Madagascar, where plague is prevalent. Then, in 2004, the year when PCR methods were challenged, Pusch and other researchers from the University of Tübingen and the Pasteur Institute in Madagascar used this method to look for the F1 capsular antigen of *Yersinia pestis* in ancient dental pulp. The samples in question were taken from the teeth of skeletons from the seventeenth century buried in the church of St. Germanus in Stuttgart in southern Germany. Tests were carried out on dental pulp from twenty-four skeletons, twelve of known plague victims, twelve of those known to have died of other causes, as a control. Both PCR and F1 antigen tests were carried out, with interesting results. PCR detected plague in only two of the twelve samples, but dipstick assay produced ten positive results. The twelve control samples tested negative in both types of assay. The research team was cautious, however, and not prepared to state definitively that plague alone had caused the death of the individuals whose dental pulp had tested positive for the F1 *Yersinia pestis* antigen. Other pathogens such as *Salmonella enterica* are known to carry similar plasmids, and the tests may have produced false-positive results. Nevertheless, they concluded that dipstick assay was a useful complement to PCR in identifying *Yersinia pestis* at low levels in historical evidence, but that more tests and more evidence were needed.[26]

Data followed apace. In 2007 Raffaella Bianucci and others published the results of a rapid dipstick assay for the F1 antigen in dental pulp from eighteen teeth taken from skeletons of putative plague victims from cemeteries in south-eastern France: at Lambesc (1590); Draguignan (1649–50); Martiques (1720–1);

Yersinia pestis to Pulmonary Antimicrobial Peptides such as Cathelicidin', *Infection and Immunity*, lxxvi (2008), 1456–64.

[25] For a detailed description of how it works, see S.X. Leng *et al.*, 'ELISA and Multiplex Technologies for Cytokine Measurement in Inflammation and Aging Research', *Journals of Gerontology, Series A, Biological Sciences and Medical Sciences*, lxiii (2008), 879–84.

[26] Suzanne Chanteau *et al.*, 'Development and Testing of a Rapid Diagnostic Test for Bubonic and Pneumonic Plague', *The Lancet*, ccclxi (2003), 211–16; C.M. Pusch *et al.*, 'Yersinial F1 Antigen and the Cause of the Black Death', *The Lancet Infectious Diseases*, iv (2004), 484–5.

and Marseilles (1722). Samples from the bones and teeth of another eighteen skeletons from the Chapel of the Cordeliers (Franciscan friars) at Besançon (Hautes Alpes) were used as a negative control. F1 plague antigens were found in twelve of the eighteen teeth from suspected plague victims (67 per cent) and not at all in any of the teeth in the control sample. In the same year (2007) Nichole Cerutti and others confirmed the presence of *Yersinia pestis* in skeletons from the fourteenth-century cemetery at the Bastione dell'Acquasola in Genoa, while in 2009 Bianucci and her colleagues reported the results of their tests on dental pulp taken from the teeth of the skeletons of four Benedictine nuns from Saint-Croixe abbey in Poitiers and two priests from the church of St. Nicholas in La Chaize-le-Vicomte in central France. The skeletons of these putative plague victims were dated to between 1500 and 1700, and rapid dipstick tests were carried out on bone and dental pulp samples from them. All six were positive for the *Yersinia pestis* F1 antigen, and the team concluded that their hypothesis that the six religious were afflicted by *Yersinia pestis* during the plague outbreaks in central France between 1587 and 1632 had 'independent biological support'.[27] Finally, in 2010 Stephanie Haensch and an international team from Germany, France, Italy, the Netherlands, Ireland and Britain used both PCR and RDT to identify *Yersinia pestis* in the dental pulp and bone samples taken from seventy-six human skeletons excavated from plague pits in England (Hereford), the Netherlands (Bergen-op-Zoom), France (St-Laurent-de-la-Caberisse, Languedoc and Roussillon), Germany (Augsburg, Bavaria, and Bosfeld, Nord-Rhine-Westphalia) and Italy (Parma, Emilia-Romagna). The investigators were firm in their conclusions: 'Together with prior analyses from the south of France and Germany, our data from widely distributed mass plague pits ends the debate about the etiology [sic] of the Black Death and unambiguously demonstrates that *Yersinia pestis* was the causative agent of the epidemic plague that devastated Europe in the Middle Ages.' They went even further than this, however, and used genotyping to argue that the strains that caused the Black Death were unrelated to either the *Antiqua* or the *Orientalis* biovars.[28]

Few medieval historians would be quite as trenchant in their judgements as these paleomicrobiologists, but it is important to note here that their results were obtained by a combination of molecular (aDNA/PCR) and protein (F1 antigen/ELISA or RDT) tests. One of the main problems with the latter is the degradation of ancient antigenic proteins and the limited number of specific antigens for which it could test, while the drawbacks of traditional PCR procedures have already been discussed. The obvious answer was to combine the two, which is what Takeshi Sano, Cassandra Smith and Charles Cantor had proposed in 1992. They developed a system known as immuno-PCR in which a specific antibody-DNA conjugate was used to detect antigens, a conjugate being a bacterium or cellular organism temporarily united with a DNA marker in order to exchange

27 Raffaella Bianucci *et al.*, 'Détection de l'antigène F1 de *Yersinia pestis* dans les restes humans anciens à l'aide d'un test de diagnostic rapide', *Comptes Rendus Biologies*, cccxxx (2007), 747–54; Nichole Cerutti *et al.*, 'La peste dans les restes anciens: un approche immunologique', in *Peste: entre Épidémies et Sociétés*, ed. Michel Signoli (Florence, 2007), 237–42; Raffaella Bianucci *et al.*, 'Plague Immunodetection in Remains from Religious Exhumed from Burial Sites in Central France', *Journal of Archaeological Science*, xxxvi (2009), 616–21.

28 Stephanie Haensch *et al.*, 'Distinct Clones of *Yersinia pestis* Caused the Black Death', *PloS Pathogens*, vi (2010), 1–8 and especially 5.

genetic information. The antibody detects antigens and the DNA functions as a marker to be identified and multiplied by PCR.[29]

There are two main reasons why this new technology did not produce an immediate sea-change in the detection of *Yersinia pestis* and other pathogens. Combining the antibody and the DNA marker proved difficult, and PCR was still a very slow and sometimes inaccurate process. But, by 2005–7, Christof Niemeyer, Michael Adler and Ron Wacker, the first an academic microbiologist, the other two microbiologists working for a chemical company set up to manufacture the compounds, published two articles describing further technical advances and the introduction of what is known as immuno or real time PCR. It allows the detection of antigens using one or more specific antibodies labelled with double-stranded DNA. The first article describes the new technology involved in constructing the sandwich of antigen and DNA, the second the application of the new PCR technique in which, thanks to the use of fluorescent dye markers or fluorescent DNA probes, the reaction between antibody and antigen can be observed and 'quantitated' (quantified) as it happens. The result is a 10–10,000 fold increase in the sensitivity of detection compared with an ELISA test.[30] This was a considerable step forward in microbiology and in medical clinical research, and, of course, it could be applied to the analysis of ancient DNA, where one of its main attractions is that it can test for the antigens of several pathogens at the same time, using much smaller samples.

The research group from the University of the Mediterranean/Aix-Marseilles II soon grasped the advantages of this new technique. In 2011 its members published their findings from an investigation into plague in medieval Venice, where they tested simultaneously for seven highly transmissible pathogens in 175 dental pulp samples from forty-six graves. One of these pathogens was, obviously, *Yersinia pestis*, the others being *Bacillus anthrax* (anthrax); *Borrelia recurrentis* (louse-borne relapsing fever); *Bartonella quintana* (louse-borne trench fever); *Rickettsia prowazekii* (epidemic typhus); *Salmonella enterica typhi* (typhoid fever); and pox virus (smallpox). For once, the results were just as staggering as the investigators claimed. Low levels of *Yersinia pestis* were detected in three samples, two from the fourteenth century and one from the sixteenth, hence the 'successive waves of plague', while *Bartonella quintana* was identified in five samples. Previously unreported data also confirmed *Yersinia pestis* and *Bartonella quintana* co-infections in individuals excavated from a burial site near Paris that had been used from the eleventh to the fifteenth centuries. Trench fever is a louse-borne disease and the importance of lice as a vector for the plague will be discussed further below. A 2012 article by the same team proclaimed that the combination of DNA and antigen-based methods 'allows the resolution of [all] controversies concerning the plague agent'. Dental pulp from thirty-four teeth from five archaeological plague graves was tested by immuno-PCR, standard PCR and ELISA. Of the three

[29] Takeshi Sano *et al.*, 'Immuno-PCR: Very Sensitive Antigen Detection by Means of Specific Antibody-DNA Conjugates', *Science*, cclviii (1992), 120–2.

[30] Christof Niemeyer *et al.*, 'Immuno PCR: High Sensitivity Detection of Proteins by Nucleic Acid Amplification', *Trends in Biotechnology*, xxiii (2005), 208–16; *idem*, 'Detecting Antigens by Quantative Immuno-PCR', *Nature Protocols*, ii (2007), 1918–30. A clear description of these techniques is given by Jeanene Swanson, 'The Rise of Immuno PCR', *Genome Technology* (www.genome-web.com, September 2007).

methods, immuno-PCR was found to be the most effective, isolating *Yersinia pestis* in fourteen of the total sample or 41 per cent, PCR in ten of the thirty-four or 29 per cent and ELISA in three of the thirty-four. In reality this was a comparative process to determine the most effective method of detecting *Yersinia pestis* in the dental pulp of teeth taken from ancient skeletons, rather than any great breakthrough in the identification of the cause of the Black Death. But, taken with the evidence gathered from twenty-seven sites across five countries in Europe using various types of microbiological tests, it now seems certain that *Yersinia pestis* was the pathogen responsible for the second great plague pandemic.[31]

Questions still remain, however, about the virulence and origins of this deadly bacterium and how and why it spread so rapidly across Europe between 1347 and 1351. It has been suggested that the strain of *Yersinia pestis* that caused the Black Death was particularly virulent, and that this was the reason for the notably high death rates from the disease. This now seems unlikely, given the investigations carried out on skeletons found during the excavation of a London cemetery known from historical evidence to contain the graves of victims of the first outbreak in the city in 1348-9.[32] Samples taken from their bones and dental pulp allowed the reconstruction of ten full human mitochondrial genomes and the full pPCP1 virulence associated plasmid.[33] Comparisons with the DNA of the modern *Yersinia pestis* strain confirmed, again, that it was the pathogen responsible for the Black Death, but also that it was of a previously unknown strain. Moreover, the genetic data carried in its pPCP1 plasmid made it no more virulent than ancient or modern forms of *Yersinia pestis*. Given that two of the research teams had previously argued against *Yersinia pestis* as the cause of the medieval plague, this was a major breakthrough, but more was to come.[34]

A second study of the East Smithfield evidence, carried out by much the same group of scientists, reached four important conclusions. The first was that the ancient organism was very close to the ancestral node of all *Yersinia pestis* associated with human infection so far discovered; the second that the Black Death of 1347–51 was the main historical event responsible for the widespread dissemination of the ancestor to all currently circulating strains pathogenic to humans; the third that contemporary (twentieth- and twenty-first-century) strains have their origins within the medieval era; and fourthly that the presumed

[31] Thi-Nguyen-Tran *et al.*, 'High Throughput, Multiplexed Pathogen Detection Authenticates Plague Waves in Medieval Venice, Italy', *PLoS One*, vi (2011), online, e16735; Nada Malou *et al.*, 'Immuno-PCR – a New Tool for Palaeomicrobiology: the Plague Paradigm', *PLoS One*, vii (2012), online, e31744; Thi-Nguyen-Tran *et al.*, 'Review Article. Beyond Ancient Microbial DNA: Nonnucleotidic Biomolecules for Palaeomicrobiology', *BioTechniques*, l (2011), 370–80.

[32] Benedictow, *The Black Death*, 21–2; Ian Grainger, Duncan Hawkins, Lynne Cowal and Richard Mikulski, *The Black Death Cemetery, East Smithfield* (Museum of London Archaeology Service Monograph, xliii, 2008), 1–3.

[33] Mitochondrial DNA carries the genes and functions for the transmission of hereditary information. Plasmids are circles of DNA independent of the genome of the bacterium but contained within it. They contain genes not vital to the growth or survival of the cell itself. During its evolution, the *Yersinia pestis* gene acquired three plasmids which gave, and give, it its virulence: pPCP1 is one of these – see below, p. 26.

[34] V.J. Schuenemann *et al.*, 'Targeted Enrichment of Ancient Pathogens Yielding the pPCP1 Plasmid of *Yersinia pestis* from Victims of the Black Death', *Proceedings of the National Academy of Sciences of the USA, Early Edition* (2011), www.pnas.org/cgi/doi/10.1073/pnas110510718.

increased virulence of the disease may not have been due to its bacterial phenotype.[35] Significantly, it is also argued that factors other than microbial genetics, such as environment, vector dynamics (transmission of the disease) and host susceptibility (lowered resistance) should be at the forefront of future epidemiological discussions regarding *Yersinia pestis* infections.[36]

These are important findings, but not quite as definitive in respect to the virulence of the *Yersinia pestis* pathogen as the authors would wish us to believe. An earlier (2010) study trying to characterize pPCP1 plasmids of *Yersinia pestis* found in states of the Former Soviet Union stressed that much more research was still needed before the virulence traits of these modern strains could be fully understood, and distinctions drawn between those that were highly virulent and those of lower virulence.[37] Whilst the debate on virulence may be on-going, it would be as well for us to take note of environmental and vector influences on the spread and effects of *Yersinia pestis* in late medieval England, on which this study will now focus. But of one thing we can now be certain, that the ancestral home of *Yersinia pestis* lies in northern China. The genome of *Yersinia pestis*, that is, the complete set of genetic material in the organism, was first sequenced in 2001, opening the way for comparisons to be made between the various strains of the pathogen to establish evolutionary changes, and by phylogenetic analysis (gene genealogy) to construct a family tree of the disease. An international team of twenty-four scientists undertook this huge task and published their results in 2010. This was done by a comparison of seventeen whole genomes of *Yersinia pestis* isolates (pure strains) and the screening of 286 further isolates for 933 SNPs, or single nucleotide polymorphisms. SNPs are building blocks of DNA and provide genetic markers that can identify changes in its genomic sequences. Screening allows such changes to be identified and mapped, and the results are fascinating. *Yersinia pestis* emerged in, or near, northern China from *Yersinia pseudotubercolosis*, a soil-based (telluric) bacterium between 1,500 and 20,000 years ago. From there it spread on multiple occasions to Mongolia, Siberia and central regions of the Former Soviet Union; along the Silk Road to East China and Kurdistan and thence to Europe (200 B.C.–1400 A.D.); from China to Africa by the ships of the Great Admiral Zheng He (1409 and 1433); from Yunan to Hong Kong in 1894, and then on to Calcutta, Hawaii and San Francisco by 1899, and to South America; while Madagascar, still a plague hot-spot, was infected from India by 1898.[38]

This might seem to be the end of the historian's problems with the Black Death. There can be little doubt now, in 2013, that its cause was *Yersinia pestis* and nothing else, but, alas, the arguments are not at an end. One of the main objections

---

[35] A phenotype is the observable physical or biochemical characteristic of an organism as determined by its genetic makeup (its genotype) and environmental influence.

[36] K.I. Bos *et al.*, 'A Draft Genome of *Yersinia pestis* from Victims of the Black Death', *Nature*, ccclxxviii (2011), 506–10.

[37] Chythanya Rajana *et al.*, 'Characterisation of pPCP1 Plasmids in *Yersinia pestis* Isolated from the Former Soviet Union', *International Journal of Microbiology* (2010), online article ID760819.

[38] Julian Parkhill *et al.*, 'The Genome Sequence of *Yersinia pestis*, the Causative Agent of Plague', *Nature*, ccccxiii (2001), 533–7; Giovanna Morelli *et al.*, '*Yersinia pestis* Genome Sequencing Identifies Patterns of Global Phylogenetic Diversity', *Nature Genetics*, xlii (2010), 1140–5; Dongshen Zhou and Ruifu Yang, 'Molecular Darwinian Evolution of Virulence in *Yersinia pestis*', *Infection and Immunity*, lxxvii (2009), 2242.

to accepting that bubonic plague caused the second great pandemic is the speed at which the disease spread across Europe. The by now traditional explanation of how *Yersinia pestis* is spread relies on the rat-flea-human relationship. According to this model, the rats or, better, rodents, carry the disease in their blood stream. Fleas, usually identified as being of the species *Xenopsylla cheopis*, the oriental rat flea, live and feed on them and in their blood meals ingest the plague bacilli. These bacilli multiply and form a block in the flea's proventriculus, or gizzard, the thick-walled muscular expansion of the oesophagus above the stomach. This block, and hence the term 'blocked flea', prevents further ingested blood meals reaching the flea's stomach and it begins to starve. The resulting increase in the number of feeding attempts by the blocked flea, combined with regurgitation of ingested blood, makes them dangerous pathogen vectors. When their rodent host dies, the fleas can transfer themselves to human hosts and so pass on *Yersinia pestis* through their bites.[39]

This is the theory. What experimental science has shown is that blocked rat fleas transmit the plague inefficiently because of the long extrinsic incubation period of twelve to sixteen days before blockage formation and subsequent transmission. Because the blocked fleas themselves die shortly after becoming infectious, they are not sufficiently long-lived to drive epizootics, when they constantly infect or re-infect their rodent hosts, unless the number of fleas per rodent is very high indeed.[40] Given the amount of time needed for fleas to block, and the relatively short span of two or three days when they are infectious, it is easy to see why scientists regard this means of transmitting plague as inefficient. The whole cycle from the flea's first infected blood meal to the death of the human can take up to thirty-two days, according to one epidemiologist, which means that the Black Death should have been a slowly moving disease.

This argument lies at the heart of attempts to show that the Black Death was caused by anything but *Yersinia pestis*. Because it relies on rats and fleas as vectors, it is inefficient in spreading to and through human settlements and is slow moving. First, it must kill off most of its resident reservoir of rats before attacking human populations via the rat flea. Even when humans are bitten by a blocked flea, transmission of the *Yersinia pestis* bacillus from the flea's gut to the human occurs in less than 13 per cent of cases. Because of this complex and inefficient mode of transmission, as opposed to person to person transfer, mortality rates are generally low, despite the extreme virulence of *Yersinia pestis*. By contrast, late-medieval and early-modern contemporaries recognized their plague as being distinctly different from any previous disease or epidemic. They not only commented on the disease's extraordinary lethality and the swiftness of death from it, but also on the speed at which it moved through towns and over vast territories. No human epidemic has travelled as swiftly as the Black Death did across Europe from 1347

---

[39] See, for example, R.S. Gottfried, *The Black Death. Natural and Human Disaster in Medieval Europe* (1983), 6–9.

[40] R.J. Eisen *et al.*, 'Early Phase Transmission of *Yersinia pestis* by Unblocked Fleas as a Mechanism Explaining Rapidly Spreading Plague Epizootics', *Proceedings of the National Academy of Sciences of the USA*, ciii (2006), 15380–5. A disease is said to be enzootic when it regularly affects animals in a particular district or at a particular season. It becomes epizootic when there is, for some reason, a sharp rise in the level of the disease in the animal population. Epizootics are the precursors of outbreaks of plague and other diseases in humans.

to 1351, not even the influenza pandemic of 1918, and certainly not the bubonic plague pandemic in nineteenth- and twentieth-century India and China. For these, and for other reasons that will be discussed later, the Black Death could not have been caused by *Yersinia pestis*.[41]

Here we have what appears to be an insoluble conundrum. Microbiologists and palaeomicrobiologists have shown us, after a somewhat bumpy ride, that *Yersinia pestis* was the cause of the Black Death. They have also suggested that it was an unknown strain or strains of the bacterium that caused the pandemic, but that they were no more virulent than current strains. Historians have argued otherwise, basing their case on the inefficiency of the rat-flea-human cycle of transmission compared to the speed with which the plague spread between 1347 and 1351. They have also noted that the Black Death did not occur again within a year or two of the first infection, since the next major outbreak was not until 1361–2, and that such a long interval between epidemics is atypical of bubonic plague in modern times. The fact that references to rats and fleas are not to be found in either contemporary accounts of the plague or in modern archaeological evidence has also been noted by the scientists, but they remain convinced that *Yersinia pestis* caused the second great plague pandemic. It might seem that stalemate has been reached, due to an irreconcilable clash of cultures, but that is not the case. The key to understanding how the plague moved so swiftly and why death rates were so high in 1347–51 lies in identifying the vector or vectors of the disease, since virulence is held to be a function of the efficacy of the vector and not necessarily of the pathogen itself. This is the approach now being taken by microbiologists studying the transmission of the disease in modern societies where plague is both epizootic and epidemic, and their findings are equally applicable to medieval society.

The first line of enquiry has been into the role of unblocked fleas in the transmission of the bacillus. The flea used in the experiments in the United States was not *Xenopsylla cheopis* but *Oropsylla montana*, the prime vector of *Yersinia pestis* in North America, which naturally infests and infects the highly plague-susceptible California ground and rock squirrels which form part of the epizootic reservoirs in the western states. The microbiologists found that after a blood meal on an infected host the unblocked fleas were *immediately* [my italics] able to transmit the plague bacillus and continued to be able to do so for at least four days and possibly longer, since they did not suffer block-induced mortality. The method of transmission was not clear: the authors of the study suggest that it might be mechanical, through the presence of *Yersinia pestis* on flea mouth parts, but

---

[41] This all-too-brief summation of Professor S.K. Cohn's distinguished contribution to the history of pandemic disease and its consequences in medieval and early modern Europe is taken from Guido Alfani and S.K. Cohn, Jnr., 'Catching the Plague: New Insights into the Transmission of Early Modern Plague', *Princeton Working Papers*, http://iussp2009.princeton.edu/papers/90564; George Christakos *et al.*, 'Recent Results on the Spatiotemporal Modelling and Comparative Analysis of Black Death and Bubonic Plague Epidemics', *Public Health*, cxxi (2007), 700–20. For a more comprehensive discussion of the thesis than can be given here see Lars Walløe, 'Medieval and Modern Plague: Some Clinical Continuities', in *Pestilential Complexities*, ed. Nutton, 59–73. This is a more reasoned critique than that by Ole Benedictow, *What Disease was Plague? On the Controversy over the Microbiological Identity of Plague Epidemics of the Past* (Leiden, 2010). Professor Cohn's many books and articles on plague, the response to it and the long-term consequences of it in Italy are essential reading.

regurgitation of the infectious remains of previous blood meals seemed 'the most likely scenario'. Although their conclusions were based upon a laboratory experiment on mice, the authors announced that 'our finding of efficient early-phase transmission of *Yersinia pestis* by unblocked fleas calls for a paradigm shift in concepts of how *Yersinia pestis* is transmitted during rapidly spreading epizootics and requires further studies to elucidate the mechanism by which early phase transmission occurs'.[42]

There is also a strong suggestion here that the role of other fleas in the transmission of *Yersinia pestis* should be considered, including, of course, the human flea *Pulex irritans*, hitherto regarded as an unlikely candidate. There has long been controversy on this issue. Field research undertaken between 1986 and 2004 in Tanzania, in a group of twelve villages in the western Usambara Mountains where there were no rats, concluded that in all of them *Pulex irritans* may have played a major role in plague epidemiology. The investigators noted the research into transmission by unblocked fleas and concluded that, during the second plague pandemic in Europe, *Pulex irritans* would have been a suitable vector because it was abundant on persons and in their homes. The World Health Organisation agrees with these modern findings. In its *Plague Manual* it states that the human flea has been considered as a possible or probable vector of plague in Angola, Brazil, Burundi, the Democratic Republic of Congo, Iran, Iraq, Nepal and, of course, Tanzania.[43] This conclusion has led the Norwegian physiologist and statistician Professor Lars Walløe to argue that 'Most (or all) of the historical European plague epidemics did not involve rats as intermediate hosts. The mode of transmission was from *human to human* [my italics] via an insect vector. *Pulex irritans* may have been the most important arthropod vector in Europe prior to the late nineteenth century.'[44]

If there was human-to-human infection via *Pulex irritans*, then it would help to explain the rapid spread of the second pandemic. More likely candidates as the prime vectors of plague, however, are the human body louse, *Pediculus humanus*, and the head louse, *Pediculus humanus capitis*. Yet again, research on this potential mode of transmission was undertaken by the team from the University of Marseilles/Aix-Marseilles II. They conducted a laboratory experiment to evaluate lice as a vector for plague by allowing the ectoparasites to feed on *Yersinia-pesti-*infected rabbits. High mortality rates were observed in all the lice two or three days after infection and all of them remained infected during their life span. They excreted viable organisms from day one and were able to transmit the *Yersinia pestis* bacterium to uninfected rabbits which rapidly became septicaemic and died of plague. This was strictly an experimental model, to test the efficiency of lice as a plague vector, but it shows that as few as ten of them could transmit plague to a host while they were feeding. The authors stressed again that *Xenopsylla cheopis*, the oriental rat flea, was not encountered in Europe during the Middle Ages, as it is not adapted to the European climate, while the northern rat flea, *Nosopsyllus fasciatus*, very rarely feeds on humans. Bubonic plague was likely to have been

---

[42] Eisen *et al.*, 'Early Phase Transmission of *Yersinia pestis*', 15380–5.

[43] D.T. Dennis *et al.*, *Plague Manual*: *Epidemiology, Distribution, Surveillance and Control*, http://www.who.int/csr/resources/publications/plague/WHO_CDS_CSR_EDC_99_2_EN/en/, 66–7.

[44] Walløe, 'Medieval and Modern Bubonic Plague', 72–3.

transmitted through a variety of vectors, but, they concluded, human lice must be considered as one of the most effective among them.[45]

In the same year, 2006, the Marseilles research team published another article that took the whole question of the persistence and transmission of *Yersinia pestis* to another level, this time drawing not only on their own findings but those of a distinguished group of French biologists working in North Africa and the Middle East in the 1930s, 1940s and 1950s, led by Dr. Marcel Baltazard. They argue that the traditional rat-flea-human model may well fit with observations of sporadic and limited outbreaks, but can hardly explain the *persistence* [my italics] of plague foci for millennia or the epidemiological features drawn from descriptions of historical pandemics. Instead, we should look to soil as a reservoir of the plague pathogen, burrowing rodents as a first link and human ectoparasites as the main driving force in pandemics. Plague is characterised by 'decades of silence' in fixed geographic foci, where its re-emergence should be linked to continuous low-level circulation of *Yersinia pestis* in rodent populations. Environmental changes lead to a sudden and rapid expansion of the rodent population and the ectoparasites they carry, so that increased human contact with rodents may explain the re-emergence of human plague.[46] The two key issues here are that soil acts as a reservoir for *Yersinia pestis* and that, in epizootics and pandemics, human ectoparasites, fleas and body and head lice, are the prime vectors. Other experimental and field research does suggest that *Yersinia pestis* can survive for between seven and eleven months in burrows where a rodent has died and where there were no living fleas. The presence of the pathogen in the soil meant that other animals could acquire it by burrowing, and thereby initiate a new cycle of rodent-flea infection. This could lead to sporadic or isolated cases of plague, to small outbreaks or, at times, to major epidemics. If we can add to this model, for that is what it is, two further pieces of research, the first on the ability of fleas to carry and transmit the pathogen over long periods of time, and the second on sylvatic or endemic plague in the United States in the twentieth and twenty-first centuries, then it begins to take a much clearer shape. Jeffrey Wimsatt and Dean Biggins acknowledge that the preservation of the plague pathogen in the soil may be important, but argue that in the field infected unblocked fleas can carry the disease for up to 130 days, whilst in the laboratory, with sufficient high quality blood meals, they can live up to 411 days. They conclude that fleas and their larvae offer important advantages in provisioning and preserving *Yersinia pestis* reservoirs that enhance plague survival during the endemic period.[47]

---

[45] Linda Houhamdi *et al.*, 'Experimental Model to Evaluate the Human Louse as a Vector of Plague', *Journal of Infectious Diseases*, cxciv (2006), 1589–96; their findings were further reported in Saravanan Ayyaduri *et al.*, 'Body Lice, *Yersinia pestis Orientalis* and Black Death', *Emerging Infectious Diseases*, xvi (2010), 892–3.

[46] Michel Drancourt *et al.*, '*Yersinia pestis* as a Telluric, Human Ectoparasite Borne Organism', *The Lancet Infectious Diseases*, vi (2006), 234–41; for Baltazard's important work see http://www.pathexo.fr/documents/BaltaWeb/Balta.pages for a list of his publications and particularly no. 58.

[47] Jeffrey Wimsatt and D.E. Biggins, 'A Review of Plague Persistence with Special Emphasis on Fleas', *Journal of Vector Borne Diseases*, xlvi (2009), 85–99; see also K.L. Gage and M.Y. Kosoy, 'Natural History of Plague: Perspectives from more than a Century of Research', *Annual Review of Entomology*, l (2005), 505–28.

The other study concerns the conservation of two known plague-carriers in the United States, the black-footed ferret and the prairie dog, both endangered species. Most of the evidence comes from field rather than laboratory studies and it shows that in the western states some rodent species act as enzootic hosts because they are highly vulnerable to the disease. Plague cycles between these hosts and their fleas, without causing high death rates in either of them. The geographical location of the plague foci is of the most interest, however. Within the United States there is an internal frontier of sylvatic or endemic infection, running roughly along the 100th meridian, from Texas in the south to North Dakota on the Canadian border. To the west of the meridian *Yersinia pestis* is preserved in the extensive burrows of the prairie dogs and carried over longer distances by carnivores such as the coyote. To the east of the meridian, in the area of intensive arable farming, plague is largely unknown. Ploughing breaks up the burrows and nests and keeps the soil clear, with the result that endemic *Yersinia pestis* does not survive there.[48]

Habitat, environment and climate are clearly all-important for the continued survival of plague foci from which occasional, local, regional, national and international outbreaks can spread. So far, little research has been undertaken or published on these important issues in the context of late medieval England, but within and surrounding most settlements there were ample areas of meadow, pasture and woodland that could have provided the habitat for enzootic colonies of *Yersinia pestis*. Bearing this fact in mind, it is now time to propose a new model for the persistence and transmission of the plague from the welter of microbiological and palaeomicrobiological evidence already considered above, and then to see if it can be applied to England between 1348 and about 1500. It accepts that the aetiological cause of the Black Death was *Yersinia pestis*; that wild rodents and their fleas preserve the disease in its epizootic state, and that the pathogen can also be preserved in the soil; that during an epidemic or pandemic bubonic plague spreads quickly because the main vectors between humans are the human flea and the louse; and that because of the efficacy of the large numbers of vectors, as much as the virulence of the strain or strains, death rates could be very high. As will be seen, this model cannot provide answers to all the questions raised by the historical evidence, but it comes much nearer to doing so than traditional explanations that rely on the rat-flea-human cycle, or suggest that what swept western Europe in the late Middle Ages was an entirely different disease.

It will explain why the plague spread so rapidly across Europe and the British Isles between 1347 and 1351, since it was almost certainly transmitted from human to human by ectoparasites, notably the human flea and the louse. The pre-existing levels of population, which had reached their peak of ± five million at the turn of the thirteenth century, and established arteries of communication certainly helped the spread of the disease. Indeed, in 2010 Bruce Campbell argued that the pattern of spread implied strongly that humans were the key agent of dissemination.[49] Death rates were high, perhaps as high as 50 per cent of the population on

---

[48] M.F. Antolin *et al.*, 'The Influence of Sylvatic [enzootic] Plague in North American Wildlife at Landscape Level with Special Emphasis on Black-tailed Ferret and Prairie Dog Conservation', in *Transactions of the Sixty-Seventh North American Wildlife and Natural Resources Conference, 2002*, ed. Jennifer Rahm (Washington, D.C., 2002), 104–27.

[49] B.M.S. Campbell, 'Nature as Historical Protagonist: Environment and Society in Pre-industrial England', *EcHR*, 2nd series, lxiii (2010), 309.

aggregate. In his recent works Ole Benedictow has urged us to think more in terms of 60 per cent, but he does not seem to have taken fully into account widespread local variation. In one settlement two-thirds of the inhabitants might die and in another less than a third. The best English evidence for such variation comes from John Mullan's study of plague on the Hampshire estates of the bishopric of Winchester during the second outbreak of the disease in 1361–2. At Bishop's Waltham there was a 65 per cent mortality rate, but on the manors in the Taunton group in Somerset it was much lower.[50] This pattern is likely to have been repeated elsewhere and, as a result, an aggregate death rate of 50 per cent in 1348–9 does not seem unreasonable. Jens Röhrkasten, in his careful study of London wills, suggests this figure for the city and although it is often argued that levels of mortality were higher in town than in the countryside, that simply does not seem to have been the case.[51]

This variability in death rates, and in some cases no deaths at all from the first wave of plague, can be seen all over Europe. David Mengel has challenged the trustworthiness of the famous map accompanying Élisabeth Carpentier's classic 1962 article on the spread of the Black Death. It offers, he says, 'no evidence that the mortality rates might have varied across the vast majority of Europe's area that falls under the epidemic's coloured or shaded sway [on this map]'. His study shows that the plague was not severe in Bohemia in 1349–50, with Prague being scarcely touched at all, and that the same was true of Nuremberg, Passau, Regensburg, Munich, Ingolstadt, Augsburg, Würzburg, Trier, Frankfurt-am-Main, Göttingen, Düsseldorf, Duisburg and probably Berlin. Local studies from the Low Countries and France also point to uneven mortality rates elsewhere in Europe, from the Black Death as well as from subsequent outbreaks of the plague.[52]

This is a salutary story and should remind us of the dangers of making blanket statements about the consequences of the plague for medieval Europe in general. Yet the English evidence does suggest that 50 per cent aggregate mortality was likely in 1348–9, and raises this interesting but as yet unresolved question: were death rates so high because there was rural overpopulation in the late-thirteenth and early-fourteenth centuries, accompanied by severe famines and national outbreaks of sheep and cattle disease and lack of protein in the diet that weakened the long-term resistance of the mass of the population to epidemic disease? There has been much debate on this issue, led by Campbell in his 2010 article and by Philip Slavin in a study of the consequences of the livestock plagues of 1319–20 that followed the Great Famines of 1315–17. Slavin argues that the lack of milk, butter and cheese, all staples of the peasant diet, was instrumental in weakening the human immune system, making the mass of the population more prone to the pestilence that followed some thirty years later.[53] This is an interesting and in many ways

[50] John Mullan, 'Mortality, Gender and the Plague of 1361–2', *Cardiff Historical Papers* (2007–8) http://www.cardiff.ac.uk/hisar/research/projectreports/historicalpapers/index.html, 18–20.

[51] Jens Röhrkasten, 'Trends of Mortality in Late-Medieval London (1348–1400)', *Nottingham Medieval Studies*, xlv (2001), 184–90.

[52] Élisabeth Carpentier, 'Autour de la Peste Noire: Famines et épidémies dans l'histoire du XIVe siècle', *Annales*, xvii (1962), 1062–92; D.C. Mengel, 'A Plague on Bohemia? Mapping the Black Death', *Past and Present*, ccxi (2011), 7, 31.

[53] Campbell, 'Nature as Historical Protagonist', *passim*; Philip Slavin, 'The Great Bovine Pestilence and its Economic and Environmental Consequences in England and Wales, 1318–50', *EcHR*, 2nd

compelling argument were it not for the fact that *Yersinia pestis* attacks the young and healthy more readily than the elderly and infirm, as will be seen.[54]

What is more certain, and far too often overlooked, is that plague was here to stay for the rest of the Middle Ages and beyond. The list of national outbreaks is ominous: 1360–2, 1367–9, 1373–5, 1389–93, 1400, 1405–7, 1413, 1420, 1427, 1433–4, 1438–9, 1457–8, 1463–4, 1467, 1471 and 1479–80. In addition, there were serious famines in the 1390s and in 1438–9, which hit northern England hard and forced the mayor of London to send ships to Danzig for grain, the flux or dysentery in 1473 (and *Yersinia pestis* is a close cousin of *Yersinia enterocolitica*), the sweating sicknesses of 1485 and 1489, which may or may not have been influenza, and the outbreak of the 'French pox' in 1475, brought back by the English troops returning from France after the Treaty of Picquigny.[55] These were national epidemics, however. Little is known about the more localised outbreaks which are sometimes only mentioned casually in records made for other purposes. The year 1438–9 was a national plague year and this affected the opening of parliament at Westminster on 17 November 1439. A common petition requested that, given the presence of plague in the realm, MPs who held by knight service might be dispensed from the customary kiss of homage to the king, for the sake of preserving his health. Three years later there is no mention of plague in the London chronicles, but between 1 April and 29 September 1442 Federico Corner and Carlo Conterini, Venetian merchants, were certified as having neither bought nor sold any merchandise since, because of pestilence in the city, they had stayed in the countryside.[56]

The reasons why the plague did not go away have already been discussed in scientific terms. *Yersinia pestis* had become sylvatic or endemic, ever present among a range of wild and domestic animals in the countryside and in colonies of rodents in towns. Most potential hosts could, and still can, survive for long periods with low levels of the plague pathogen in their bloodstreams. The bacterium cannot kill unless it can multiply rapidly in the bloodstream of its host, which helps to explain why case mortality from bubonic plague in humans is only 60 per cent of those who actually catch the disease. Fleas can re-infect new hosts and so keep the

---

series, lxv (2012), 1239, 1263; see also Ian Kershaw, 'The Great Famines and Agrarian Crisis in England', *Past and Present*, lix (1973), 3–50; B.M.S. Campbell, 'Physical Shocks, Biological Hazards and Human Impacts: the Crisis of the Fourteenth Century Revisited' and Philip Slavin, 'The Fifth Rider of the Apocalypse: the Great Cattle Plague in England and Wales and its Economic Consequences, 1319–50', both in *Le interazioni fra economia e ambiente biologico nell'Europa preindustriale, secc. XIII–XVIII*, ed. Simonetta Cavaciocchi (Florence, 2010).

[54] See below, pp. 35–6.

[55] John Hatcher, *Plague, Population and the English Economy, 1348–1530* (1977), 57; J.L. Bolton, '"The World Upside Down". Plague as an Agent of Economic and Social Change', in *The Black Death in England*, ed. W.M. Ormrod and P.G. Lindley (Stamford, 1996), 30, 32; *idem, Money in the Medieval English Economy, 973–1489* (Manchester, 2012), 231–2 and n. 13; R.S. Gottfried, *Epidemic Disease in Fifteenth-Century England: the Medical Response and the Demographic Consequences* (New Brunswick, N.J., 1978), 43, 106; Edward McSweegan, 'Anthrax and the Etiology of the English Sweating Sickness', *Medical Hypotheses*, lxii (2004), 155–7.

[56] *Rot. Parl.*, v. 39a; TNA, E101/128/30, rot. 10, translated in *The Views of the Hosts of Alien Merchants 1440–1444*, ed. Helen Bradley (London Record Society, xlvi, 2012), no. 47; Carole Rawcliffe, *Urban Bodies: Communal Health in Late Medieval English Towns and Cities* (Woodbridge, 2013), appendix, for a chronological survey of national, regional and urban epidemics between 1250 and 1530.

disease going from year to year at a low level until, and perhaps for climatic reasons, it breaks out again among humans at local, regional and then national levels. Recent scientific research, already discussed and factored into the model above, has also shown that, even when animal hosts die, fleas and other ectoparasites can act as reservoirs of plague for periods of over a year, probably over winter, in time to infect new hosts in the following spring. We have also seen that *Yersinia pestis* can survive for long periods in the soil itself, thus providing another reservoir of plague.[57]

Scientific theory needs empirical evidence for historians to be convinced, however. Here, re-examination of Robert Gottfried's earlier work on epidemic disease in fifteenth-century England, first published in 1978, is timely. He argued that localised and largely unrecorded outbreaks of plague were as important as national epidemics as a brake on population recovery, and that there were villages in East Anglia where death rates were constantly well above average levels in the surrounding areas. In Norfolk and Suffolk these villages could be linked together in two broad geographic locations, a long coastal strip from Great Yarmouth to Aldeburgh, and on the border region between the two counties stretching along the Waveney valley from Beccles to Bungay. These he saw as unhealthy areas of endemic disease or plague reservoirs. Interestingly, most of these 'plague' villages lay outside the prime arable areas in both counties. They had either extensive coastal pastures or were situated near woodland and heath, precisely the habitats where *Yersinia pestis* can survive in burrows and nests, although Gottfried himself does not make this point. His study was much criticised at the time for over-reliance on the vagaries of testamentary evidence, but in the light of recent scientific research it now needs careful re-consideration. Plague reservoirs from which further outbreaks could spread were clearly to be found in late-medieval East Anglia, then one of the country's most densely populated and prosperous regions. Were they not also likely to have been present elsewhere?[58]

Late-medieval England was a plague-ridden society. There may well have been lower death rates from a less virulent bacterium during the national outbreaks after 1348–51, although that remains to be proved, but what they and other largely un-noticed localised outbreaks did was prevent population recovery. 'Disease was prevalent at all levels of society, and even relatively affluent groups such as Benedictine monks were afflicted, so that mortality cannot be assigned an economic cause. Deaths from hunger must have been very rare as basic foodstuffs were relatively cheap and plentiful.' This is Christopher Dyer's most recent conclusion, and he goes on to argue, convincingly, that in the 1520s the English population was probably in the region of 2.2 to 2.3 million, which, with Wales, would mean about 2.5 million, based on evidence from lists of taxpayers under the new assessments of the early sixteenth century. These estimates are supported by the studies of death rates in the communities of Benedictine monks cited by Dyer, which also suggest, alarmingly, that life expectancy actually fell in the second half of the fifteenth century. If this finding can be applied to the population generally,

---

[57] See above, pp. 30–1; the evidence for plague reservoirs is conveniently summarised by R.J. Eisen and K.L. Gage in 'Adaptive Strategies of *Yersinia pestis* to Persist during Inter-Epizootic and Epizootic Periods', *Veterinary Research*, xl (2009), *passim*.

[58] Gottfried, *Epidemic Disease in Fifteenth-Century England*, 126–37.

then it came at a time when plentiful food and vacant lands available at low rents should have encouraged early marriage, rising birth rates and the survival of more children, which should have led to steady population growth. This did not happen. The population did not recover, and in 1520 it stood at the same level that it had been 400 years earlier, in the reigns of William I and William II.[59]

Most modern historians consider this catastrophic population decline – and catastrophic is the right word to use here – to be the result of a crisis in mortality caused by high death rates from persistent plague. The scientific evidence supports an alternative, or rather an additional, explanation: that plague led to later marriage, with fewer children being born of the marriage and even fewer surviving, so that the population, having fallen to new, low levels, could barely replace itself. This is a contentious issue, yet the idea of a changing north-west European marriage pattern has had considerable, if indirect, support from the bacteriologists. Their studies of how *Yersinia pestis* works within humans, mammals and ectoparasites have shown that the bacterium must multiply rapidly in the bloodstream before it can overwhelm existing immune defence systems and kill its host. It does this by the acquisition of ferric iron (Fe^{3+}) through its own built-in iron uptake mechanism, Yersiniabactin, a siderophore-dependent[60] that is widespread among pathogenic bacteria, including *Yersinia pestis*. Ferric iron is literally hoovered-up from haemoglobin, transferrin, lactoferrin and ferritin. If sufficient ferric iron cannot be found in the host, then the bacterium cannot multiply and, if it cannot multiply, it cannot kill.[61]

This phenomenon had been extensively studied in the 1980s by S.R. Ell, who, very unusually, had trained both as a medieval historian, with a Ph.D. from the University of Chicago, and as a radiologist, and published a series of articles on plague and leprosy before he died in 1997 at the early age of 48. In 1985 his study of 'Iron in Two Seventeenth-Century Plague Epidemics' was published, the two epidemics being those in St. Botolph's parish, London, in 1603 and 1625. His conclusions were quite clear. There was a significant preponderance of male victims over females, and males in the healthiest age-group of 15–35 were most affected. Except for those who were pregnant, women were relatively spared, while children over the age of five were also at relatively greater risk than some groups in the population of the parish. Adult sex ratios in iron status are established around the time of puberty. Adult males have a favourable iron balance and a low incidence of iron deficiency, but females of child-bearing age are at tremendous

[59] Christopher Dyer, *A Country Merchant, 1495–1520. Trading and Farming at the End of the Middle Ages* (Oxford, 2012), 5–6; John Hatcher, 'Mortality in the Fifteenth Century: Some New Evidence', *EcHR*, 2nd series, xxxix (1986), 19–38; Barbara Harvey, *Living and Dying in England, 1100–1540: the Monastic Experience* (Oxford, 1993); Mark Bailey, 'Demographic Decline in Late Medieval England: Some Thoughts on Recent Research', *EcHR*, 2nd series, xlix (1996), 1–19; Pamela Nightingale, 'Some New Evidence of Crises and Trends of Mortality in Late Medieval England', *Past and Present*, clxxxvii (2005), 33–68; John Hatcher, A.J. Piper and David Stone, 'Monastic Mortality: Durham Priory, 1395–1529', *EcHR*, 2nd series, lix (2006), 677–87; R.M. Smith, 'Measuring Adult Mortality in an Age of Plague: England 1349–1540', in *Town and Countryside in the Age of the Black Death. Essays in Honour of John Hatcher*, ed. Mark Bailey and S.H. Rigby (Turnhout, 2012), 43–85.

[60] A siderophore is a compound of low molecular mass with a high affinity for ferric iron.

[61] R.D. Penny and J.D. Fetherston, 'Yersiniabactin Iron Uptake Mechanisms and Roles in *Yersinia pestis* Pathogenesis', *Microbes and Infections*, xx (2011), 1–10.

risk, so that 'most women in medieval Europe can be assumed to be iron deficient when not overtly anaemic'.[62]

Ell's work on the importance of iron in plague pathogenesis has been amply supported by recent scientific research, and the implications are obvious. *Yersinia pestis* thrives on ferric iron. Males between 15 and 35 are the best source of such iron and death rates from the plague in this group were, and are, higher than those in any other group, male or female, in both medieval and modern society. As a result, there was a shortage of young adult males at all levels in late-medieval England and women were able to step in, albeit temporarily, and fill gaps in the labour force, either through life-style servant-hood or even through apprenticeships. Marriages were later and fewer children were born of them, and in some cases none at all. Such choices were offered to women by the nature of plague itself, since in order to multiply and kill *Yersinia pestis* must find sufficient supplies of Fe^{3+} in the bloodstream of its hosts.[63] Medievalists are usually wary of chronicle evidence. Bias and inaccuracy are commonplace, yet chronicles do provide us with the only contemporary narrative evidence of events, even if some of their stories were half-remembered, written up in old age or copied from other sources. When chroniclers in England, France and Spain all record that the plagues of 1361–2 and 1369 struck at infants and young men, then perhaps more notice should be taken of them. Thomas Walsingham described the outbreak of 1361–2 as a great pestilence which struck more at men than women, and that of 1369 as a pestilence of men and the larger animals. By the fifteenth century chronicle evidence in England scarcely mentions the plague, alas, but that it was both gender and age specific can surely no longer be doubted.[64]

Most scientists are not good historians and most historians are even worse scientists. The purpose of this study has been to try to bring the two disciplines together to confirm that *Yersinia pestis* was the cause of the pandemic that swept through Europe from 1347 onwards and to explain how and why bubonic plague persisted through the late-medieval and early-modern periods, with such devastating consequences. In so doing, it has become clear that yet more scientific research is badly needed, by historians that is, in certain areas. Was this simply a pandemic of bubonic plague? Pneumonic plague has scarcely been mentioned, although it is well known that if and when *Yersinia pestis* reaches the lungs it can cause secondary pneumonic plague which can then be transmitted to other humans directly through droplets in the breath causing primary pneumonic plague. This strain of the disease results in much higher death rates and even today it is difficult to control or cure, but as yet there seems to be no agreement among scientists or historians as to whether pneumonic plague played any part at all in the second great pandemic.[65] The need for more historical local studies to determine the

---

[62] S.R. Ell, 'Iron in Two Seventeenth-Century Plague Epidemics', *Journal of Interdisciplinary History*, xv (1985), 445–57; see also Vern Bullough and Cameron Campbell, 'Female Longevity and Diet in the Middle Ages', *Speculum*, lv (1980), 317–25.

[63] The debate on the north-western European marriage pattern and life-style female servant-hood is usefully discussed by Deborah Youngs, *The Life-Cycle in Western Europe, c.1300–c.1500* (Manchester, 2006).

[64] There is a detailed discussion of these issues in Bolton, '"The World Upside Down"', 26–40.

[65] J.L. Kool, 'Risk of Person to Person Transmission of Pneumonic Plague', *Clinical Infectious Diseases*, xl (2005), 1165–72; W.W. Lathem *et al.*, 'Progression of Primary Pneumonic Plague: a

presence of plague foci is self-evident, and a greater accommodation between those who argue that the fall in population was due to a continuing crisis of mortality rather than of fertility is overdue, but perhaps beginning to happen.

Most of all, we need a greater sense of perspective, a recognition that the plague had consequences for economy and society reaching far beyond the later Middle Ages. In his letter of 24 October 1348 to all the clergy in his diocese, lay and regular, Bishop Edendon of Winchester may have been guilty of overstating his case, but not by much. Basing his warnings on Matthew 24.18, he wrote that 'A voice has been heard in Rama and much lamentation and mourning has echoed through various parts of the world. Nations, bereft of their children, alas, in the days of unprecedented pestilence, refuse to be comforted.'[66] It is scarcely surprising that the refrain from the Office of the Dead, *'Timor mortis conturbat me'*, was taken up so readily in the art and literature of the late Middle Ages. A simple graph by a modern demographer and a stanza from a poem by the late-fifteenth-century Scottish poet, Robert Henryson, can help us to re-establish the Black Death for what it was, a catastrophic event with very long-term consequences. The graph (overleaf) shows that in 1100 the population of England and Wales stood at between 2 and 2.5 million. It reached its medieval peak of between 4.5 and 5.5 million in about 1300, perhaps began to decline in the early fourteenth century and by 1450, because of plague, had fallen back to the levels of the early twelfth century. It was not until the mid eighteenth century that it again reached the five million mark, some 400 years after the Black Death first arrived in England. The plaintive verse by Henryson helps us understand why this was so:

We beseech thee, O Lord of Lords all,
Thine ears incline and hear our great distress.
We ask of thee aid in general
That is, aid and comfort to those who are destitute.
Unless from pity you restore our hearts,
Without thy mercy we are merely dead.
We thee exhort on bended knees,
Preserve us from this perilous pestilence.[67]

Mouse Model of Infection, Pathology and Bacterial Transcriptional Activity', *Proceedings of the National Academy of Sciences of the USA*, cii (2005), 17786–91; S.T. Smiley, 'Immune Defence against Pneumonic Plague', *Immunological Reviews*, ccxxv (2008), 256–71; David Wong *et al.*, 'Primary Pneumonic Plague Contracted from a Mountain Lion Carcass', *Clinical Infectious Diseases*, xlix (2009), e33–e38; Wang *et al.*, 'A Dog-Associated Primary Pneumonic Plague', 185–90; Röhrkasten, 'Trends of Mortality', 184–8 for plague in London in the winter of 1348–9.

[66]   *The Black Death*, ed. Rosemary Horrox (Manchester, 1994), no. 33, pp. 115–16.
[67]   Robert Henryson, 'Ane Preyr for the Pest', stanza two, in *The Poems of Robert Henryson*, ed. C.G. Smith (3 vols., Scottish Text Society, Edinburgh, 1908), iii. 165.

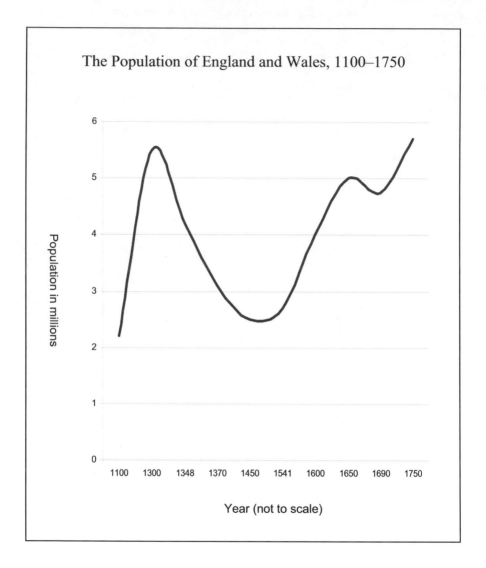

PESTILENCE AND POETRY: JOHN LYDGATE'S *DANSE MACABRE*

Karen Smyth

O Ye folks hard hearted as a stone,
Whiche to this worlde geue al your aduertence,
Lyke as it should euer lasten in one, –
Where is your wit, where is your prouidence
To seen aforne the sodayn violence
Of cruel death, that be so wyse and sage,
Which slayeth, alas, by stroke or pestilence
Both yong and olde of lowe and high parage?[1]

Death is the active subject in this fifteenth-century poem and is portrayed as a multi-faceted character, being both perceptive and learned but also tactile and aggressive.[2] Plague is the agency, or form of attack, by which Death's desires appear to be fulfilled. His targets: everyone. John Lydgate translated this text, he tells us in the '*Verba tanslatoris*' or prologue to the poem, from a French original '*Danse macabre in cimetière des Innocents*', which it is presumed he saw when he was in Paris (as a member of the earl of Warwick's administrative staff) in 1426.[3] A

---

[1] John Lydgate, 'The Daunce of Machabree', in *Lydgate's Fall of Princes*, ed. Henry Bergen (4 vols., EETS, extra series, cxxi–cxxiv, 1923–7), lines 1–8, 1025 ff. I use this edition throughout as it is based on conflations of the A version of the poem (there are two versions or stages of the poem, known as A and B, but the A group is fuller, and there is greater uniformity in the ordering and labeling of figures in it). This edition of the poem is specifically based on Tottel's edition: *Fall of Princes*, ed. Richard Tottel (1554) (f. 220 to the end of f. 224), collated with BL, MS. Harley 116 and, in part, with MS. Lansdowne 669. In what follows, references to the poem are given by line in brackets after citations in the text.

[2] Philippa Tristram outlines the problems in entitling this poem: *danse macabre* implies a dance of death, whereas *danse des morts* suggests a plural significance, 'of the Dead', and that it is the dead who dance while the living are frozen in fear. Tristram notes that Lydgate employs the phrase '*de la danse*' in relation to one specific figure, 'Machabree the Doctour': *Figures of Life and Death in Medieval English Literature* (New York, 1976), 125–7. I have used the term 'Dance of Death' throughout, as it has become the customary way of describing this genre.

[3] The reference is to a depiction of the *Danse Macabre* at the cemetery of the Holy Innocents in Paris. This mural is the earliest known dateable example of the *danse*. See Sophie Oosterwijk, 'Death, Memory and Commemoration: John Lydgate and "Macabrees daunce" at Old St. Paul's Cathedral, London', in *Memory and Commemoration in Medieval England, Proceedings of the 2008 Harlaxton Symposium*, ed. Caroline Barron and Clive Burgess (Donington, 2010), 190–9. For a discussion of how Lydgate translated and adapted the French text, see Oosterwijk, '"Owte of the frensshe": John Lydgate and the Dance of Death', in '"Fro Paris to Inglond?": The Danse Macabre in Image and Text in Late-Medieval England' (Leiden University Ph.D. thesis, 2009), ch. 3. The scheme at St.

slightly revised version was inscribed and decorated with painted images on the cloister walls of the circular Pardon churchyard at St. Paul's cathedral in London, in about 1430, following a request by John Carpenter, the city's common clerk.[4] It was destroyed about 120 years later during the Edwardian Reformation, in 1549.[5] The text, nevertheless, remains extant in twelve manuscripts.[6] In the majority of these manuscripts the figures with whom Death interacts are: a pope, emperor, cardinal, king, patriarch, constable, archbishop, baron, princess, bishop, squire, abbot, abbess, bailiff, astronomer, burgess, canon secular, merchant, Carthusian, sergeant, monk, usurer, poor man, physician, lover, youthful squire, gentlewoman, man of law, Master John Rykill, fool, parson, juror, minstrel, labourer, friar minor, child, young clerk and hermit. Lydgate makes six additions to his French source: the four women, a juror and a conjuror (Master Rykill).[7]

A monk of the Benedictine abbey of St. Edmund at Bury in Suffolk, Lydgate (1371–c.1449) is notionally England's first poet laureate and bestselling medieval poet.[8] Due to the intertwining of his religious, court and public lives and to the sheer volume of his work (that totals in excess of 140,000 lines of verse), it is natural to turn to Lydgate's poetry for an insight into perceptions of, and reactions to, the constant threat of plague. Admittedly, the original epidemic had taken place

---

Paul's was vividly described by Sir Thomas More in *The Four Last Things*: J.M. Clark, *The Dance of Death in the Middle Ages and the Renaissance* (Glasgow, 1950), 12–13.

[4] It is uncertain as to whether all the new additions are by Lydgate. The material relating to the new juridical characters scans differently (being decasyllabic with octosyllabic verses) while still in rhyme royal, and this is wholly uncharacteristic of Lydgate's style. For a recent overview of research in this area and possible ways of reading, see Oosterwijk, "'Owte of the Frensshe'".

[5] The destruction was recorded by the 16th-century antiquarian John Stow: 'in the yeare 1549, on the tenth of Aprill, the said Chappell by commaundement of the Duke of Summerset, was begun to bee pulled downe, with the whole Cloystrie, the daunce of Death, the Tombes, and monuments: so that nothing thereof was left, but the bare plot of ground'. John Stow, *A Survey of London*, ed. C.L. Kingsford (1908), 310. James Simpson considers the motives behind the destruction to have been less a matter of doctrine and more to do with the fact that the message, as well as the religious roles and social estates of the characters, seemed out of date: *Reform and Cultural Revolution, 1350–1547*, *The Oxford English Literary History*, II (Oxford, 2004), 55.

[6] From these 12 manuscripts it is clear that there were different stages of composition and revision. More belong to the A category, which has one additional character and the translator's opening stanzas (leading most commentators to conclude that the B version was revised to accompany the images at St. Paul's). In the B version, nine figures from the A version are replaced with eight new ones, more of whom belong to the world of urban culture, while the order and labeling of the characters also differ. A.C. Seymour goes further in suggesting that there were also C and D groupings: 'Some Lydgate Manuscripts: Lives of SS. Edmund and Fremund and Dance Macabre', *Edinburgh Bibliographical Society Transactions*, v (1985), 20–4. Much critical attention has been paid to the variants, but this debate is not of primary concern in my study. Discussion of the manuscripts and early prints can be found in Oosterwijk, "'Owte of the Frenssh'"; and, for the confusion in creating any kind of textual history, see Derek Pearsall, 'Signs of Life', in *Zeit, Tod und Ewigkeit in der Renaissance Literatur*, ed. James Hogg (Salzburg, 1987), 58–71. For a parallel text of the 'A' and 'B' versions, see *The Dance of Death*, ed. Florence Warren (EETS, original series, clxxxi, 1931).

[7] Critics have been unable to ascertain why Rykill is singled out as a named character, beyond the suggestion that Lydgate desired to make an explicit connection to Henry V's court. See Oosterwijk for a discussion of the possibility that Rykill was Henry V's conjuror: 'Death, Memory and Commemoration', 198.

[8] Today his work survives in more manuscripts and prints than that of any other medieval author. For a documented life history, see Derek Pearsall, *John Lydgate, 1371–1449: A Bio-bibliography* (Victoria, B.C., 1997).

almost a century earlier, and to witness initial literary responses one could turn to William Langland's fourteenth-century 'C-version' of *Piers Plowman* (which reveals a constant state of fear and flight). However, pestilence still struck repeatedly during Lydgate's lifetime: between his birth and the approximate date of the composition of this verse, there were at least twenty-four significant outbreaks of plague in England.[9] Therefore, to explore the development of a tradition of literary tropes on the theme of endemic plague we would do better to study literature in the fifteenth century. This is not an attempt to claim that the Dance of Death genre is a direct response to the plague and the plague alone. Rather, it adopts an endogenous model: that a pre-disposed culture found refuge in a specific range of responses, such as the Dance of Death, that gained prominence after the effects of the plague had made an indelible mark on society, religion and culture.[10] Yet, apart from a few passing references and one practical set of verses on how to avoid catching the disease, pestilence rarely features overtly in Lydgate's work. The exception is this one poem, which clearly professes to be a direct response to the most pervasive, recurrent and determined predator of the age.[11] Even so, in this poem there are no buboes, fevers, or delirium; instead there is a constant interplay and discussion between the figure of Death and the people who represent an assortment of religious orders, professions and social groups. These figures, as stated above, range from the emperor to the lowliest of individuals – religious and secular positions alternating – which schools us in, as well as taunting us with, the lesson that all are equal in the face of death and all must join the dance; all must prepare to meet their maker.[12]

---

9   For a chronology of plague outbreaks in England, see Carole Rawcliffe, *Urban Bodies: Communal Health in Late Medieval English Towns and Cities* (Woodbridge, 2013), appendix, which documents national and major urban epidemics in 1374–5, 1377, 1378–9, 1380, 1382, 1383, 1384, 1387, 1389, 1390, 1391, 1393, 1399–1400, 1407, 1410, 1413, 1417–18, 1419, 1420, 1421, 1423, 1426–7, 1428 and 1429. I am grateful to Carole Rawcliffe for granting me access to this material before its publication.

10   For a more detailed discussion of this theory see Paul Binski, 'The Macabre, the Black Death and Cultural "Causation"', in his *Medieval Death: Ritual and Representation* (1996), 126–34.

11   There are a couple of references to the 'Daunce of Poules', another name by which the 'Dance of Death' became known, across the country (reflecting the impact of the St. Paul's version), in two of Lydgate's later lyrics. The first is to be found in 'Tyed with a Lyne', which is a meditation on the transitory nature of life, and a reminder that everyone must soon join the dance of St. Paul's: *The Minor Poems of John Lydgate, Part II, Secular Poems*, ed. H.N. MacCracken and Merriam Sherwood (EETS, original series, cxcii, 1934), no. 74, lines 66–7. The second reference appears in a poem that is often accredited to Lydgate – 'Prohemy of a Mariage betwixt an Olde Man and a Yonge Wife', in which the old man is cautioned about the progress he has already made in his personal 'Dance of Macabre': *A Selection from the Minor Poems of Dan John Lydgate*, ed. J.O. Halliwell (1842), 34. The practical verse is *The Dietary*, which is less of a poem than a vernacular advice manual based upon Latin plague *consilia*. It comprises recommendations about diet, exercise and personal conduct derived from the *Regimen sanitatis*, as well as some commonplace proverbs (but no lengthy moralizing), designed to offer protection against pestilence: John Lydgate, *The Dietary*, ed. George Shuffleton, in *Codex Ashmole 61: A Compilation of Popular Middle English Verse* (Kalamazoo, Mich., 2008); below, notes 37 and 38.

12   A study of the macabre genre allows Amy Appleford to envisage the strategies whereby a city might represent itself to itself in a socially useful manner: 'The Dance of Death in London: John Capgrave, John Lydgate, and the Daunce of Pulys', *Journal of Medieval and Early Modern Studies*, xxxvii (1998), 285–314. For more on the representation of plague, see Pamela Berger, 'Mice, Arrows and Tumours: Medieval Plague Iconography North of the Alps', in *Piety and the Plague from Byzantium*

This poem is typical of Lydgate's vast oeuvre (he wrote about three times as much as Chaucer), in that we do not encounter frequent or graphic imaginings of the horrific death brought about by plague.[13] Instead, we are invited to contemplate the idea of human existence transcending time, while being playfully pitched against the ceaseless teasings and tauntings of mortality; we encounter a tension between the *ubi sunt* theme of transience and a consciousness of the mutability not simply of the flesh but also of the soul. Another lyric of Lydgate's – 'That now is Hay some-tyme was Grace' – encapsulates this duality, since it opens with the theme of regret for the natural and inevitable transience of mortal life, but then moves to focus on the unnatural duplicity of Fortune and the cruel arbitrariness of her sharp spear. This thematic shift is accompanied by a stylistic one, with a transition from a natural rhythmic cadence in the lyric to unnatural feminine rhymes and emphatic caesura: transience is accepted but mutability causes resistance and disruption. In this one lyric we can observe, writ small, the change in the English literary landscape concerning writings on death in an age of plague: while a desire to affirm and celebrate the positive value of the resurrection of the body lingered, the dominant effect of pestilence was to heighten anxiety about the ruthless, unpredictable and indiscriminate hand of mutability.

Nonetheless, exposure to the effects of death from epidemic disease (not only plague, but also dysentery, tuberculosis and typhus), as well as from famine and war, also produced a certain fascination in literature with morbid imaginings of processes of decay and decomposition: worms, hideous bodies and raggedy skeletons feature in many lyrics from about the middle of the fourteenth century onwards.[14] Lydgate indulges such macabre fantasies in his grisly visualisation of black bones standing upright in their graves in 'The Fifteene Tokyns aforn the Doom'.[15] However, generally in Middle English texts from the late fourteenth and fifteenth centuries, more prominence is given to themes of mutability than to graphic descriptions of specific ailments or of the dying process.[16]

---

to the Baroque, ed. Franco Mormando and Thomas Worcester (Kirksville, Mo., 2007), 23–63; and Elina Gertsman, 'Visualizing Death: Medieval Plagues and the Macabre', in *ibid.*, 64–89.

[13]   Such horrific imaginings can be found, but more often in continental verse, such as the 27 stanzas by Heinrich von Mülgen (c.1320–72), in which he delights in describing plague deaths, or in the songs of the flagellants which reveal the 'plague mentality': Edelgard du Bruck, 'Death: Poetic Perception and Imagination, Continental Europe', in *Death and Dying in the Middle Ages*, ed. Edelgard du Bruck and Barbara Gusick (New York, 1999), 296.

[14]   Tristram demonstrates in a wide-ranging survey that 'a concern with decay is more apparent in writing after the Black Death': *Figures of Life and Death*, 159. Many scholars have warned, however, that a fascination with the macabre cannot be attributed wholly to the outbreak of 1348–9: 'as representations of the three living and the three dead reveal, there was a lively sense of the macabre before the plague. Conversely, the "classic" representations of the macabre in funerary art, the development of shroud brasses and the representations of the cadavers in transi tombs, do not develop until significantly after the plague. The representation of Death as an armed, attacking corpse also seems, in England at least, to postdate the plague': Rosemary Horrox, 'Purgatory, Prayer and Plague: 1150–1380', in *Death in England: An Illustrated History*, ed. P.C. Jupp and Clare Gittings (Manchester, 1999), 115. The changes mentioned here took place well into the 15th century, but, as noted above, plague outbreaks were then far from over and these tropes belong to the age of endemic plague, rather than to the immediate aftermath of the Black Death.

[15]   John Lydgate, 'The Fifteene Tokyns aforn the Doom', *The Minor Poems of John Lydgate, Part I, Religious Poems*, ed. H.N. MacCracken (EETS, extra series, cvii, 1911), no. 18.

[16]   For a survey of contemporary responses to disease and warfare – including the prevalence of the Boethian transcendent ideal, personifications of Fortune, imaginings of grisly corpses and decay, and

This tendency is clearly apparent in Lydgate's religious and secular poems, where themes and images of change and transience predominate. They include the recurrent seasonal imagery of decay and rejuvenation that reminds us of the cyclical and transitory forces of change in nature; the images of heaped bodies on the battlefield in the epic pseudo-historical poems, such as the *Troy Book* and *Siege of Thebes*, symbolizing the capricious nature of warfare; the focus on the tragic deaths of individuals, caused by Fortune's vengefulness and volatility, especially in his *Fall of Princes*; and the consciousness of Lydgate's own need to prepare for death as exemplified in his poetic 'Testament'.[17] Throughout his corpus, life is repeatedly represented as an arduous pilgrimage towards one's own shrine of mortality. Death is, however, also portrayed as a craft that can be learnt, as in 'Deth giveth me no warning', which belongs to the *ars moriendi* genre.[18] A contemporary fifteenth-century text, which was originally ascribed to Lydgate (although his authorship is now disputed), entitled 'The Assembly of Gods', focuses, in a similar fashion, on a wide range of ideas about death and imaginings of, and reactions to, mortality, with the result that fear of death is not only articulated but also analyzed and debated.[19] Throughout its 301 seven-line stanzas, familiar motifs and images recur, reinforcing the message so forcefully conveyed by Lydgate elsewhere: despite the efforts of expert physicians, 'deth al consumyth which may nat be denyed'.[20]

If, therefore, we are to view the long-term effects of plague upon the poetic imagination less in terms of an external and specific physical threat than of an internal state of being, then the principal question raised by Lydgate's *Dance of Death* concerns the light it can shed upon emotions and attitudes during this challenging time. What can it tell us about the challenge of living constantly in the face of random and indiscriminate death? To formulate an answer we need to establish how far this poetic response belongs to a literary tradition already surrounding the figure of Death in the age of plague.

The Dance of Death is a genre akin to the English Morality play, in portraying an allegorical journey, or a metaphorical stripping of both society and the individual, and was a widespread phenomenon across Europe (particularly in the north). A common representative mode and narrative emerged, whereby at least one, but usually several, emaciated corpses, sometimes clothed in burial robes, were painted (or, more rarely, carved) dancing along with one or more characters from various walks of life, on the outside walls of cloisters, of ossuaries and of

---

the development of such genres as *contemptus mundi*, and the *poema morale*, see Tristram, *Figures of Life and Death*; for both English and continental works, see du Bruck, 'Death: Poetic Perception and Imagination'.

[17] See Elizabeth Salter and D.A. Pearsall, *Landscapes and Seasons of the Medieval World* (1973); and K.E. Smyth, *Imaginings of Time in Lydgate and Hoccleve's Verse* (Turnhout, 2011).

[18] For a discussion of the literary genre on 'how to die well', which evolved from a c.1415 collection of Latin texts about Christian attitudes to death and gave rise to one of the most popular printed manuals of the second half of the 15th century, see N.L. Beaty, *The Craft of Dying: A Study in the Literary Tradition of the* Ars moriendi *in England* (New Haven, 1970).

[19] John Lydgate, *The Assembly of Gods*, ed. Jane Chance (TEAMS Middle English Texts; Kalamazoo, Mich., 1999).

[20] This is the final line of Lydgate's rhyme royal translation of the *Secrees of Old Philosoffres* and is thought to have been the last that he wrote before his death: *Lydgate and Burgh's Secrees of Old Philosoffres*, ed. Robert Steele (EETS, original series, lxvi, 1894), line 1491.

family vaults, or inside some churches.[21] Below or above the images, verses were
often inscribed in which Death in a threatening, cynical or even charming manner
addresses each of his victims (and in that sense exercises a little more agency than
the universal abstract of Death in the morality plays). The response of the victim
follows, full of remorse and despair, and crying for mercy, but Death is unyielding
and leads everyone into the dance. Such frescoes range in scope from one to as
many as thirty-six scenes. There is considerable debate as to the origins of the
genre – it has been suggested that such verses were first composed either in Latin,
French or German, but that the Dance itself might have originated in Denmark or
another Scandinavian country.[22] Despite this uncertainty there were clearly
precursors: from the Roman revelry of the souls in the Elysian fields (which was a
rather jollier affair), to various pagan rituals, or folk traditions, such as the death
dances in the Mummers' plays, or schemes relating to the Ages of Man, or the
drawings that sometimes illustrated sermons on Death.[23] By the thirteenth century
there was also a literary genre of French origin called *Vado-mori* (I prepare myself
to die).[24] In these Latin poems, male representatives of various social classes
lament, mostly in two verses, the fact that they will soon have to die. However,
Death does not appear to summon them and nobody answers their prayers.

By contrast, in depictions of the Dance of Death after the 1348–9 pandemic,
dilapidated skeletons dance about centre stage, teasing and tugging at people:
thoughts on the impermanence of life now have to share mental space with an all-
encompassing exposure to death and a vivid consciousness of its arbitrary
character. This imagery does not, however, present death as the antithesis to life;
on the contrary, death enjoys an inherent inter-relationship with the living (even if
it is like an unwelcome relative). What critics do agree upon is that the Dance of
Death rose to prominence as an identifiable genre in both verse and pictorial form
(the two sometimes co-existing but, on occasion, remaining independent from one
another) from the fourteenth century onwards in Europe, and that it continued up to
the eighteenth century through the medium of graveyard poems. There are
suggestions that the Dance of Death was also performed as a play in the fifteenth
and sixteenth centuries, particularly on feast days or in association with guild
dramas.[25] In the fourth and fifth decades of the nineteenth century the topos was

---

[21] Edelgard du Bruck suggests that the Dances were a very specific response to the plague: 'The
     frescoes and woodcuts themselves are said to have evolved from the vision of a Dominican, who
     saw the victims of the plague dance, while Death piped a melody', though she does qualify this
     statement by adding that 'there are many other theories': du Bruck, 'Death: Poetic Perception and
     Imagination', 299.
[22] J.M. Clark, 'The Dance of Death in Medieval Literature: Some Recent Theories of its Origins',
     Modern Language Review, xlv (1950), 336–45.
[23] For speculations on the origins of the genre, see *The Dance of Death*, ed. Warren, pp. xiii–xvi; also
     Der tanzende Tod: Mittelalterliche Totentänze, ed. Gert Kaiser (Frankfurt, 1983), 55–8; and
     Christoph Morgeli and Uli Wunderlich, 'Tanzende Tote in einer Aargauer Handschrift des 14.
     Jarhunderts', *L'Art Macabre*, iii (1999), 144–61.
[24] For a discussion of this genre, see Hellmut Rosenfeld, 'Vadomori', *Zeitschrift für deutsches Altertum
     und deutsche Literatur*, cxxiv (1995), 257–64.
[25] See E.K. Chambers, *The Medieval Stage* (2 vols., 1903), ii. 253. For links with the N-Town play, see
     Gail McMurray Gibson, *The Theater of Devotion: East Anglian Drama and Society in the Late
     Middle Ages* (Chicago, 1989). For links with the Chester cycle, see Sophie Oosterwijk, 'Lessons in
     "hopping": the *Dance of Death* and the Chester Mystery Cycle', *Comparative Drama*, xxxvi (2002),
     249–87.

reinvigorated by revolution and social upheaval, as seen in English and German satirical versions, such as Alfred Rethel's great series, *Auch ein Todtentanz*.[26]

Lydgate's translation, which brought the scheme to England in verse form for the first time, dates from the third decade of the fifteenth century, and is therefore somewhat late, both in terms of the origins of the tradition and in response to the Black Death and subsequent national epidemics. There cannot, however, be any doubt that Lydgate's poem was not only influenced by earlier precursors that pre-date the 1340s, but was also a direct response to the continuing threat of plague and other diseases. Indeed, Sophie Oosterwijk draws our attention to line 483, where 'noble Henry king of Engelond' is named, observing that Henry V had recently been toppled by the Wheel of Fortune, coming to an early, sudden and cruel death through some strain of pestilence, which we now know to have been dysentery.[27] In addition, while the sins of each of the living figures that Death taunts are stereotypical, being the vices of Everyman in relation to the profession or the social or religious group that the figure represents, there are enough hints of topical relevance concerning the specific nature of the sins and of the anxieties voiced by Death's victims to suggest direct allusions to the reign of Henry V and the concerns raised by contemporary commentators and members of parliament.[28] As we shall see below, many of these concerns were all too predictable in a society buffeted by recurrent waves of plague.

But perhaps more indicative of the fifteenth-century date of composition is the fact that there are no graphic horrors describing the realities of death from pestilence in the opening lines of the poem (cited at the start of this essay). Instead we find the late medieval impulse for intellectualizing death through allegory, and for familiarizing it through personification. Here, the personification of Death is engaged in the act of slaying, while a representative group of 'people', irrespective of estate or age, are the victims. The agent of Death is clearly identified as the plague. The opening declaration also suggests that Death is an active force that uses whatever instruments are expedient: plague in itself is no more than a convenient weapon; to take effect it requires an active mediator that is both brutal and sagacious, in the form of the figure of Death. Plague thus becomes more recognizable yet terrible through the concept of personification.

Concomitant with this powerful figure of violence and social leveling comes a suggestion that one cardinal virtue – that of prudential foresight – can be a tool in the hands of those whom Death strikes.[29] This tool cannot help to defeat, or even to

---

[26] For a survey of this genre and theories about its origins, see Clark, *Dance of Death*, 1–7. For a detailed list of all known surviving remnants of medieval Dance of Death schemes, see Oosterwijk, 'Lessons in "hopping"'; and for a fine example in Rouen, Elma Brenner, below p. 127. For a study of how the medieval legacy continued up to the 18th century, see R.H. Bowers, 'Iconography in Lydgate's Dance of Death', *Southern Folklore Quarterly*, xii (1948), 111–28. For adaptations of the genre in more recent centuries, see Anon., *The Dance of Death from the XIIth to the XXth Century: The notable collection of Miss Susan Minns of Boston Mass. Auction Catalogue* (New York, 1922).

[27] Oosterwijk, 'Death, Memory and Commemoration', 185.

[28] For a detailed discussion of the topical aspects of Lydgate's scheme, see Appleford, 'Dance of Death in London', 285–314.

[29] Cicero's definition of the cardinal virtue of prudence in *De officiis* was commonly adopted in the Middle Ages (and is a central theme throughout Lydgate's verse): to cultivate prudence was to 'perceive consequences, to comprehend the cause of things, their precursors and their antecedents, so to speak; to compare similarities and to link and combine future with present events'. Quoted in

defend, oneself against, the enemy; rather it prepares one for the event, providing that one's emotions (as signified by the heart) have not been trivialized or hardened; that they have not grown inflexible or numb because of the transitory vain glories of the secular world. The process of learning the steps (of prudential foresight) so that we may meet this leveler on an equal footing is the lesson that the poem promises to teach. The didactic tone (the advice poem was, after all, the predominant text of the Lancastrian era) is clearly established from the beginning, as in just three short lines the French clerks ask the poet to 'avyse ... cownseille ... [and prompt] sterynge ... and mocioun' (lines 25–7). Although the poem is not an example of the *ars moriendi*, it still instructs and teaches. Lydgate even adds to his French source an exhortation that his readers should themselves learn how to 'trace the daunce of Machabree' (line 46), and at the end encourages them to revise or alter his verses if they wish.

There is, however, a reminder of the fascination with visceral decomposition akin to the characteristic of the more gruesome lyrics from earlier plague years, in that perishable human flesh still graphically succumbs to decay. The closing sequence is spoken by the 'Kynge ligging eten of Wormes', which, we are warned, is also our fate:

> Ye folke that loke vpon this purtrature,
> Beholding here all estates daunce,
> Seeth what ye been & what is your nature:
> Meat vnto wormes; nought els in substaunce.
> And haueth this mirrour aye in remembrauce,
> Howe I lye here whylom crouned a kynge,
> To al estates a true resemblaunce,
> That wormes foode is fine of our liuyng.[30]

Even so, less emphasis is placed upon the final stage of the life-cycle than upon the need to prepare for this inescapable fate. Lydgate's brief, but disturbing, reference to the King's rotting corpse, in a poem that has as its focus more transcendent thoughts, is emblematic of a duality encouraged, if not directly inspired, by endemic plague. John Aberth illustrates this phenomenon vividly by describing such products of the macabre as transi tombs and Dance of Death schemes on the one hand, while, on the other, detecting a fervent hope of resurrection, salvation and eternal life in the cultural artifacts of the day.[31] Rather than cataloguing the dangers of being caught out by Death, Lydgate's poem concentrates upon the energy and supple emotions required to engage with the dance of death while one is still alive.

While the vivid image of worms digesting human flesh might signal the end not only of the King and of us, the readers, but also of the poem, the elaborate and verbose rhetorical processes of Lydgate's writing style constitute a more prominent

---

James Simpson, '"Dysemol daies and fatal houres": Lydgate's *Destruction of Thebes* and Chaucer's *Knight's Tale*', in *The Long Fifteenth Century: Essays for Douglas Gray*, ed. Helen Cooper and Sally Mapstone (Oxford, 1997), 15–16.

[30] Lines 633–40.

[31] John Aberth, *From the Brink of the Apocalypse: Confronting Famine, War, Plague and Death in the Later Middle Ages* (2001), 107–78.

and persistent feature throughout the rest of the verse. A grammar of French gnomic style involving summaries of predictable proverbs, mostly from Biblical or classical sources, is employed, each instance being appropriate to the social role or profession represented by a particular speaker. Such rhetorical devices are in themselves one of the ways by which the moral lesson that all must prepare to die is constructed in the poem. As Derek Pearsall explains, 'in the *Danse Macabre*, what Lydgate had to do for once happily coincided with what he could best do. There is no need for any development of ideas, no narrative, no exposition, only variation, reiteration and insistence on the call of death and man's reply, a prolonged and varied antiphon – "You must die": "I must die".'[32] The mechanical, almost android nature of the extended antiphons reflects the character of the Dance's protagonist: Death 'is personified yet lacks personhood; its form is the form of the cadaverous body, and not the soul, and this lends to it its uncanny robotic quality and its automaton's attribute of irresistible yet terrible inexpressive power'.[33]

Thus Death never does anything else but in the space of one stanza ask, in some way, its subject to dance and refer to the (stereotypical) life that he or she has led. Variation and repetition appear not so much in the dialogue initiated by Death, as in relation to its tone and the emotions associated with it. This can be seen in the extended and varied opening conceit of Death, in which it is introduced by the narrator across some twenty lines. Death may seem robotic, but it is not abstract: it still has plenty of character. It is presented in the act of slaying, invoking the post Black Death 'language rich in weapon imagery ... [of] bows and arrows, swords, and lancets ... as symbols of plague-causing agents', as, with a spear, it strikes down its victims.[34] We also encounter a variation on the theme of the aggressor, with the specific reference to pestilence, reminding us of its insidious and highly infectious presence spreading wilfully among us all. Yet another variation is the idea of the memorial, with reference to the Paris scheme (lines 18–21). What is most indicative of fifteenth-century attitudes is how resigned acceptance of the transience of life is apparent from this evocation of Death, but vies with resentment over the arbitrariness of Fortune's cruel abandonment of those spinning on her wheel. As Tristram comments, 'the harsh, generalised moral, that all men are equal in death, all subject to the fall of Fortune's wheel, is modified by the natural freshness and tenderness, equally typical of Lydgate, of those images of transience – flower, sun, shower and shadow'.[35] As we have seen, these different responses reflect the tension between capricious mutability and meaningful transience that is the trademark of literature in the age of plague.

That Lydgate wishes to emphasize this tension should not be underestimated. Oosterwijk has demonstrated that many of Lydgate's additions to his French source, within the descriptions of individual characters, as well as the translator's preface and envoy, comprise further references to the Wheel of Fortune or comparisons on the theme of '*ubi sunt*'.[36] Complications in our understanding of

---

[32]   Pearsall, 'Signs of Life', 63.
[33]   Binski, *Medieval Death*, 158.
[34]   Berger, 'Mice, Arrows and Tumors', 45.
[35]   Tristram, *Figures of Life and Death*, 169.
[36]   Oosterwijk, '"Owte of the Frensshe"', ch. 3.

transience and capacity to act upon it are underlined, for instance, in the dance with the Physician, when Death affirms that:

> Mans lyfe is nought els, platly for to thinke,
> But as a winde which is transitory,
> Passing ay forth, whether he wake or winke,
> Toward this daunce, haueth this in memorye,
> Remembryng aye there is no better victory
> In this life here than fle syn at the least;
> Than shal ye reygne in paradise with glorye.
> Happy is he that maketh in heauen his feast![37]

While the instability and temporality of life are invoked here, more than passive acceptance is required of Death's victims. An awareness of this transience should be ever-present in the memory: the dance must remain steadfast and constant in every waking and sleeping moment, requiring continuous preparation for salvation and the reward of eternal life. This sentiment is echoed time and time again throughout the dance, whether we encounter those of high or low estate, rich or poor, man or woman, old or young. Lydgate's repetitive narrative about the brevity of life focuses upon the fact that when death is the subject it has the privilege of stasis and fixity, whereas every individual has to remain in a flexible state, constantly being ready to meet the change and the challenge that death brings.

The core tension of the poem is eloquently articulated in the exchange between Death and the Physician. Medical practitioners interested Lydgate; they are mentioned in a number of his works, such as *The Dietary*, where one might expect them to take centre stage, with their remedies and advice on how to avoid infection.[38] Given Lydgate's penchant for lengthy moralizing digressions, the absence of such asides in *The Dietary* is notable. Instead, Lydgate provided simple practical instructions on how to remain healthy, rather than reflecting on divine retribution. Does this mean that the role of the physician assumed primary importance in any discussion of plague? After all, in the *Dance of Death*, the Physician is also at the heart of the complex rehearsal of attitudes towards transience and death. Paradoxically, although there are several passages in *The Dietary* that praise the work and learning of physicians, the advice on offer about prevention is aimed at men and women who sought 'well-being without doctors', not least on grounds of cost.[39] Like many religious, Lydgate presents in simplified, vernacular form the type of material hitherto confined to Latin *regimina* and plague *consilia*, along with more basic recommendations about personal conduct.[40] In a

---

[37] Lines 641–8.

[38] This treatise against the pestilence was, at the time, the most widely read of Lydgate's poems (surpassing even his large scale histories, *The Troy Book* and *The Fall of Princes*, or his romances, fables and religious poems). *The Dietary* survives in 57 manuscripts, only exceeded in the Middle Ages by *The Pricke of Conscience* and *The Canterbury Tales*, and was printed by each of the three early printers – Caxton, de Worde and Pynson. For details about the manuscript and early print contexts, see *The Dietary*, ed. Shuffleton, 1.

[39] Faye Getz, *Medicine in the English Middle Ages* (Princeton, N.J., 1998), ch. 5.

[40] For the translation of texts, see Faye Getz, 'Charity, Translation and the Language of Medical Learning in Medieval England', *Bulletin of the History of Medicine*, lxiv (1990), 1–15; and for Lydgate's sources, Carole Rawcliffe, 'The Concept of Health in Late Medieval Society', in *Le*

similar fashion, in the *Dance of Death*, the exchange with the Physician does not focus on his academic expertise (in contrast to most of Death's other confrontations, where a specialist vocabulary relevant to the victim's craft or profession is employed, no technical medical terms are used here). This ambiguity (of dual presence and absence) is a rhetorical ploy. By including a physician, but neither advertising his skill nor overtly mocking him, what role, we might ask, did Lydgate assign to medical men in the battle against plague? The answer is ambivalent: they are present, they practise, they perform an important function in the physical world, where they are valued, but, as this one stanza in the *Dance of Death* demonstrates, their training and wisdom are irrelevant to the dance of the soul. The medical, corporeal process of healing and curing is largely divorced from the spiritual one, as signified by the absence of specialist vocabulary (in the *Dance of Death*) or moralization (in *The Dietary*). A different language, which, in the *Dance*, is about negotiating and understanding transience, and, in *The Dietary*, is about how to prepare for eventual death by living well, predominates.

Although there is not much movement in terms of rhetorical style in Lydgate's *Dance of Death*, this cathartic exploration of the constant flux of emotions that exposure to death in life creates is expressed, ostensibly, in dance form. Dancing, by its very nature, requires considerable movement and vitality. The visual representations of the skeletons in these Dance schemes are usually full of energy, as their movements appear to be extremely accentuated, even disjointed. Consequently, we can assume that the skeletal figures depicted in St. Paul's churchyard would have been similar to those found in Holbein's repertoire of wood engravings.[41] It is surely no coincidence that the peculiar gestures of the skeletons mimic the involuntary actions of the victims of plague, whose bodies were violently energised just before death with random movements when poisoned by cell necrosis.[42] The significance of the fact that the pictorial representation of such movements was contentiously described as a form of *dance* should not be underrated. As Paul Binski has noted, the depiction of Dance of Death schemes in graveyards challenged ecclesiastical prohibitions on dancing there, as such activity was deemed to be both disorderly and sensual and therefore sinful. In a similar fashion, the Dances portrayed on walls and windows inside churches challenged the sacred notion of the dead at rest, as enshrined in the requiem mass. Conversely, dance was also becoming an allegorical means of explaining and categorising social customs and the stages of life.[43] As Binski again observes, 'the Dance of Death is thus at one level a tableau of class norms. The living step cautiously, the dead with uncannily enthusiastic high kicks: the dead by virtue of their movement are another order, another class.'[44]

Death's gestures and movements in Lydgate's Dance are revealing. Death varies its demeanour, from being tantalizing (in relation to the proud and greedy rulers) to becoming demure (with the Hermit and Labourer) and even protective (of the

---

interazioni fra economia e ambiente biologico nell'Europa preindustriale secc. XIII–XVIII, ed. Simonetta Cavaciocchi (Florence, 2010), 321–38.

[41] Hans Holbein, *The Dance of Death*, intro. Austin Dobson (London and New York, 1892), plates VI–XXXIX, XLII–XLIX.

[42] Aberth draws our attention to this phenomenon: *From the Brink*, 206.

[43] Binski, *Medieval Death*, 154–8.

[44] *Ibid.*, 156.

Child). Death's mutability is heard as well as seen, as it changes the register it uses in relation to whoever it is seducing. For example, when conversing with the Juror it employs a measured legal tone, whereas it adopts the discourse of magic with the Astronomer: Death is able to morph and mutate.[45] James Simpson explains how Death unnervingly targets and defeats his subjects by explicitly challenging society's sources of comfort, ease and power, be it through the fragility of the legal system, the impermanence of military conquest, or the illusive freedom of cities once feudal powers had been undermined.[46] Perhaps, though, most striking is the fact that a whole gamut of emotions is also run by Death. Indeed, a close reading of its gestures and emotive strategies, as we shall see here, reveals that this poem is not just about the depiction of class hierarchies, not just a satire on the greedy and sinful, not just a moral admonition concerning the universality of death, but a performative index (in rhetorical terms) of attitudes towards death in this age of plague.

For example, the most frequent refrain employed by Death is one of mentoring, encouraging its victims to 'learn the dance', professing to be a teacher or cheering them on to heed its instructions. This suggests a desire to make death meaningful as a craft or skill that can be learnt, and to emphasise the potential benefits to be gained from an encounter with this frightening force. At other times, however, Death reveals a much more strident personality, as it variously insists that its followers obey, or chides their sins and foibles. It gains satisfaction in mockery, is dismissive as it instructs them to forget their earthly lives, and harshly questions, chastises or delights in warning them of looming tribulations. The moral message of repentance and atonement is forcefully conveyed by this personality, but so too is a feeling that everyone is defenceless, and that this secular world is a transient, pointless one. There is also a brutal, dark side of Death that emerges in a number of the dialogues, as it asserts its right to compel a reluctant victim to dance, threatens its prey with Judgement Day, talks of stabbing and slaying, and boasts that its steely grip will not let anyone go or that its weight will crush them all. The mutability and savagery of Death is given a distinct personality, presenting the otherwise incomprehensible in a familiar guise as a bully and a tyrant, and giving fear of death a voice. One more aspect of Death's multifaceted character emerges in some of the exchanges, being arguably more cunning and eloquent: it denies the alternative reality of dream worlds, it flatters, it presents the dance as a communal one with enticing company, and it cajoles its victims by begging them to learn the steps, or tempts with promises of an exciting journey or with an outreached hand. It even claims that a transformation can happen during the dance, while also planting seeds of doubt about the attractions of the secular world with references to the Wheel of Fortune. A sense of manipulation develops, as if mutability is sweeping onwards and acquiring a force of its own. At one point Death (who is also a comedian) expresses some reluctance at the thought that its dance partner might be heavy and stout, but it constantly insists that it is ready, willing and able to start at any given moment, and that any hour could be the last. The sense of urgency suggests an undercurrent of panic concerning the need to be instantly ready and a

---

[45] See Oosterwijk, '"Owte of the frensshe"', ch. 3, for a figure-by-figure description of Death's responses and discourses.

[46] Simpson, *Reform and Cultural Revolution*, 54.

sense of regret that death will take anyone, even those who may not seem to be ideal partners.

The significance of gesture and emotion in this genre thus crucially provides an additional narrative through which to understand attitudes to mortality in an age of plague. Lydgate presents us with an extended scale by which to measure these reactions, for it is not only Death but all of the other figures as well who are constructed as emotional signifiers. Before turning to their responses, a brief consideration of another visual source will offer a further insight into this aspect of the Dance.

A stained-glass panel in St. Andrew's church in Norwich, dating from about 1510, depicts a scene from the Dance of Death that shows a skeleton accosting a bishop. Its origins are unknown, and although the iconography suggests that it could be French, many of the details are similar to those exhibited in local glass and in a number of printed primers from the end of the fifteenth century, as David King has discovered. King has established that, in 1500, around the same time as an unusually virulent outbreak of plague in London, Nicholas Goldwell, then dean of the college of St. Mary in the Fields, designed and initiated the building of St. Andrew's nave to accommodate the proposed glazing for an entire Dance of Death scheme:

[the scene] depicting Death leading a bishop away, now in the south aisle, was in the north clerestory, part of a series of what could have been thirty-three panels across eleven windows, showing Death leading off men of all degree, from an emperor, pope, cardinal and bishop to a carpenter and other tradesmen, as Kirkpatrick noted. This series is unique in English medieval glass, and must have provided an impressive display and a continual *memento mori* to the members of the congregation.[47]

As can be seen in the image reproduced here (see plate 1), the skeleton, while leaning in towards the bishop in what may be a vague imitation of the gesture known as *syndesmos*, is, however, met with resistance.[48] The bishop's body is arched away from Death, straining to be free, while the head, which is the vessel containing the mind, is tilted as far away from his assailant as possible. But the bishop's eyes appear to be magnetically drawn back, staring towards his captor. That we should read this stance figuratively is not in question, largely because of the symbolism of the chess board on which Death is standing: amid outbreaks of plague, a popular metaphor was that life was a game of chess, and to be struck by pestilence was check-mate. (This conceit is employed by one of the subjects of Lydgate's poem: an amorous gentlewoman refers to herself as being 'checke-mate'

47 David King, 'Norfolk: Norwich, Parish Church of St Andrew. O.S. TG232087', *Corpus Vitrearum Medii Aevi of Great Britain*: http://www.cvma.ac.uk/publications/digital/norfolk/sites/ norwichstandrew/history.html [accessed July 2012]. King refers here to the antiquarian John Kirkpatrick, who recorded his observations on St. Andrew's church in September 1712. Norfolk RO, Fitch Collection, MC 500/14, 761X7, 39–43. The epidemic of 1500 may have spread to other cities, including Norwich, and certainly reached Bury St. Edmunds: Rawcliffe, *Urban Bodies*, appendix.

48 This gesture is typically associated with God, when He faces the beholder with arms outstretched. See Pamela Sheingorn, 'The Visual Language of Drama: Principles of Composition', in *Contexts for Early English Drama*, ed. M.G. Briscoe and J.C. Coldewey (Bloomington, Ind., 1989), 173–91.

by the plague.)[49] The bishop's gesture of defiance and resistance, as expressed in the body's movement and by an intellect that wishes to distance itself from the inevitability of death, is contradicted by his eyes, which, as the popular proverb of the day explained, are the mirrors of the soul.

Is it surprising that a bishop is cast in such a pose? No, for the Dance schemes are widely recognised as satires, not only of secular rulers but also of rich and powerful religious figures, who, being human, were subject to the same sins and foibles as the lowlier members of society. During plague epidemics the clergy were particularly vulnerable to infection because they were responsible for performing funeral rites and administering confessions, which had led by the fifteenth century to a decline in the number of ordinands and, in turn, to a lowering of standards among the newly admitted. The alleged failure of the clergy to discharge their obligations because of falling numbers and a general lack of vocation resulted in the stereotypical corrupt and greedy cleric becoming a common trope in literature at this time. Lydgate's Bishop is also resistant to Death's embrace, as he covets his worldly goods above the prospect of heaven and fears that the food provided at his lavish feasts will rot and decay. Even Lydgate's Friar is criticised for abandoning the path to salvation, by focusing on horrific depictions of the macabre in his sermons rather than on the Christian lessons of how to learn to die. Everyone, as Lydgate's most senior religious figure – the Pope – warns us, needs to 'prudently see' the dance that awaits (line 72). It is worth noting that the audience for the scheme in St. Andrew's was socially mixed, in that it included mayors and aldermen, as well as craftsmen, among its members. Significantly, a Dominican friary stood opposite the church.[50]

Tristram maintains that throughout Lydgate's Dance the powerful and rich seem proud and do not shield their faces; nor do they feel terror. The poor and the good are at peace with God, the old are weary for the grave and the innocent child is protected and unafraid.[51] This interpretation has been rarely challenged, although, on closer inspection, a more nuanced narrative of emotions can be read. Just like Death, its many victims express a range of telling sentiments. Anxiety and fear in the face of mortality are perhaps the most obvious of these human responses, but that it is the senior religious figures who most often and most intensely react in this way is less expected. The adjectival phrase of being in 'grete distresse', or a variation on it, such as 'gret drede', of experiencing a desire to 'fle' or nursing a 'gret greuaunce' feature predominantly in the Cardinal's, Patriarch's, Archbishop's and Abbot's responses. Like the bishop in the stained-glass panel in St. Andrew's church, they are resistant to, if not overtly afraid of, Death. By comparison, the most powerful secular figures convey a more measured sense of regret and disappointment. Any resistance is expressed not as the raw emotion of terror but as denial, in attempts to postpone, reason or negotiate. The Emperor has a 'querel' (line 83) in his own mind and feels constrained, while the King refuses at first to dance but then becomes desperate for counsel, while the Bailiff grumbles about the hard journey to come. Does this behaviour imply that the eminent religious figures are only too conscious of the day of reckoning ahead, whereas their secular

---

[49]   Line 459.
[50]   King, 'Parish Church of St Andrew'.
[51]   Tristram, *Figures of Life and Death*, 167.

counterparts are completely immersed in vain glories, harbouring a naive belief that they can restrain and bargain with Death? This is unlikely, for Death attacks the pride and greed of all of the senior religious figures; they are not presented as perceptive members of the Dance. The Pope is shown myopically to believe Death's satiric hyperbole concerning his sovereignty. The Cardinal is mocked for his pride in his red hat, as is the Abbot with regard to his great hat (echoes of Geoffrey Chaucer's caricature of the Miller, and, indeed, of Bishop Beaufort's celebrated confrontation with his nephew, Henry V, are not far from the surface here).[52] Meanwhile, the Archbishop and Bishop are guilty of treasuring worldly goods rather than preparing their souls for heaven. These religious subjects are not overwhelmed by fear of the Day of Judgement; rather they are too preoccupied with material possessions and achievements to contemplate it as they should. While the secular figures are subject to the same robust satire, and are also denounced by Death, the difference in their emotional responses suggests that Lydgate criticises religious figures who profess good deeds and thoughts but behave very differently, in a far more trenchant fashion than those in secular life, whose hearts have become numb and who have grown oblivious of, or defiant towards, the inevitability of the Dance.

By contrast, a second group, whose religious and lay members rank a little lower in clerical, professional or social status than those of the first, elicits a more accommodating response. These individuals, nonetheless, still differ in their reactions to Death's call. There is, for instance, a sub-group that demonstrates an intense and extreme repugnance when faced with the contemplation of death: cries of pain and protests that their hearts are fraught with emotion, as well as noisy laments about their inability to defy death, emanate from these characters. This time they are not powerful prelates, but perhaps it should be no surprise that they include figures such as the Merchant, Usurer of the poor, Man of Law, Amorous Squire, Minstrel, Young Clerk and Parson: all of whom are (stereotypically) greedy and covetous, or consumed with the youthful delights (and vices) of life. Their despair in the face of *mors improvisa* reflects their refusal to learn how to die, while their resistance marks a failure to comprehend the mutability of life when no thought is given to its inherent and meaningful transience. Yet at times such laments are employed in a more positive way as a means of signifying compliance without true understanding. This alternative sub-group comprises figures such as the Man of Law, the Astronomer, the Juror and the Friar, each of whom uses his verbal skills or specialist vocabulary in an attempt to make the Dance appear comprehensible, sometimes in a doomed effort to defy death but in others simply as a way of acknowledging it. An almost 'neutral', matter-of-fact response reveals a pragmatic desire to rationalise and familiarise death.

A poignant sadness is also felt, especially by the Burgess, Constable and Monk, each of whom in some way experiences 'sorowe and eke sweteness' at the prospect of death. While there are still moments of anguish among this group, as exemplified by the Monk's overdue yearning after contemplation, melancholy is tinged with self-awareness, with consciousness of past vices and a recognition of

---

[52] Geoffrey Chaucer, *The Canterbury Tales*, in *The Riverside Chaucer*, ed. L.D. Benson (3rd edn., Oxford, 1998), 66, line 16; K.B. McFarlane, 'Henry V, Bishop Beaufort and the Red Hat, 1417–21', *EHR*, lxix (1945), 316–48.

the futility of life. Several of these responses are similar to refrains in the literature of the *ars moriendi*. Learning the craft of dying, while undertaken reluctantly and with sadness, is still a better option than to resort to recriminations and a futile desire to flee, as we saw in the case of the prelates. Simpson briefly draws attention to this development, observing that 'the lower we go, the more moving become the encounters', and citing the humble labourer's sense of regret tinged with resignation, and the affectionate, blissfully ignorant child's inarticulate but pitiful cry: 'A a a, a woorde I cannot speake; / I am so younge; I was borne yesterday'.[53]

Pity for the Child is all the more intense because of the changing demographics of plague, for 'chroniclers across Europe agree that, while the Black Death of 1348–9 hit a broad cross-section of society, children were the major victims of plague in the later fourteenth century and fifteenth century'.[54] In England, in the last four decades of the fourteenth century alone, there were at least six major outbreaks of pestilence that appear to have killed far more youngsters than adults. One such epidemic occurred in 1361–2, taking a particular toll in East Anglia; in 1378–9 another began in York and spread across the north; in 1382 London was afflicted; in 1383 disease again ravaged children in Norfolk; in 1390 the young died in considerable numbers throughout England; and at the turn of the century, in 1399–1400, another child-centred epidemic spread across the country.[55] Adam of Usk's terse reference to the 1399–1400 pestilence is typical in its response to such 'foul death'. He notes that the disease 'prevailed through all England, and specially among the young, swift in its attack and carried off many souls'.[56] Whereas chroniclers tended to dwell upon the unbearable pain, spasms or stench when adults were the main victims of plague, in descriptions of the children's fate the focus is invariably on the rapidity and clinical efficiency of death. It is little wonder, then, that in Lydgate's poem emphasis is placed on how short a time the Child has spent in this world.

That the Child has not yet learnt how to speak is significant. A metaphorical stripping of the body's functions occurs throughout the various responses. The Pope may begin by urging us to use our eyes prudently, but they and other parts of the body cease to work as the verse progresses. As the Baron is struck down by Death his legs grow lame. Vain to the very end, the Princess welcomes her escape from wrinkly skin. The Abbess imagines that her whole body has become a vessel for Death, a boat for his journey. Meanwhile, the Poor Man has no voice and the Usurer is blind. If the physical attributes are stripped away, all we are left with are emotions. That the warmest and most gentle responses to Death are more collectively positioned towards the end of the poem, and thus among the lower echelons of the social hierarchy, is no accident. A number of these figures welcome death. The Old Man weary of life is relieved to embrace it. The young Child, too innocent for this world, is oblivious and happy. The Carthusian and the Hermit, however, who are already dead to this world, and actively chose to be so, are the calmest and most humble. The Hermit is the only figure to whom Death

---

[53] Simpson, *Reform and Cultural Revolution*, 54; lines 585–6.

[54] Deborah Youngs, *The Life Cycle in Western Europe, c.1300–c.1500* (Manchester, 2006), 25.

[55] For chronicle entries relating to each of these epidemics, see Rawcliffe, *Urban Bodies*, appendix; and for Italian evidence, below, p. 205.

[56] *Chronicon Adae de Usk*, ed. E.M. Thompson (1904), 46, 207, quoted in Rawcliffe, *Urban Bodies*, appendix.

actually replies, when it praises him by asserting 'that is wel sayd ... A better lesson there can no clerke expresse, / Than til to-morow is no man sure to abide.'[57]

Death is at once feared and desired, an object of disgust and horror, but also of pleasure. By describing these diverse, sometimes contradictory attitudes, Lydgate permits us to escape the profane banality of death. Thoughts about meaningful transience co-exist with deeper anxieties concerning the arbitrariness of Fortune, mutability and decay. The wide range of moving responses to Death cannot be dismissed by modern commentators as no more than a laboured rhetorical exercise in variations on a theme: Death may be the protagonist in Lydgate's poem, presenting different faces to different people, but, through an analysis of their socially conditioned reactions, a moral form of resistance to mortality is created. The striking array of emotions enacted by Death and its victims is not intended to suggest that, in the end, we all are destined to become non-signifying cadavers. Rather, Lydgate conveys the more positive, if disconcerting, message that each of us has a dance to learn and to perform during life.

[57]   Lines 625, 631–2.

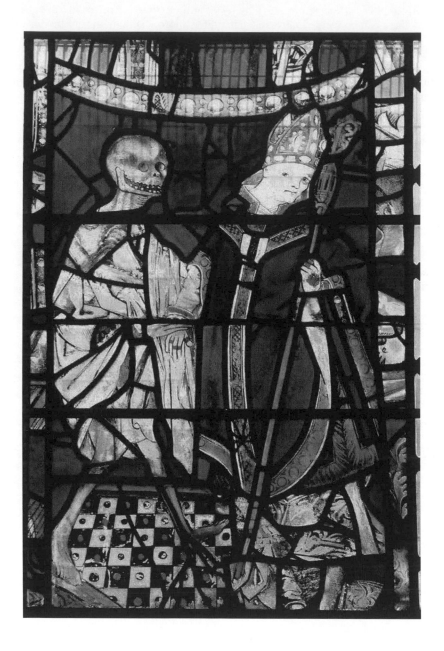

Plate 1: Death leading a bishop away: stained-glass panel in St. Andrew's church, Norwich. Photograph: David King.

PILGRIMAGE IN 'AN AGE OF PLAGUE': SEEKING CANTERBURY'S 'HOOLY BLISFUL MARTIR' IN 1420 AND 1470

Sheila Sweetinburgh

As Carole Rawcliffe has reminded us, in medieval culture the close linkage between the Church and healing with respect to both body and soul was widely understood, and pilgrimage was a principal means of seeking such aid.[1] Even though the greatest collections of miracle cures at English shrines belong to the high Middle Ages, miracles continued to be recorded in various ways until the shrines were destroyed in the sixteenth century. Pilgrimage, too, was recognised for its penitential value, the shrine of St. Thomas of Canterbury being one of the four major destinations; and, as well as encouraging personal initiatives, certain bishops seem particularly to have favoured its imposition.[2] Nor was the potential for bodily and spiritual healing confined to the individual pilgrim, or for those on whose behalf s/he was acting, because processions (and pilgrimages) were at times staged by entire communities in order to seek collective relief from specific dangers and disasters. In these circumstances, the Church often sanctioned a variety of pious activities, including the bearing of relics, in an attempt to avert divine wrath or retribution, notwithstanding the belief that such events might have been sent by God to punish or test mankind.[3]

The upsurge in income received at English shrines in the fourteenth century, and especially about the time of the Great Famine and in the aftermath of the Black Death, would seem to represent a significant increase in the number of pilgrims acting individually and collectively in response to these crises.[4] The apparent desire by so many to go on pilgrimage might even suggest that there were widespread apocalyptic fears; and, although such fears may have abated somewhat for

---

[1] Carole Rawcliffe, 'Curing Bodies and Healing Souls: Pilgrimage and the Sick in Medieval East Anglia', in *Pilgrimage: The English Experience from Becket to Bunyan*, ed. Colin Morris and Peter Roberts (Cambridge, 2002), 108.

[2] As Diana Webb has noted, Bishop Hamo's register from Rochester furnishes numerous examples: Diana Webb, *Pilgrimage in Medieval England* (London and New York, 2000), 235–6. See also Paul Booth, 'The Last Week of the Life of the Black Prince', in *Contact and Exchange in Later Medieval Europe: Essays in Honour of Malcolm Vale*, ed. Hannah Skoda, Patrick Lantschner and R.L.J. Shaw (Woodbridge, 2012), 242–3.

[3] For example: *The Black Death*, ed. Rosemary Horrox (Manchester and New York, 1994), 111–12; and Rita Tekippe, 'Pilgrimage and Procession: Correlations of Meaning, Practice, and Effects', in *Art and Architecture of Late Medieval Pilgrimage in Northern Europe and the British Isles*, ed. Sarah Blick and Rita Tekippe (Leiden and Boston, 2005), 731–2.

[4] Ben Nilson, *Cathedral Shrines of Medieval England* (Woodbridge, 1998), 241.

succeeding generations, the sense that they were justified evidently remained.[5] This is not to imply that the fifteenth century should be seen in terms of Johan Huizinga's *Waning of the Middle Ages*, but that an awareness of 'last things' was part of that century's cultural capital, whether in terms of contemporary art, literature, drama, or piety, including pilgrimage.[6]

Recent English scholarship on late medieval pilgrimage has focused on what are seen as its different characteristics when compared to those of pilgrimage during the pre-Black Death era, and especially the twelfth and thirteenth centuries. Thus, Eamon Duffy has highlighted the importance of localism (while not totally discounting national shrines such as Walsingham and Canterbury), where the distance travelled was no more than a visit to the nearest market, and also the general shift away from old thaumaturgic relics to specific Marian images and Christocentric cults, from the great Rood of Boxley to lesser roods, as at Blythburgh or Bramfield.[7] Ronald Finucane had already observed this development; and he, too, acknowledged that certain older shrines, in particular St. Thomas of Canterbury, remained popular among pilgrims throughout the Middle Ages: an assessment qualified by Ben Nilson on the ground that saints' cults were often the victims of fashion.[8] From his analysis of English cathedral shrines Nilson concluded that pilgrims turned away from many established cults, once they had achieved their optimum popularity, in search of new attractions, and that, in addition to images and other wonders, political martyrs became a significant focus of devotion in the fourteenth and fifteenth centuries. This latter phenomenon has been the subject of a recent study by Danna Piroyansky, who sees the growth of Thomas of Lancaster's and Henry VI's cults as being driven by popular appeal.[9] Yet, as she and others have recognised, the promoters of some of these cults were still keen to link their miracle-working martyr to older saints, particularly St. Thomas the Martyr, which served further to enhance the Canterbury saint and his Christ-like sacrifice.[10] Nonetheless, the proliferation of such new cults did not always meet with official approval, especially when opposition to the ruling regime might gather around the 'saint'. Additionally, as Diana Webb and others have

---

[5]   L.A. Smoller, 'Of Earthquakes, Hail, Frogs, and Geography: Plague and the Investigation of the Apocalypse in the Later Middle Ages', in *Last Things: Death and the Apocalypse in the Middle Ages*, ed. C.W. Bynum and Paul Freedman (Philadelphia, 2000), 156–87; Miriam Gill, 'Monastic Murals and *Lectio* in the Later Middle Ages', in *The Culture of Medieval English Monasticism*, ed. J.G. Clark (Woodbridge, 2007), 64–7.

[6]   Johan Huizinga, *The Waning of the Middle Ages*, trans. F.J. Hopman (1924). For an appraisal, see Margaret Aston, 'Huizinga's Harvest: England and The Waning of the Middle Ages', *Medievalia et Humanistica*, new series, ix (1979), 1–24. For example: *The Pilgrimage of the Lyfe of the Manhood*, ed. Avril Henry (EETS, original series, ccxcii, 1985); *Everyman and Medieval Miracle Plays*, ed. A.C. Cawley (1974); Pamela Berger, 'Mice, Arrows and Tumors: Medieval Plague Iconography North of the Alps', in *Piety and the Plague from Byzantium to the Baroque*, ed. Franco Mormando and Thomas Worcester (Kirksville, Mo., 2007), 42–61; and Elina Gertsman, 'Visualizing Death: Medieval Plagues and the Macabre', in *ibid.*, 64–89.

[7]   Eamon Duffy, 'The Dynamics of Pilgrimage in Late Medieval England', in *Pilgrimage: The English Experience*, ed. Morris and Roberts, esp. 166, 172.

[8]   R.C. Finucane, *Miracles and Pilgrims: Popular Beliefs in Medieval England* (Basingstoke, 1977), 191–202; Nilson, *Cathedral Shrines*, 178.

[9]   Danna Piroyansky, *Martyrs in the Making: Political Martyrdom in Later Medieval England* (Basingstoke, 2008).

[10] *Ibid.*, 32, 43, 48.

noted, those accused of heresy were often fierce critics of pilgrimage, and especially of what they saw as the worship of relics comprising no more than dead sticks and stones.[11]

From the evidence of offerings to St. Thomas at Canterbury in the fourteenth century, particularly in the immediate aftermath of the Black Death, again during the 1370s, and, to a lesser extent, in the years following the Great Famine, it would appear that the shrine then drew an increasing number of pilgrims.[12] Indeed, notwithstanding the problem posed by several unquantifiable variables, it is conceivable that, during the post-Black Death period, the percentage of the population visiting St. Thomas' shrine may not have been significantly lower than that reached at the height of the saint's international popularity in c.1220.[13] This suggests that the growing appeal of saints especially revered for their aid against plague did not impinge on Becket's standing, and that people viewed pilgrimage to his shrine during a period of devastating plague epidemics and other disasters as highly worthwhile, perhaps specifically in penitential terms for the pursuit of salvation.[14] But if this was true in the late 1300s, was it still the case in the following century? Trying to answer this question is problematic; and, to a degree, the difficulties involved have coloured assessments of St. Thomas' cult in the later Middle Ages, especially when Canterbury is compared to various newer sites of veneration.[15] This essay's modest aim is to offer an alternative approach to the widely used tactic of concentrating on the income from shrine offerings, supplemented by disparate references to individual Canterbury pilgrims. Here, the emphasis is upon case studies, with a specific focus on fifteenth-century sources from the city and its hinterland, for, even though St. Thomas may have continued to draw pilgrims from other parts of England, and also from overseas, the miracles recorded by Benedict and William in the late twelfth century indicate that his greatest impact was always in the local area, even during the initial decades.[16]

Although the reasons for going on pilgrimage were almost as diverse as the pilgrims themselves, the pattern of offerings, noted above, would imply that considerable numbers of people responded to crises in this way, seeing St. Thomas

---

[11] Webb, *Pilgrimage*, 233, 239, 242–4, 246, 248. See also Margaret Aston, *Lollards and Reformers: Images and Literacy in Late Medieval Religion* (1984), 149, 151–2, 161, 165.

[12] Nilson, *Cathedral Shrines*, 214–15, 234.

[13] Even rough estimates of population are notoriously difficult to establish for the medieval period, but, if the sum of approximately £1,000 collected at the tomb, shrine and site of martyrdom in 1219–20 included more offerings from foreign pilgrims and donations worth more than the traditional symbolic penny than in 1350–1, when almost £700 was given, the fact that England's population was then lower (on Hatcher's estimate) would suggest a continuing level of popularity: *ibid.*, 212, 214, 241. In the early 16th century an offering of one penny was still deemed appropriate: Thomas Bencher bequeathed 20*d.* in 1520 for a man to take an offering penny to the Rood of Grace for him: Kent History Centre [KHC], PRC 17/14, f. 309.

[14] John Aberth, *From the Brink of the Apocalypse: Confronting Famine, War, Plague, and Death in the Later Middle Ages* (2nd edn., London and New York, 2010), 125–6.

[15] Probably one of the most negative is presented by C.E. Woodruff, 'Financial Aspects of the Cult of Thomas of Canterbury', *Archaeologia Cantiana*, xliv (1932), 13–32. Yet, as Barrie Dobson has demonstrated, among English monastic churches on the eve of the Dissolution only the offerings to Our Lady of Walsingham were greater than those to St. Thomas' shrine: R.B. Dobson, 'The Monks of Canterbury in the Later Middle Ages', in *A History of Canterbury Cathedral*, ed. Patrick Collinson, Nigel Ramsay and Margaret Sparks (Oxford, 1995), 136.

[16] Finucane, *Miracles*, 164.

as a particularly appropriate protector and advocate. Consequently, the first part of this analysis will consider whether conditions during the fifteenth century were sufficiently challenging to provide comparable motivation for new generations of men and women among whom fear of the Apocalypse continued to enjoy at least some currency.[17] The second section will examine how those in Canterbury sought to attract pilgrims to the shrine in the fifteenth century, and especially in 1420 and 1470. The conclusion will establish what is known about the incidence of pilgrimage to Canterbury in order to convey some sense of the level of support, especially regionally, for Becket's cult in 'an age of plague' and of attempts to promote it.

The Four Horsemen in Canterbury?[18]

John Stone's chronicle has recently been re-edited by Meriel Connor and her text has been used here.[19] Stone was a monk at Christ Church priory from 1417 until his death at some point shortly before 1480. His chronicle, which ends in 1472, fits the time frame required, providing the means for us to explore the incidence of catastrophic events which may have seemed to those in Canterbury and its hinterland to herald the 'last things', including, perhaps, the horsemen of Plague, Famine and War, bringing Death to their city. As John Hatcher found when analysing the record of events kept by Thomas Cawston, a near contemporary of Stone, the list of obits at the priory reveals that Canterbury suffered from a series of plague outbreaks in the fifteenth century, during which there was at least one particularly bad year per decade.[20] After 1420 the next major epidemic was in 1431; thereafter the city enjoyed some respite before it was again hit in 1447, and then a decade later.[21] There was a similar interval before the next major outbreak in 1467.[22] Yet, two years earlier, a Christ Church monk had died of 'raging plague', and after the 1470 Jubilee, as in 1420, pestilence again returned to Canterbury.[23] Worst of all was 1457. Stone noted that there was then a great and serious plague

---

[17] Smoller, 'Of Earthquakes', 185–6. Although the evidence relates to France rather than England, it is worth noting that, in the late 15th century, Duke Louis of Anjou's tapestries of the Apocalypse were given to Angers cathedral, where they were displayed on major feast days in the nave and choir: Margaret Manion, 'The Angers Tapestries of the Apocalypse and Valois Patronage', in *Prophecy, Apocalypse and the Day of Doom. Proceedings of the 2000 Harlaxton Symposium*, ed. Nigel Morgan (Donington, 2004), 235.

[18] Borrowing from Aberth, *From the Brink*, 4–5.

[19] *John Stone's Chronicle, Christ Church Priory, Canterbury, 1417–1472*, selected, trans. and intro. Meriel Connor (Kalamazoo, Mich., 2010); *eadem*, 'John Stone, Monk of Christ Church, Canterbury and his Chronicle, 1417–1472' (London Univ. M.Phil. thesis, 2001).

[20] John Hatcher, 'Mortality in the Fifteenth Century: Some New Evidence', *EcHR*, 2nd series, xxxix (1986), 19–38. See also Joe Connor, 'Profession and Death at Christ Church Priory, Canterbury, 1207–1534', *Archaeologia Cantiana*, cxxxi (2011), 282, 288, 289. For a recent reassessment of monastic mortality and the implications of the data: Richard Smith, 'Measuring Adult Mortality in an Age of Plague: England, 1349–1540', in *Town and Countryside in the Age of the Black Death. Essays in Honour of John Hatcher*, ed. Mark Bailey and S.H. Rigby (Turnhout, 2012), 43–85.

[21] Connor, 'John Stone', 147, 153–4, 186, 188, 214–16.

[22] *Ibid.*, 246–7.

[23] *Ibid.*, 240, 263–4.

in the city of Canterbury and in various other parts of the kingdom.[24] The severity of the epidemic can also be gauged from the response of the prior and convent. Following the death of an eighth monk on 15 August, the brethren staged a procession nine days later through the monastic cemetery carrying a reliquary of St. Ouen, a saint known to protect against plague.[25] To honour further this powerful intercessor on his feast day, the prior personally celebrated at high mass. The monastic community once again enlisted St. Ouen's protection in 1471, which may indicate the success of the first appeal, although it was only on the second that Stone recorded the plague's cessation after the procession.[26] Nevertheless, recourse to such measures highlights the fear still occasioned by plague, both at Canterbury and more widely, a sense of foreboding that seems totally justified in the context of Hatcher's analysis of the Christ Church evidence. No fewer than fifteen cathedral monks died in 1457.[27]

The horseman symbolising Famine might be envisaged in terms of extreme weather and worsening economic conditions.[28] As noted above, medieval chroniclers are well known for their attention to such phenomena, but Stone's interest in these matters does reflect the problems likely to have affected agricultural production locally and regionally, and even nationally in some instances. Exceptionally severe winters in terms of heavy and prolonged snow or unseasonably late snowfalls in April were reported in 1434–5, 1449 and twice in the 1460s, that is in both 1460 and 1464–5.[29] Nor were these the only years in which ploughing would have been difficult or impossible for several months. For example, floods lasting for over a month are noted at the beginning of 1468.[30] Obstacles to cultivation during the winter period were compounded by the likelihood that any autumn-sown crops would have succumbed to the harsh conditions. In these years the harvest must have been heavily dependent on anything planted in the very late spring, which would have drastically reduced overall grain production, as well as adversely affecting livestock farmers. Such a scenario may also have happened in 1458, when there was a severe storm in May, and again in 1465, which had already seen prolonged snowfall at the beginning of the year, followed by drought conditions in May that can only have exacerbated the situation.[31] The monks responded to this particular crisis by going on procession via the Burgate to the neighbouring abbey of St. Augustine, where they joined their fellow Benedictines in prayers for rain. The worst year for weather-related problems at harvest time was probably 1439: Stone records a severe storm in September when the greatest devastation would, potentially, have taken place.[32] However, large-scale crop damage may also have occurred in early June 1467, when there was 'a great hail such as we had never seen in our time', and at the end

[24] *Ibid.*, 213; *eadem, Stone's Chronicle*, 99.
[25] Connor, 'John Stone', 216; Tekippe, 'Pilgrimage', 731–2. It is worth noting that 24 Aug. is also the feast day of St. Bartholomew, another healing saint.
[26] Connor, 'John Stone', 267; *eadem, Stone's Chronicle*, 131.
[27] Hatcher, 'Mortality', 26, 30.
[28] Compare: Bruce Campbell, 'Grain Yields on English Demesnes after the Black Death', in *Town and Countryside*, ed. Bailey and Rigby, 152–6.
[29] Connor, 'John Stone', 160, 191, 225, 239; *eadem, Stone's Chronicle*, 65, 85, 103, 112.
[30] Connor, 'John Stone', 250; *eadem, Stone's Chronicle*, 120.
[31] Connor, 'John Stone', 221, 240; *eadem, Stone's Chronicle*, 102.
[32] Connor, 'John Stone', 166; *eadem, Stone's Chronicle*, 69.

of the month, when disaster struck again.[33] Thus, in common with plague epidemics, there seems to have been at least one incidence of seriously adverse weather per decade. Overall, in terms of agricultural production, the 1460s appear to have been an especially challenging decade, since, as Bruce Campbell has remarked, it is the cumulative effect of poor harvest yields that is the most catastrophic, particularly when the livestock sector is also disrupted.[34]

Famine as a consequence of harsh economic conditions is more difficult to chart in Canterbury and its hinterland. However, Hatcher's assessment of the mid-century depression confirms that life was then generally grim, as does the work of Jim Bolton and others.[35] Canterbury would not have been immune to these prevailing circumstances: indeed, as Andrew Butcher has demonstrated in his comparison between Oxford and Canterbury, the Christ Church priory rental evidence for the later fifteenth century reveals the ubiquity of arrears among the priory's tenants, as well as a number of empty properties.[36] Although they are slightly later in date, city ordinances tell of problems with Canterbury's cloth trade, manufacturing having already begun to move away from the city to the Weald.[37] Commercial life may have been more widely affected; the lists of *intrantes* (that is individuals ranking below the freemen who paid an annual licence fee to trade in the city) reveal a distinct fall in the numbers entering Canterbury during the third quarter of the fifteenth century.[38] Whether the same period was also marked by an upsurge in the proportion of the city's population classed as paupers is unclear, but over a third of local testators remembered the poor and bedridden.[39]

The next horseman, War, may not have been as busy in Canterbury as he was along the Kent coast, but the city did experience at first-hand the damaging effects of political instability. Not that the civic authorities were unwilling to take advantage of the crown's weakness: the city charters secured first from Henry VI and later Edward IV imply otherwise, but in many ways Canterbury was still vulnerable. Stone provides some indication of this mood of insecurity, noting that in May 1439 the cathedral monks joined members of other religious houses in a procession through the city to the church of the Blackfriars, where prayers were said 'for peace, for good weather and for various other intentions'.[40]

Stone describes the murder of the duke of Suffolk and, of even greater concern to this Canterbury monk, the transportation of his body from Dover to London,

[33] Connor, 'John Stone', 247; *eadem, Stone's Chronicle*, 117.

[34] Bruce Campbell, 'Agriculture in Kent in the High Middle Ages', in *Later Medieval Kent, 1220–1540*, ed. Sheila Sweetinburgh (Woodbridge, 2010), 48, 50.

[35] John Hatcher, 'The Great Slump of the Mid-Fifteenth Century', in *Progress and Problems in Medieval England*, ed. Richard Britnell and John Hatcher (Cambridge, 1996), 237–72; J.L. Bolton, '"The World Upside Down". Plague as an Agent of Economic and Social Change', in *The Black Death in England*, ed. W.M. Ormrod and P.G. Lindley (Stamford, 2003), 64–6.

[36] A.F. Butcher, 'Rent and the Urban Economy: Oxford and Canterbury in the Later Middle Ages', *Southern History*, i (1979), 37–44.

[37] Canterbury Cathedral Archives and Library [CCAL], CC/AB/1, ff. 7–8.

[38] *Intrantes. A List of Persons Admitted to Live and Trade within the City of Canterbury, 1392–1592*, ed. J.M. Cowper (Canterbury, 1904).

[39] Sheila Sweetinburgh, 'Clothing the Naked in Late Medieval East Kent', in *Clothing Culture, 1350–1650*, ed. Catherine Richardson (Aldershot, 2004), 114, 115.

[40] Connor, 'John Stone', 164; *eadem, Stone's Chronicle*, 68.

including its time in Canterbury cathedral.[41] He also reports the arrival of John Mortimer (*alias* Jack Cade) and his four thousand followers just over a month later on 3 June 1450, an event that must have been deeply worrying for the civic authorities, as well as the priory, because the rebels were encamped in the western suburbs.[42] An indication of the danger this posed to the city can be ascertained from notes inserted under the year 1449–50 in the chamberlains' 'Great Book', which describe the insurrection led by the 'Hermit Bluberd' and then Cade's Rebellion, the latter involving the decapitation of Lord Saye and *'multi alii magnati apud London'*.[43] Such entries bring home the instability of royal government as perceived from below, the king's weak hold on the country being further exemplified by the charter gained soon after from Henry VI by the civic authorities.[44] Recording the aid provided by the ruling elite with the backing of the commonalty against his enemies, Henry's new charter demonstrates his dependence on Canterbury, because he had only recently, in 1448, allowed the city to elect its own mayor. The exploitation of such shifts in the relationship between king and people may have been envisaged locally as an essential component in the city's continuing good governance. Stone's description of a violent incident at Sandwich in his chronicle entry for 1450 clearly reflects the deep uncertainty that had taken hold across the region.[45]

In the dynastic struggle of the next decade and beyond, the Christ Church community seems to have favoured the Lancastrian cause, although Stone's only reference to political events in the 1450s is to the first battle of St. Albans, when he names several prominent Lancastrian casualties.[46] War, in terms of the 1457 French raid on Sandwich, did merit an entry in his chronicle, as he records that the port was captured and plundered of all its goods.[47] In addition to the personal and commercial connections that were maintained between individuals living in the two places, Christ Church priory had its own links to Sandwich, where it still retained property and wharfage. Consequently, the port's fate mattered on various levels, the horseman being only one stride away from Canterbury. In 1460 he came far closer. The arrival of the three Yorkist earls and their followers in defiance of Henry VI was important to Stone, as it was to the city more generally. This must have been a tense time for the mayor and senior townsmen, at least until the immediate crisis was averted by the desertion to the earls of the three courtiers who had been sent to Canterbury by the royal party to stop their advance.[48] Nonetheless, a sense of danger persisted, and in March 1461, instead of simply processing

---

[41]   Connor, 'John Stone', 194; *eadem, Stone's Chronicle*, 87.

[42]   Connor, 'John Stone', 194; *eadem, Stone's Chronicle*, 87–8.

[43]   Since he was a traitor, Bluberd's head was set on Canterbury's Westgate: CCAL, CC/FA/1, f. 27v.

[44]   CCAL, CC/AA/33. This charter reflects the crown's continuing reliance on Canterbury, already apparent in that of 1448: CCAL, CC/AA/32.

[45]   This dramatic event involved the capture of Ralph Cheker of Dover on 1 Sept. at Sandwich and his decapitation near St. Bartholomew's hospital in the town: Connor, 'John Stone', 195.

[46]   *Ibid.*, 211; *eadem, Stone's Chronicle*, 98; *eadem*, 'The Political Allegiances of Christ Church Priory 1400–1472: the Evidence of John Stone's Chronicle', *Archaeologia Cantiana*, cxxvii (2007), 383–406.

[47]   Connor, 'John Stone', 216; *eadem, Stone's Chronicle*, 100.

[48]   Connor, 'John Stone', 226–7; *eadem, Stone's Chronicle*, 104. See, in comparison, *An English Chronicle of the Reigns of Richard II, Henry IV, Henry V, and Henry VI*, ed. J.S. Davies (Camden Society, original series, lxiv, 1856), 94.

through the cathedral, the prior and convent led another procession for peace through the city.[49]

The inter-relationship between English and continental politics meant that Stone's report of the stalling of the peace negotiations at Canterbury between the French and English, in August 1467, was followed almost immediately by his observation that the earl of Warwick had thereafter not crossed to France with the earl of Northumberland and his wife.[50] Warwick's activities were next recorded by Stone in 1469, when the earl's ship, *The Trinity*, was blessed by three senior churchmen, including the prior of Christ Church; this was only one of several references to the earl in that tumultuous year.[51] Stone also mentions some events concerning Edward IV's recovery of the crown in 1471, but it is the omission, or rather the 'loss', of perhaps two relevant folios which is even more telling.[52] Connor presumes that they contained material about the summary execution of the city's mayor on Edward's orders following the failure of the Fauconberg Rebellion, a reminder to those inside and outside the cathedral precincts that he would not tolerate traitors.[53] Even though the execution occurred after 1470, the terminal point of this essay, we should bear in mind that the mayor and several other senior citizens had been part of Warwick's affinity for some time, and that the years before and after the Readeption were extremely precarious for those in Canterbury who became caught up in national politics.[54]

The apparently vigorous activities of the horsemen of Plague, Famine and War in and around Canterbury meant that Death was even busier. Stone's chronicle contains numerous references to the deaths and funeral arrangements of his monastic brethren, while occasionally recording similar events at St. Augustine's abbey. Cawston's list of obits provides an even fuller register of the Christ Church community; and from these sources Hatcher concludes that life expectancy among the Canterbury monks was particularly low in the second half of the fifteenth century. He is cautious about the implications of this evidence for the population at large, but his conclusions do seem more widely applicable during the period from about 1450 (and perhaps earlier) to 1470, which can be regarded from a historical perspective as 'an age of death'.[55] Whether contemporaries viewed it in this way remains difficult to establish, but, as noted above, there is some evidence to support such a belief. Notwithstanding the problems of establishing a causal link between an impending sense of 'last days' and the incidence of pilgrimage to St. Thomas' shrine, it seems worthwhile to consider the efforts of the priory and city, especially in 1420 and 1470, to attract pilgrims.

---

[49] Connor, 'John Stone', 230.

[50] *Ibid.*, 249; *eadem, Stone's Chronicle*, 119.

[51] Connor, 'John Stone', 258; *eadem, Stone's Chronicle*, 125.

[52] Connor, 'John Stone', 265; *eadem, Stone's Chronicle*, 130.

[53] *Eadem*, 'Political Allegiances', 401.

[54] Sheila Sweetinburgh, 'A Revolt too Far: Paying the Price in Late Medieval Canterbury', in *Kent, the South-East and War 1000–1450*, ed. Paul Dalton and Charles Insley (forthcoming).

[55] Hatcher, 'Mortality', 28, 36.

Promoting the 'hooly blisful martir'

Both Ben Nilson and R.B. Dobson have discussed some of the promotional activities of the Christ Church monks regarding the cult of St. Thomas in the fifteenth century, but it is important to extend this investigation to include Canterbury's citizens, both corporately and individually.[56] The following section will approach this topic in three ways: first, with respect to the shrine itself, then in terms of the personnel associated with the cathedral and priory, and finally by discovering what the city sought to offer visitors to Canterbury.

In a world that so often measured the power of sanctity through material display, the sheer physical splendour of St. Thomas' shrine, as recorded by certain late medieval visitors, would have provided a forceful attraction for those contemplating a pilgrimage.[57] In addition to the gold, jewels and other precious objects which were still being augmented by the bequests of local citizens into the sixteenth century (Alice Byng offered a gold ring with a sapphire, William Chilton another with a 'poynt diamond'), the shrine and its precincts were adorned with candles.[58] The symbolic implications of these massed ranks of tapers, smaller candles and the twelve large square ones on the beam above the shrine – all lit daily at the start of the mass of St. Thomas – would have been widely understood and appreciated by pilgrims.[59] The citizens similarly valued such items, and among those bequeathing wax, candles or tapers to the shrine in 1471 were Roger Rydle and John Grey.[60] Gifts of wax in the form of votive offerings representing body parts or other objects were equally important to pilgrims, and were prominently displayed around the shrine.[61] Among them was the Dover candle (measuring the circumference of the town) on its great reel that the townspeople gave to St. Thomas every three years. This gift presumably marked a special relationship which was prized by both parties, and, although its purpose is unknown, it may have been intended to secure protection against plague.[62]

Even though most pilgrims would only have been allowed to gaze at the magnificent *feretrum* as they knelt and perhaps rubbed the shrine base, the early-fifteenth-century customary indicates that the two Becket shrine keepers and their assistants were expected to enrich the pilgrims' experience as far as possible

---

[56] Nilson, *Cathedral Shrines*, 127, 133, 172, 185; Dobson, 'Canterbury', 139–40.

[57] For example, an Italian diplomat seems to have been overawed by the Régale, Louis VII's famous ruby, which was set to the right of the altar: *A Relation, or Rather a True Account, of the Island of England*, ed. C.A. Sneyd (Camden Society, original series, xxxvii, 1847), 30. See also Desiderius Erasmus, *Pilgrimages to Saint Mary of Walsingham and Saint Thomas of Canterbury*, trans. J.G. Nichols (2nd edn., 1875), 49; Sarah Blick, 'Reconstructing the Shrine of St Thomas Becket, Canterbury Cathedral', in *Art and Architecture of Late Medieval Pilgrimage*, ed. Blick and Tekippe, 407–11.

[58] KHC, PRC 17/14, f. 196; 17/9, f. 2.

[59] Peter Rowe, 'The Customary of the Shrine of St Thomas Becket, a Translation of the Customary with Notes' (London Univ. M.A. dissertation, 1990), app. 4, p. 3.

[60] Rydle gave an impressive 100 pounds of wax to be made into 13 large tapers: KHC, PRC 17/2, f. 46.

[61] Blick's reconstruction of the shrine from depictions on contemporary pilgrim badges is particularly valuable because of its total destruction under Henry VIII: 'Reconstructing', 419–41.

[62] Sheila Sweetinburgh, 'Wax, Stone and Iron: Dover Town Defences in the Late Middle Ages', *Archaeologia Cantiana*, cxxiv (2004), 185, 187–8; Rowe, 'Customary', app. 4, pp. 21–2.

without disrupting the liturgical life of the priory.[63] Consequently, among other things, they had to ensure that visitors were aware when the cathedral first opened early in the morning, and were supposed to aid, when necessary, those 'who [might] be cold or wearied by their journey'.[64] To a degree, sick pilgrims received preferential treatment, but all were to be 'spoken to and answered with friendly gentleness and care'; and during the day the shrine was generally only closed over lunchtime.[65] Although these requirements may represent an ideal, the number of staff involved and the detailed nature of the ordinances reveal an understanding on the part of Christ Church that such care was necessary. Similarly, although they were an earlier development, Anne Harris has argued that the miracle windows encircling the shrine were intended to enhance the atmosphere of devotion.[66]

Furthermore, the exalted position of the feast days of St. Thomas' martyrdom (passion) and translation within the liturgical life of Canterbury provided considerable scope for those wishing to visit the shrine at auspicious times. For as well as being spaced almost six months apart, one within the twelve days of Christmas and the second in early July, the feast days themselves offered additional opportunities for access. For example, pilgrims waiting overnight on 28 December were allowed into the shrine when the bell for matins was sounded and were also given sustenance in the form of bread, cheese and ale.[67] This provision was probably not new in the fifteenth century, but nevertheless may have been seen as an effective means of extending the bounty of St. Thomas, especially because, in addition to those attending on the two principal feast days and their vigils, large crowds were anticipated on the feast day of the return of St. Thomas (2 December), the octave of the martyrdom and the quinzaine of the translation, as well as on Tuesdays because of their association with the saint.[68]

The greater elaboration of the liturgy at such times, the presence of the prior, and sometimes the archbishop or other senior clerics, the use of special vestments and the increased number of candles were all important in terms of the monastic community's veneration of God and St. Thomas, yet they presumably also attracted pilgrims to the shrine.[69] Similarly, the time and effort spent on cleaning everything connected with the shrine before the feast of the translation, 'so that the holy church of Canterbury and particularly this place [shrine] may appear to the faithful and pilgrims as beautiful as the face of Rachel, and not unattractive like Leah', were valued beyond their theological merits.[70]

---

[63] Nilson, *Cathedral Shrines*, 99–100; Tim Tatton-Brown, 'Canterbury and the Architecture of Pilgrimage Shrines in England', in *Pilgrimage: The English Experience*, ed. Morris and Roberts, 106. Yet it is interesting that, in a continuation of Chaucer's *Canterbury Tales*, which is considered by some to have been written by a monk, the pilgrims are allowed to kiss the relics under the watchful eye of a keeper: *The Tale of Beryn*, ed. F.J. Furnivall and W.G. Stone (EETS, original series, cv, 1909), pp. vi, 6, 120, 137, n. 1.

[64] Rowe, 'Customary', app. 4, p. 3.

[65] *Ibid.*, 4, 9.

[66] A.F. Harris, 'Pilgrimage, Performance, and Stained Glass at Canterbury Cathedral', in *Art and Architecture of Late Medieval Pilgrimage*, ed. Blick and Tekippe, 245, 255–6, 260–5.

[67] Rowe, 'Customary', app. 4, pp. 14–15, 21.

[68] *Ibid.*, 5–6, 10–12, 14–15, 20–3.

[69] Tekippe, 'Pilgrimage', 695–7, 700–1, 748–51.

[70] Rowe, 'Customary', app. 4, p. 21.

These feast days and other lesser, but still perhaps more locally significant, occasions were part of the annual cycle at Canterbury which was comparable to arrangements at other shrines in England. However, the Christ Church monks had also acquired the privilege of seeking plenary indulgences for the jubilees of St. Thomas that had begun at the time of his translation in 1220.[71] Two hundred years later they were again successful, and, in their bid to publicise this inducement to attend the jubilee celebrations, letters announcing the list of newly-available indulgences and a poem composed by a monk were nailed to several church doors. In addition to the poem, a four-verse schedule was fixed to the door of St. Paul's cathedral in London. Interestingly, the schedule also referred to St. Thomas of Lancaster, a juxtaposition that may have bolstered Lancaster's following, but in the aftermath of Agincourt would have seemed mutually beneficial.[72] Among the other places chosen to advertise these papal indulgences were the pilgrim hospital at Ospringe, a house under royal patronage conveniently sited on Watling Street, and Canterbury cathedral itself.[73] A detailed letter and a schedule were attached to the cathedral door, while the monk's poem was displayed at several places around the cathedral, no doubt to intensify the devotion of the pilgrims gathered there.

Whether John Oxney, the prior in the late 1460s, intended to emulate his predecessor is unclear, but the priory's bid to gain indulgences for the 1470 jubilee, which had started as early as 1460, enjoyed limited success. First, the requisite papal bull was not issued until a month before the jubilee of 1470, and secondly the plenary indulgence it contained was only available to those who visited St. Thomas' shrine and attended services at the feasts of the Nativity (8 August) and Assumption (15 August) of Our Lady, and of St. Michael the Archangel (29 September).[74] Nevertheless, it seems likely that the prior would have tried to publicise this concession during the summer of 1470, and again the following year once the political situation had become more stable, because the indulgence was still available under the same conditions.

Even though St. Thomas' thaumaturgical powers seem rarely to have been deployed by 1400, late-fifteenth-century priors were able to announce that miracles still took place. A letter distributed in 1445 to several churches told of the miraculous cure of a lame man from Aberdeen, while a poem, copied by Stone into his chronicle, records St. Thomas' intervention to abate a storm, thereby saving the pilgrims on board ship.[75] The poem's refrain refers to other new miracles that the saint had performed, without vouchsafing further details, yet how widely it was

---

[71] Webb, *Pilgrimage*, 66, citing Raymonde Foreville, *Le Jubilé de saint Thomas Becket du XIIIe au XVe siècle, 1220–1470* (Paris, 1958). See also Foreville, 'L'Idée de Jubilé chez les théologiens et les canonistes (XIIe–XIIIe siécle) avant l'Institution de Jubile Romain (1300)', reprinted in *Thomas Becket dans la Tradition Historique et Hagiographique* (1981), 401–23.

[72] Foreville, *Le Jubilé de saint Thomas Becket : Étude et documents* (Paris, 1958), 129, 134–5. Like Becket, Thomas of Lancaster was linked to St. George, such chivalric associations being of particular significance during Henry V's reign: Piroyansky, *Martyrs in the Making*, 40, 44.

[73] Foreville, *Le Jubilé: Étude et documents*, 134–7.

[74] J.J. Zeiger, 'The Survival of the Cult of St Thomas of Canterbury in the Later Middle Ages' (Kent Univ. M.A. dissertation, 1997), 20. Stone recorded this indulgence and also noted that Edward and his queen had spent several days in Canterbury in early June 1470: Connor, 'John Stone', 262; *Literae Cantuarienses: The Letter Books of the Monastery of Christ Church, Canterbury*, ed. J.B. Sheppard (3 vols., 1887–9), iii. 253–5.

[75] HMC, v. 462; ix. 114; Connor, 'John Stone', 248; *eadem, Stone's Chronicle*, 117–18.

disseminated is uncertain. Interestingly, occasional miracles were also recorded in the priory archive, although once again there is nothing to indicate if they were broadcast elsewhere.[76]

Events that may have generated far more publicity and interest were pilgrimages by royalty, by members of the lay and ecclesiastical aristocracy, and by eminent foreigners. As Stone indicates, such important personages were favoured by the monks, the prior meeting his honoured guests and conducting them personally to the shrine, while the ordinary public was presumably kept at some distance.[77] Nonetheless, knowledge of the arrival of distinguished pilgrims may well have attracted crowds to the shrine, especially on the occasion of Henry V's pilgrimage shortly after his success at Agincourt and on his return to Canterbury in August 1416, when he was accompanied by the Emperor Sigismund.[78] Similarly, Henry VI's young queen (her pious husband was particularly devoted to St. Thomas) may have drawn pilgrims to Canterbury when she visited the shrine in 1446; and, for entirely different reasons, so may Edward IV and Queen Elizabeth when they received a plenary indulgence there at Michaelmas 1471.[79] In addition to these royal pilgrims, it is conceivable that the experiences of the fictional characters described in the prologue to *The Tale of Beryn* provided an incentive to less devout souls contemplating a journey to St. Thomas' shrine.[80]

As well as the shrine, it seems likely that other features of the cathedral would have attracted pilgrims in the fifteenth century, even though parts of the precinct must at times have resembled a building site; it was not until about 1500 that the rebuilding programme was completed.[81] The early-fifteenth-century visitor would have entered the newly-rebuilt nave from the south-west porch, on which there was a fine relief carving of Becket's murder.[82] The visually impressive perpendicular nave with its great Rood at the east end would have been enhanced by the several nave chantry chapels, including one established by Archbishop Arundel, who intended that pilgrims should hear the mass celebrated there.[83] They might also have profited from sermons preached from the pulpit in the nave, as happened at the 1420 jubilee when Thomas Tynwyth, an Austin friar, was called upon to repeat his sermon twice more by the throng of pilgrims who had been unable to hear because of the crowds.[84] From 1438 onwards they might also have heard the boys' choir in the Lady Chapel in the north nave aisle, and after 1455 perhaps have done

---

[76] C.E. Woodruff, 'Notes on the Inner Life and Domestic Economy of the Priory of Christ Church, Canterbury, in the Fifteenth Century', *Archaeologia Cantiana*, liii (1940), 14.

[77] In 1441 the duke of Gloucester was met at the cathedral entrance by the prior and convent in green copes: Connor, *Stone's Chronicle*, 72.

[78] Dobson, 'Canterbury', 143.

[79] Connor, 'John Stone', 184, 268; *eadem, Stone's Chronicle*, 80, 131. In addition to his frequent pilgrimages, Henry VI recorded his devotion to the saint in his charter to the city: CCAL, CC/AA/33.

[80] *The Tale of Beryn*, ed. Furnivall and Stone, 1–24.

[81] Keith Blockley, Margaret Sparks and Tim Tatton-Brown, *Canterbury Cathedral Nave: Archaeology, History and Architecture* (Canterbury, 1997), 127; Tatton-Brown, 'Canterbury', 101.

[82] Tatton-Brown, 'Canterbury', 101.

[83] Blockley, Sparks and Tatton-Brown, *Canterbury Nave*, 126, 137.

[84] Foreville, *Le Jubilé: Étude et documents*, 142. See also William Urry, 'The Jubilee of St Thomas, 1420: Billetting and Rationing Problems in the Fifteenth Century', *Canterbury Cathedral Chronicle*, xlii (1947), 24.

so more clearly when they approached the site of the martyrdom, because the Chapel moved to its new location that year.[85] This assault upon the pilgrims' senses may have been especially intense as they approached the east end of the nave, because, as Tim Tatton-Brown has noted, the unusual deployment of openwork iron screens and gates was seemingly intended to provide visitors with a view of the shrine from afar as they gazed eastwards and upwards from the nave.[86] Moreover, the use of incense and candles and the introduction of polyphonic music must have heightened the affective sensory experience for those nearing the shrine.[87] Such experiences may also have had a reassuring physiological impact, because, as the *Regimen sanitatis* taught, it was important to avoid corrupt air and instead to seek out pleasant odours, uplifting sights and harmonious sounds. Plague treatises endorsed such ideas, incense and perfumes being recommended not merely to mask bad smells, but also to combat infection by strengthening the body's vital spirits.[88]

Among the other building works undertaken in the fifteenth century that may have attracted pilgrims to Canterbury, as well as enhancing their route through the cathedral to the shrine and other places associated with St. Thomas, were the construction of the tomb of Henry IV and his queen and the remodelling of the area to the west of the monks' quire. As Tatton-Brown observes, the development of the crossing area between the western transepts was extremely complicated, but the newly-built passage under the steps would have facilitated the pilgrims' approach from the nave (south-east) to the site of martyrdom, and thence to St. Thomas' tomb and Our Lady Undercroft in the crypt.[89] The rest of their route from the crypt to the Corona and finally the shrine itself primarily used the south ambulatory.[90] This layout greatly improved circulation, which was especially valuable when there were very large crowds, but also provided opportunities to see and even examine several archiepiscopal tombs, as well as the Black Prince's magnificent monument and that of his nephew, the first Lancastrian king.[91]

The priory was further able to promote Canterbury through the provision of hospitality. This was mainly offered to high status guests, although the poor were probably given some aid through the almonry.[92] Within the precincts were several buildings, including the cellarer's guesthouses and guest hall, and the newly-built

---

[85] Roger Bowers, 'The Liturgy of the Cathedral and its Music, c.1075–1642', in *A History of Canterbury Cathedral*, ed. Collinson, Ramsey and Sparks, 419–20.

[86] Tatton-Brown, 'Canterbury', 102.

[87] Bowers, 'Liturgy', 420. Yet again it is interesting (and perhaps more 'realistic') that some fictional pilgrims seem to have shown little respect for their sacred surroundings: *The Tale of Beryn*, ed. Furnivall and Stone, 6.

[88] Carole Rawcliffe, *Medicine and Society in Later Medieval England* (Stroud, 1995), 39, 41–2; and for divine intervention through scent, *ibid.*, 17.

[89] Tatton-Brown, 'Canterbury', 102–3; Blockley, Sparks and Tatton-Brown, *Canterbury Nave*, 138–9.

[90] M.F. Hearn's proposed route for 13th-century pilgrims was still largely applicable in the 15th-century cathedral: Harris, 'Pilgrimage', 272.

[91] Tatton-Brown, 'Canterbury', 104–5; Sheila Sweetinburgh, 'Canterbury's Martyred Archbishop: the "Cult" of Simon Sudbury and Relations between City and Cathedral', in *Monuments and Monumentality in Later Medieval and Early Modern Europe*, ed. Michael Penman (forthcoming, Donington, 2013). The north ambulatory was the monks' principal processional route: Connor, 'John Stone', 171.

[92] Julie Kerr, *Monastic Hospitality: The Benedictines in England, c.1070–c.1250* (Woodbridge, 2007), 3, 5–6, 23–8, 32, 48–9.

Meister Omers, that were used to accommodate visitors, prominent among whom was Queen Margaret.[93] Such hospitality was especially lavish on important occasions, as at the banquet given by the archbishop on the feast day of the translation in 1470.[94] The prior is also known to have provided entertainment in the form of minstrels and plays, while the giving of gifts was another valued means of promoting Canterbury's saint.[95]

For centuries gift-giving in the form of confraternity had been a valued aspect of Benedictine life. As well as extending the offer of perpetual commemoration in the community's prayers to other religious orders, the monks also awarded letters of confraternity to certain members of the laity. The ever-expanding community of the living and the dead based at Canterbury cathedral seems to have continued during the fifteenth century to attract senior churchmen, such as Cardinal Beaufort, who was a regular visitor there, along with members of the aristocracy, including those who additionally sought burial in the cathedral.[96] For the priory these relationships often extended beyond the individual to encompass his or her kindred and associated persons of similar rank, constituting a network of benefaction, prayerful provision and influence that was valued by all parties, especially during the factional disputes and other uncertainties of the mid fifteenth century.[97] Nor were these reciprocal gifts confined to the upper echelons of society. Even though the evidence is limited, it appears that some local townspeople and clerics wished to be admitted into the monastic confraternity, while burial within the priory's lay cemetery was also a prized mark of favour.[98] This particular privilege extended to poor pilgrims (provided they were not lepers) who died while staying at the pilgrim hospital of St. Thomas by the city's Eastbridge, although the numbers involved are impossible to ascertain.[99]

According to *The Tale of Beryn*, the last act of the pilgrims before they leave the cathedral is to purchase 'Cauntirbury brochis' (all except the miller, who steals some with his accomplice the pardoner) and attach them to their caps.[100] Given the variety and number of Canterbury pilgrim badges known from the archaeological evidence (about 1,300 have been found in England), it would seem that such items were extremely popular. In part this may have been due to their apotropaic value, because, in common with *Christus medicus* (who could cure the body as well as

---

[93]   Margaret Sparks, *Canterbury Cathedral Precincts. An Historical Survey* (Canterbury, 2007), 24, 25, 27–9, 49–50, 64, 67, 70; Nilson, *Cathedral Shrines*, 185–6.

[94]   Connor, 'John Stone', 261; *eadem, Stone's Chronicle*, 128.

[95]   Nilson, *Cathedral Shrines*, 127, 183.

[96]   Meriel Connor, 'Brotherhood and Confraternity at Canterbury Cathedral Priory in the Fifteenth Century: the Evidence of John Stone's Chronicle', *Archaeologia Cantiana*, cxxviii (2008), 149, 150.

[97]   *Ibid.*, 154–5.

[98]   Most of the lay examples were women: *ibid.*, 157. For those of even greater wealth and status, burial within the cathedral was a possibility, and among the knights who sought this privilege in the early 15th century were Sir Thomas Fogge, Sir William Septvans and Sir Edmund Haute: KHC, PRC 32/1, ff. 16, 17.

[99]   *Literae Cantuarienses*, ed. Sheppard, ii. 256; John Duncombe and Nicholas Battely, *The History and Antiquities of the Three Archiepiscopal Hospitals at or near Canterbury viz. St. Nicholas at Harbledown, St. John, Northgate and St. Thomas of Eastbridge, with some Account of the Priory of St. Gregory, the Nunnery of St. Sepulcre, the Hospitals of St. James and St. Laurence and Maynards Spittle* (1785), 330.

[100] *The Tale of Beryn*, ed. Furnivall and Stone, 7.

the soul), St. Thomas was seen by some as a physician to the sick.[101] Moreover, even though the quality of the metalwork apparently declined during the fifteenth century, these badges presumably continued to be valued by visitors as a token of a successfully completed pilgrimage, and were still useful to the priory as a means of promoting the cult of St. Thomas.[102] Nor was the cathedral the only source of such memorabilia: at least one 'brochis' maker was working in the city; and shopkeepers outside the precinct gates are known to have sold these items in the fifteenth century.[103]

Before visiting the shrine, the pilgrims in the prologue to *The Tale of Beryn* book their accommodation at one of Christ Church's inns in the city.[104] *The Cheker of the Hope* had been built in the early 1390s at a cost of over £860; another of the priory's large, high quality establishments was *The White Bull*.[105] These inns, along with others belonging to the priory, were clustered around the main route into the precinct, which must have made them especially attractive to pilgrims. The building of *The Sun Inn* in the 1430s, perhaps with a separate range of ground floor shops, suggests that the priory continued to have confidence in the pilgrim trade.[106] The construction of lodgings over shops was also a feature of one of the city's own inns, called *The Lyon*; and *The Sun*'s status ensured that, like *The Cheker*, 'many a man' knew it.[107] Whether the other inns belonging to the city and the priory were equally celebrated is less certain, but travellers to and from London, the coastal ports and other places may have transmitted information about lodgings quite widely in southern England and beyond. Evidence of this well-established network of communications survives in the reciprocal arrangement made between the hackneymen of Canterbury and Dover, which was probably replicated elsewhere.[108]

The names of some inns, both inside and outside the walls, are known from the surviving records, and from them it appears that the main topographical clusters were close to Christ Church gate around the Bullstake, in neighbouring Burgate and Mercery Lane, along the High Street, especially between Westgate and St. Andrew's church, and outside the city on the main approach road from London called Westgate Street.[109] This arrangement suggests the primacy of the western approach to the city, although pilgrims did not solely come from London, and there were several inns in Canterbury's other suburbs. What it is not clear is how many beds could be provided in total. It seems that the number was considerable, but at

---

[101] Rawcliffe, *Medicine and Society*, 17–18, 21, 94, 96. In this context the presence of pilgrim-tokens in graves is highly suggestive: Webb, *Pilgrimage*, 212.

[102] Nilson, *Cathedral Shrines*, 112; Blick, 'Reconstructing', 421–2; Marike de Kroon, 'Medieval Pilgrim Badges and their Iconographic Aspects', in *Art and Architecture of Late Medieval Pilgrimage*, ed. Blick and Tekippe, 385–6, 392, 403.

[103] Nilson, *Cathedral Shrines*, 113. In 1518 Robert Lambe bequeathed all his pins, great and small, several penny moulds, half a hundredweight of lead and his tools: KHC, PRC 17/13, f. 328.

[104] *The Tale of Beryn*, ed. Furnivall and Stone, 1.

[105] CCAL, Lit. MS C/14, f. 35v.

[106] Personal communication from Paul Bennett, Canterbury Archaeological Trust.

[107] *The Tale of Beryn*, ed. Furnivall and Stone, 1.

[108] CCAL, CC/AC/1/26; M.E. Mate, *Trade and Economic Developments, 1450–1550: The Experience of Kent, Surrey and Sussex* (Woodbridge, 2006), 19.

[109] Information about inns can be gleaned from testamentary sources, rentals, deeds and the city chamberlains' accounts. Inns in Westgate Street included *The Tabard*, *The Catherine Wheel*, *The Cornysh Chogh*, *The Hart* and *The Bell*.

times such accommodation may have been shared with the workforce employed by the priory on various construction projects inside and outside its precincts. Moreover, in years when plague visited the city there must have been significant problems regarding the availability of accommodation and care for the sick. Although the bailiffs could congratulate themselves in 1420 on providing sufficient lodging for the jubilee, in the aftermath, when plague struck, conditions were probably exceedingly difficult.[110]

Even though only a few of the poor pilgrims visiting Canterbury could ever have been accommodated at St. Thomas' hospital, on the main route from Westgate to the cathedral precincts, it would have been a welcome refuge for them, as the last in a series of pilgrim hospitals located beside the main road from London.[111] St. Thomas' hospital was expected to maintain twelve beds, the poor pilgrims being cared for by an elderly woman who received 4d. per day to cater for her charges.[112] Such provision may have been exceedingly basic, but some idea of the quality of the surroundings can be ascertained from the remains of the surviving wall paintings in the refectory. As well as the depiction of St. Thomas' martyrdom (now lost), the painting of Christ in majesty with the four evangelists would have provided a potent reminder that salvation awaited the penitent, a fitting subject for those journeying to St. Thomas' shrine.[113] Moreover, even though the able-bodied poor could only stay at the hospital overnight, the sick were allowed to remain; and, should they die there, might be buried in the cathedral's lay cemetery. An additional privilege reserved for these paupers was the provision of tapers cut from Dover's great candle for use at their burial.[114]

As noted above, distinguished pilgrims might be offered hospitality by the priory or at St. Augustine's, but increasingly their accommodation seems to have become the responsibility of the civic authorities. Among the royal guests who stayed in 'the Hale in the Blean' when on pilgrimage to Canterbury were Henry VI and later Edward IV and his queen. The first extant reference to this tented complex appears in 1447–8, when 3s. 4d. was spent on making '*unum* Hale' for Henry VI's pilgrimage.[115] However, early in Henry IV's reign, the city chamberlains had paid for bread, red and white wine and goblets to be taken into the Blean when the queen was staying there. Mention is also made of provisions being delivered '*ad palacium*', and of the construction of 'logges in le Blean' (perhaps the forerunner of 'the Hale').[116] After 1448 'the Hale' was refurbished for

[110] CCAL, CC/OA/1, f. 34v; Foreville, *Le Jubilé: Étude et documents*, 143; Urry, 'Jubilee', 26.
[111] Webb, *Pilgrimage*, 223–5; Sheila Sweetinburgh, *The Role of the Hospital in Medieval England: Gift-giving and the Spiritual Economy* (Dublin, 2004), 88–96.
[112] Archbishop Stratford revised the hospital's statutes in 1342: *Literae Cantuariensis*, ed. Sheppard, ii. 256; Duncombe and Battely, *Three Archiepiscopal Hospitals*, 331. A woman named Alice was the 'guardian of the paupers' in 1475: KHC, PRC 32/2, f. 324.
[113] The linking of subject and space has been discussed by Miriam Gill, 'The Role of Images in Monastic Education: the Evidence from Wall Painting in Late Medieval England', in *Medieval Monastic Education*, ed. George Ferzoco and Carolyn Muessig (London and New York, 2000), 125–9.
[114] Rowe, 'Customary', app. 4, p. 22.
[115] CCAL, CC/FA/2, f. 20v.
[116] Lists of expenses incurred during Richard II's and Henry IV's first pilgrimages contain no references to the Blean, but some appear in 1401–2 with regard to the queen's visit: CCAL, CC/FA/3, ff. 11, 19v; CC/FA/1, f. 61v.

each visit, which meant that the mayor and civic officers could confidently greet their honourable guests at the Westgate before escorting them through the city.[117] Such ceremony would be expected by all parties, providing an opportunity for the authorities to stage an appropriate display of prosperity, order and good government.[118]

In the early 1470s, however, the poor state of the streets was detrimental to the way in which the leading citizens wished to portray Canterbury to their royal guests, as well as to pilgrims more generally.[119] Such conditions were replicated elsewhere in England as a consequence of the economic problems then experienced by many towns, but this fact would have been of little comfort to the mayor and aldermen who sought to make the best possible impression.[120] To promote their city, the ruling elite petitioned for aid towards the cost of paving certain important streets, the most vital being the way from the Westgate to the cathedral gate via St. Andrew's church.[121] This new corporate initiative seems to have followed earlier attempts, including some work commissioned by private citizens, as is apparent from the ten loads of stone bequeathed by William Benet to pave the way between St. Andrew's church and the pillory, and the 66*s.* 8*d.* left by Roger Rydle for paving the Bullstake, provided others also contributed.[122] Nor were such gifts confined to the city: William Bigge, in 1470, bequeathed 33*s.* 4*d.* to repair the way at the 'spytel hill', which was conceivably the hill by St. Nicholas' hospital at Harbledown.[123] Initiatives such as these, alongside the provision of a public latrine by the King's Mill and the work of the official scavengers, were all part of the corporation's response to the threat of plague.[124] It was no doubt for this reason that issues of public hygiene, based on a fear of miasma and noxious fumes, came to assume far greater urgency.

Pavage was not the sole weapon in the authorities' campaign to render their city more visually attractive to pilgrims and other visitors. As they reached the top of the hill at Harbledown, the panorama of Canterbury cathedral, especially the 'Angel Steeple' that was replaced by the even more impressive 'Bell Harry' towards the end of the fifteenth century, must have inspired awe, but perhaps almost as striking was the view of the Westgate on the approach from St. Dunstan's church.[125] The Westgate, with its innovative gun loops, had been built in

---

[117] Among those preparing 'the Hale' in 1450–1 were Thomas Cok and John Stace; the provisions then included over 25 gallons of wine: CCAL, CC/FA/2, f. 34. Far more was spent in 1464–5 on 'the Hale' and the royal pilgrims in general, since in total the chamberlains paid out £28 13*s.* 8*d.*: CCAL, CC/FA/2, f. 95v.

[118] Tekippe, 'Pilgrimage', 727–8.

[119] According to the chamberlains' accounts, stone had been purchased at various times during the 15th century to repair the main streets, but conditions had deteriorated appreciably by this date: CCAL, CC/FA/1, 2.

[120] Similar problems at Strood near Rochester had provoked royal censure in the past, since they posed a danger to travellers visiting St. Thomas' shrine: Webb, *Pilgrimage*, 228.

[121] CCAL, CC/AA/36.

[122] KHC, PRC 17/1, f. 14; 17/2, f. 46.

[123] *Ibid.*, 17/1, f. 343.

[124] Rawcliffe, *Medicine and Society*, 42.

[125] Towering to a height of 235 ft. from the ground, its pinnacles being 120 ft. above the apex of the roof, the great cathedral crossing tower is one of the tallest in England. Significantly, the original height was doubled during the building campaign of the late 1490s, perhaps reflecting Christ

about 1380, and almost a century later the civic authorities commissioned the construction of an equally commanding gateway at the opposite end of the High Street.[126] Like the paving initiative, the new St. George's gate was partly funded by leading citizens whose contributions aided the chamberlains considerably.[127] The fifteenth century had also seen the rebuilding of the city wall, an imposing structure that was intended to enhance the perception of Canterbury as a well-defended and tightly regulated city, and may, indeed, have succeeded in its purpose.[128] Such features in themselves might not have attracted pilgrims to the shrine of St. Thomas, yet they may have added to the wider appeal of visiting Canterbury; and, like the knight in *The Tale of Beryn*, pilgrims may have toured the city defences.[129] Nonetheless, even though its walls and artillery were not tested, war in the form of revolt did touch the city, and may well have discouraged pilgrimage in the turbulent years of 1450, 1460 and especially 1470–1.

Another aspect of a well-ordered city was law and order, which might be demonstrated through the official scrutiny and regulation of the food supply available for both citizens and visitors. Canterbury's role as a distribution centre in east Kent was important, but for those controlling the shops, markets and fairs, including the St. Thomas fair held within the cathedral precincts, there was the added burden of finding extra provisions at particular festivals, and especially in jubilee years.[130] Even though the civic authorities shouldered much of this responsibility, the two great Benedictine houses were also involved, which at times led to jurisdictional disputes regarding the location and control of certain markets.[131] It has not been possible to correlate such disputes to the years of potential difficulty arising from harsh weather conditions, as recorded in Stone's chronicle, but these factors presumably had an impact on the number and prosperity of stall and shop holders in the city. Yet, notwithstanding such problems, a measure of the corporation's success in the early fifteenth century, at least, can be gauged from the low cost and ready availability of victuals in 1420. For, in contrast to the previous jubilee, when shortages led to high prices and serious disruption, the bailiffs reported that four loaves could be bought for 1*d.*, a gallon of ale for 1½*d.*, and a roast goose for 7*d.*[132]

Food and drink were no less important to the author of the prologue of *The Tale of Beryn*, whose pilgrims partake of dinner and supper, the latter including wine. They also seek entertainment in the city: the wife of Bath and the prioress appreciate the well-cultivated garden of the inn, the merchant and several others the many sights of Canterbury. Although no further details are provided, the

Church's confidence in its saint and in society more generally: Blockley, Sparks and Tatton-Brown, *Canterbury Nave*, 145.

[126] S.S. Frere, Sally Stow and Paul Bennett, *Excavations on the Roman and Medieval Defences of Canterbury* (Canterbury, 1982).

[127] One of them was the above-mentioned William Bigge, who left £10 to work in progress: KHC, PRC 17/1, f. 343.

[128] There is a growing literature on the value then placed on town walls, over and above their importance for defence. See, for example: J.M. Steane, *The Archaeology of Power: England and Northern Europe, AD 800–1600* (Stroud, 2001), 194–5, 202–5.

[129] *The Tale of Beryn*, ed. Furnivall and Stone, 9.

[130] Mate, *Trade and Economic Developments*, 11–12, 36–7.

[131] *Ibid.*, 24; CCAL, Lit. MS E/23, f. 117.

[132] CCAL, CC/OA/1, f. 34v; Foreville, *Le Jubilé: Étude et documents*, 143; Urry, 'Jubilee', 27.

prologue suggests that the city had much to offer its visitors. For those of a pious disposition there were the shrines of St. Augustine and St. Mildred, among others, at St. Augustine's abbey; the shrine of St. Etheldreda at St. Sepulchre's nunnery (her principal shrine was at Ely); and several relics at the Austin friary, including a piece of St. Katherine's hairshirt bequeathed by William Haute in 1462.[133] Sporting types may have preferred the chance to play various games at the city's taverns, such as tennis, closh and bowls.[134] Even though the evidence is exceedingly slim, it seems that there was an annual Corpus Christi play, performed by the city's craftsmen, which was probably a major attraction.[135] Whether the St. Thomas pageant and four other pageants, known to have been staged on the vigil of the translation from at least 1505, also took place in the late fifteenth century is unclear.[136] Nonetheless, the giant candle of Dover would have been drawn through the streets to the cathedral every third year on that day, which alone would have provided a great spectacle. Thus, even though the civic authorities and the monastic community were sometimes at loggerheads, there seems to have been a tacit agreement that they would join together to promote Canterbury's premier saint for their mutual benefit.[137]

Canterbury Pilgrims in the Fifteenth Century

On the basis of the evidence presented above, it seem feasible to suggest that conditions in the fifteenth century might still have persuaded some, at least, that fear of the Apocalypse, so apparent after the Black Death, was still justified. Although, perhaps, for more it was 'the deep insecurity' that plague caused on a personal level, with the associated terror of sudden death and an attendant focus upon 'last things', including penance, which necessitated constant vigilance.[138] Additionally, pilgrimage could be an enjoyable adventure; and what might today be called 'the pilgrim experience' was being actively promoted by different constituents in the city. Yet there remains the question posed at the start of this essay: did such feelings and activities translate into a quantifiable level of interest in pilgrimage to Canterbury?

As Nilson has indicated, a change in accounting procedures at Christ Church means that the recording of annual totals for shrine offerings did not continue after

---

[133] A 15th-century plan of the east end of the abbey church shows the various shrines: Cambridge, Trinity Hall, MS I, f. 77. In 1425 Thomas Wykes remembered Etheldreda's shrine at the nunnery, bequeathing 40s. to it: KHC, PRC 32/1, f. 19; 32/2, f. 79.

[134] Closh was a kind of skittles played with a mallet: Mate, *Trade and Economic Developments*, 164.

[135] CCAL, CC/AB/1, f. 6; *Kent: Diocese of Canterbury*, ed. J.M. Gibson (Records of Early English Drama, 3 vols., Toronto and London, 2002), i. 139.

[136] CCAL, Lit. MS C/13, f. 10; CC/FA/2, f. 411–11v; *Kent: Diocese of Canterbury*, ed. Gibson, i. 98–9, 144–5.

[137] Rebecca Warren, '"With Rewt and Ryott": Urban Conflict between Church and State in Fifteenth-Century Canterbury', *Archaeologia Cantiana* (forthcoming).

[138] *The Black Death*, ed. Horrox, 13. Sir John Heveningham was, for example, 'nevyr meryer' before nine o'clock, but dead soon after noon: *Paston Letters and Papers of the Fifteenth Century*, ed. Norman Davis, Richard Beadle and Colin Richmond (3 vols., EETS, supplementary series xx–xxii, Oxford, 2004–5), i. 39.

1384–5.[139] However, the prior's accounts for a few random years between 1410 and 1473 do offer some insight into the shrine's financial health. Not surprisingly, the best year was 1420, when over £640 was allegedly collected at the various Becket stations in the cathedral.[140] How far this sum derived from the offerings of the 100,000 pilgrims said by the city bailiffs to have attended the jubilee is a moot point, but their estimate would seem to indicate an exceedingly crowded city with far more visitors than usual.[141] Yet, even if it represents a grossly inflated figure, throughout the century the corporation and convent continued to promote St. Thomas's shrine, which suggests that they still regarded pilgrimage as a valuable part of Canterbury's economy.

It is possible to gain only a rough idea of the offerings at the 1470 jubilee, but the sum of almost £100 said to have come from jubilee gifts in the prior's accounts for 1472–3 and 1473–4 presumably represents part of a significant increase.[142] Further evidence of a growing influx of pilgrims may be found in a directive by the archiepiscopal commissary, who forbade the confessors specially appointed to shrive this army of penitents from demanding fees.[143] Nonetheless, as we have seen, the limited nature of the papal indulgence was probably a disincentive to some. So too may have been the political problems and uncertainties that had engulfed England generally during the Readeption, and Kent most particularly during the final phase involving Fauconberg's Rebellion.[144] Notwithstanding the notorious capacity of public executions to attract crowds, the sight of the mayor being hanged, drawn and quartered in the Bullstake outside the gate to the cathedral in May 1471 can hardly have been a magnet to visitors. Edward IV returned at Michaelmas that year to receive his papal indulgence at St. Thomas' shrine, an event that seemingly drew far more pilgrims than his imposition of royal justice had done four months earlier.[145] This glittering occasion, which formed part of the 1470 jubilee, was described by Sir John Paston in a letter to his brother and namesake, in which he states that there were 'neuyr so moche peple seyn in pylgrymage her-to-foor at ones, as men seye'.[146]

Diana Webb has drawn attention to a small number of fifteenth-century pilgrims who travelled to Canterbury. Her evidence derives mainly from published inquisitions *post mortem* and wills, but east Kent testators do not appear to have included the shrine of St. Thomas among their favoured destinations.[147] Not that all preferred Marian or Christocentric centres: St. Thomas de Halys in Dover, St. 'Roncon' in Scotland, and, most frequently, St. James de Compostella are mentioned.[148] Nevertheless, even if the Canterbury saint is conspicuous by his poor showing in the county's wills, his cult in 'an age of plague' was clearly far from moribund, if not, perhaps, thriving to the extent that it had done in the previous

---

[139] Nilson, *Cathedral Shrines*, 149, 215.
[140] CCAL, DCc/Register H, f. 102.
[141] CCAL, CC/OA/1, f. 34v; Urry, 'Jubilee', 26.
[142] Nilson, *Cathedral Shrines*, 150.
[143] *Literae Cantuarienses*, ed. Sheppard, iii. 252–3.
[144] Colin Richmond, 'Fauconberg's Kentish Rising of May 1471', *EHR*, lxxxv (1970), 673–92.
[145] Connor, 'John Stone', 268; *eadem, Stone's Chronicle*, 131.
[146] *Paston Letters*, ed. Davis, Beadle and Richmond, i. 443.
[147] Webb, *Pilgrimage*, 184, 186, 191, 193–5, 197, 199, 200.
[148] KHC, PRC 17/5, ff. 50, 320; 32/1, f. 32; 32/2, ff. 253, 521; 32/4, f. 137; 32/5, f. 54.

century.[149] Furthermore, it seems to have remained sufficiently viable for the promotional strategy of the city and cathedral to be still very much in evidence during the early sixteenth century; indeed, their tried and tested appeal to pilgrims may even have endured beyond the next jubilee of 1520.[150]

---

[149] Even though he was not specifically requesting a pilgrimage, Thomas Polton of New Romney wanted his executors to give 6*d*. to the shrine at Canterbury in 1487: *ibid.*, 32/3, f. 175.

[150] Sheila Sweetinburgh, 'Looking to the Past: the St Thomas Pageant in Early Tudor Canterbury', in *After Becket: The Reaction of the Plantagenet World*, ed. Marie-Pierre Gelin and Paul Webster (forthcoming).

AN URBAN ENVIRONMENT: NORWICH IN THE FIFTEENTH CENTURY

Elizabeth Rutledge

Academic interest in the medieval and later urban environment is by no means a new phenomenon and is apparent, for example, in an historical account of Norwich written by the early eighteenth-century antiquary John Kirkpatrick.[1] The final decades of the last century, however, witnessed a renewed interest in the subject in relation to both medieval and to more modern towns. Many of the resulting studies have concentrated on a specific aspect of the urban landscape and the responses this invoked, and/or on the relationship between the environment and health.[2] This paper, however, aims to look more generally at the state of one particular city in the fifteenth century, and to attempt to assess how it might have felt to live in Norwich at that time, together with how far the civic authorities sought to ameliorate environmental problems. All towns, of course, have their individual characteristics, both physical and social, but Norwich is an interesting case study. In the sixteenth century it was promoted as an exceptionally clean and healthy city and the governing body undertook new initiatives to clear the river and the streets.[3]

---

[1] John Kirkpatrick, *The Streets and Lanes of the City of Norwich*, ed. William Hudson (Norwich, 1889), 1–89.

[2] For example: D.J. Keene, 'Rubbish in Medieval Towns', in *Environmental Archaeology in the Urban Context*, ed. A.R. Hall and H.K. Kenward (Council for British Archaeology Research Report no. 43, 1982), 26–30; Alain Corbin, *The Foul and the Fragrant. Odor and the French Social Imagination* (New York, 1986); Peter Brimblecombe, *The Big Smoke. A History of Air Pollution in London since Medieval Times* (1987); I.H.H. Fay, 'Health and Disease in Medieval and Tudor Norwich' (Univ. of East Anglia Ph.D. thesis, 2007); Dolly Jørgensen, 'Cooperative Sanitation: Managing Streets and Gutters in Late Medieval England and Scandinavia', *Technology and Culture*, xlix (2008), 547–67; *eadem*, '"All Good Rule of the Citee": Sanitation and Civic Government in England, 1400–1600', *Journal of Urban History*, xxxvi (2010), 300–15, where Jørgensen examines the effect that efforts to improve the sanitary conditions in Norwich and Coventry had on the civic governmental structures; Carole Rawcliffe, *Urban Bodies*: *Communal Health in Late Medieval English Towns and Cities* (Woodbridge, 2013). The archaeological evidence for a wide range of European towns is discussed in *Lübecker Kolloquium zur Stadtarchäologie im Hanseraum IV*: *Die Infrastruktur*, ed. Manfred Gläser (Lübeck, 2004). The volume includes a contribution from Brian Ayers, 'The Infrastructure of Norwich from the 12th to the 17th Centuries' (*Lübecker Kolloquium IV*, ed. Gläser, 31–49), in which he considers several of the issues raised in this paper over a longer time-span. My thanks to Carole Rawcliffe for letting me read in draft her chapter on the urban water supply in *eadem*, *Urban Bodies*, and for taking the photograph used in plate 1.

[3] The promotion included William Cuningham's 'Prospect of Norwich' in his *Cosmographical Glasse* of 1558. See Carole Rawcliffe, 'Introduction', in *Medieval Norwich*, ed. Carole Rawcliffe and Richard Wilson (2004), p. xx; and (for a detailed assessment of Cuningham and the ideas behind his 'Prospect') Fay, 'Health and Disease', 127–77. For the 16th–century initiatives see Jørgensen, '"All

There is therefore particular value in looking back to the fifteenth century in order to examine the base on which this sixteenth-century urban environment was built, as well as in considering how far such a positive picture reflected the experience of most fifteenth-century inhabitants of Norwich.

The beginning of the fifteenth century was not a propitious time for Norwich, as it continued the struggle to maintain its position as a major provincial city. Recurrent attacks of plague, coupled with reduced immigration from the countryside, had cut the resident population from perhaps 25,000 before the Black Death to about 8,000 in 1400, compared, for instance, to a contemporary York population of 14,000 to 15,000. Nevertheless, the civic authorities can be seen taking up the challenge to redress this situation, by putting the corporate finances on a firmer footing and in asserting their independence by a royal charter of 1404 that established the office of mayor in place of the previous four bailiffs and accorded Norwich county status. In many ways their efforts were clearly successful. Although Norwich continued to suffer from plague and other epidemic diseases throughout the fifteenth century, it did not experience a major mid-century economic decline, and by 1525 it ranked as the wealthiest of English towns after London.[4]

The first notable aspect of Norwich in the fifteenth century would have been its appearance as a city of slopes and valleys (Fig. 1). Norwich developed on either side of, and along, the valley of the Wensum. North of the river the gradients are fairly gentle, but the situation to the south is quite different. The eastern section, which included the precinct of Norwich cathedral priory and that of the hospital of St. Giles, is low-lying. Away from the river and the flood plain, however, the ground rises steeply. Not surprisingly, the castle was sited at the end of a spur of particularly high land (the Ber Street ridge) which runs back to the southern corner of the city. The contours shown on Fig. 1 are taken from the 1884 ordnance survey map. By then considerable levelling and smoothing out had taken place in the eighteenth century and, although some infilling occurred earlier, the effect would have been far more pronounced in the fifteenth century. John Kirkpatrick, writing in about 1700, was very aware of differences in level, and refers to high places and low places and to lanes rising steeply.[5]

Secondly, Norwich was a city of gardens and open spaces, so much so that in 1618 Thomas Baskerville praised it for its 'gardens, orchards and enclosures', and in 1662 Thomas Fuller famously described it as 'either a city in an orchard or an orchard in a city'.[6] This comment was equally true of the fifteenth century. The area enclosed within the city walls was approximately a square mile, far larger than in any other English provincial town. Though prestige was no doubt a factor, there were two purely practical reasons for the creation of such a large circuit. One was

---

Good Rule of the Citee"', 309–11, and *Norwich's River and Street Accounts, 1556–80*, ed. Isla Fay (Norfolk Record Society, lxxvii, 2013, forthcoming).

[4] Penelope Dunn, 'Trade', and R.H. Frost, 'The Urban Elite', in *Medieval Norwich*, ed. Rawcliffe and Wilson, 213–14, 234, 236; Penny Dunn, 'After the Black Death: Society and Economy in Late Fourteenth-Century Norwich' (Univ. of East Anglia Ph.D. thesis, 2003), 341, 342, n. 12; *eadem*, 'Financial Reform in Late Medieval Norwich: Evidence from an Urban Cartulary', in *Medieval East Anglia*, ed. Christopher Harper-Bill (Woodbridge, 2005), 99–114.

[5] Brian Ayers, *Norwich: 'A Fine City'* (Stroud, 2003), 150–1; Kirkpatrick, *Streets and Lanes*, 1–89.

[6] Rawcliffe, 'Introduction', p. xxiii.

that the walls as built skirted the head of all but one of the urban tributaries of the Wensum, enabling them to be built on firm ground while contending with the minimum length of slope. Secondly, the resulting walls enclosed not only Norwich's densely populated centre but also most of its substantial ribbon development along the major access routes. This settlement pattern, despite considerable fluctuations in population, survived almost unchanged between the late thirteenth century and 1800, the only obvious effect of the Black Death being the apparent abandonment of a hitherto lightly populated area on the higher land to the south-west. The consequence was both that pre-1800 Norwich had very little in the way of development outside the walls, and that large areas of open land were to be found immediately within them.[7] Transfers of Norwich property often mention gardens both before and after the Black Death, and the feeling of space in the fifteenth-century city must have been accentuated by the drop in population to a third of its previous level.

This did not mean, however, that the mass of the urban population necessarily benefited from all these open spaces. For Norwich was also a city of flint walls.[8] The pre-eminent flint wall, of course, was the city wall itself, completed just before the Black Death. This was a massive two and a half miles in length with some forty towers, encircling two-thirds of the city, with the river acting as the boundary on the eastern side. Standing about 20 ft. high, there can be no doubt of its making a formidable impression.[9] For much of its course the city wall was set on rising ground, and in such a way that no countryside could be seen beyond. Indeed, the areas of unoccupied land just inside the walls may have made them appear even more impressive. This was partly because, subject to what follows, the walls would often have been viewed across open space, rather than being obscured by housing. But also because the mere size of the area within the walls at Norwich may, in a way, have increased the sense of enclosure. With so little urban settlement outside the walls, there was a contrast between the within and the without that may not have occurred in places where well-developed suburbs acted as an extension of the town.

Moreover, much of the undeveloped land within the city would not have been readily accessible, or even visible, to the bulk of the population. Some of the apparently open areas were the extensive precincts of major religious institutions, and by 1400 all of these had been surrounded by substantial walls. Fig. 2 shows the precincts of Norwich cathedral priory, of the four friaries (belonging to the Blackfriars, who moved across the river so that they had in effect two precincts, the Whitefriars, the Greyfriars and the Austin friars), of the Chapel in the Fields and of the hospital of St. Giles.[10] Such walls were far from negligible. Much of the cathedral priory wall still survives to the height of over 16 ft. and is shown as

---

[7] The one designated medieval suburb was Heigham to the west.

[8] Flint, which appears black when cut, or knapped, is the local building stone.

[9] Nikolaus Pevsner and Bill Wilson, *Norfolk I: Norwich and the North-East* (The Buildings of England, 2nd edn., 1997), 260–1.

[10] The latest to be built was probably the precinct wall of the Chapel in the Fields which was in the course of construction in 1374: Christopher Harper-Bill and Carole Rawcliffe, 'The Religious Houses', in *Medieval Norwich*, ed. Rawcliffe and Wilson, 116. Norwich cathedral priory had some form of precinct wall from at least the 12th century: Roberta Gilchrist, *Norwich Cathedral Close. The Evolution of the English Cathedral Landscape* (Woodbridge, 2005), 44–6.

crenellated on a plan of about 1630,[11] while an impressive section of the Greyfriars'
wall continues to face the priory precinct wall in St. Faith's Lane. In fact, far from
these precincts being immediately recognizable as open spaces, their perimeter
walls must have produced a considerable feeling of exclusion, especially when, as
mentioned above, they faced each other across the street. (Plate 1 shows the road
running between the flint walls of the bishop's palace and of the hospital of St.
Giles.) How far the same considerations applied to the other large areas of open
space around the edges of the city is impossible to say, but the Gildencroft (north
of the river), for instance, mainly belonged to the hospital of St. Giles. Its master
was presented in 1286 for making a wall there (3 ft. wide and 40 ft. long), on the
highway and for enclosing a common path through the middle, which hardly
suggests that he promoted free access.[12]

Then there were the domestic walls. Here I am not concerned with buildings,
though there were certainly flint buildings, both ancient and more recent, but
curtilage walls. Although the deeds of this period do not often give specific details,
walls are mentioned time and again. From the early 1380s, for example, come
references to a messuage and gardens with a stone wall to the east; a whole
messuage with a curtain wall; a part tenement called 'le gardyn' with walls; a
tenement with a stone wall on its south side.[13] Other walls were newly built.
Following a dispute in 1400, John Bray was to construct a new stone wall
bordering a messuage in King Street. There were also internal tenement walls. A
quitclaim of property near the Blackfriars in 1420 mentions a stone wall between
two parts of a holding.[14] This ubiquity of flint walls is cited as a characteristic of
Norwich in a piece of fifteenth-century doggerel verse.[15]

The presence of walls inevitably implied gates, and in the case of the more
prestigious establishments gatehouses. The city walls included twelve gates. The
gatehouses were all demolished between 1791 and 1808, but their substantial
proportions are apparent from a series of nineteenth-century engravings.[16]
However, the two great gateways into the cathedral priory precinct still survive, as
does the entrance to the grounds of the bishop's palace. Two-storey gatehouses
would also have guarded the approaches to the friary precincts, though all of these
have disappeared.[17] Such gateways were not only for show. Entrances could be

[11]   Gilchrist, *Norwich Cathedral Close*, plate 1, after p. 148.
[12]   Kirkpatrick, *Streets and Lanes*, 81.
[13]   Norfolk RO, MC 146/11, 624X2, cards for Norwich court roll 14 (NCR 1/14), rots. 9, 14, 19. These
       are part of a series of cards produced by the Norwich Survey summarising the information given in
       the deeds enrolled on the court rolls. They are available for 1285 to 1340 and for 1377 to 1390.
[14]   Norfolk RO, NCR 1/16, rot. 3d (John Bray); 1/17, rot. 17 (John Davy).
[15]   '*Haec sunt Norwycus .... dyrt quoque vicus flynt valles rede thek ...*' ['foul street, flint walls, reed
       thatch']: *A Norfolk Anthology. A Collection of Poems, Ballads and Rare Tracts Relating to the
       County of Norfolk*, ed. J.O. Halliwell (Brixton Hill, 1852), 55, taken from a Trinity College,
       Cambridge, Library ms. A marginally different version is quoted in full in Elizabeth Rutledge,
       'Norwich before the Black Death: Economic Life', in *Medieval Norwich*, ed. Rawcliffe and Wilson,
       157.
[16]   By Henry Ninham, taken from drawings by John Kirkpatrick. Some of the city gates were faced
       with the more prestigious freestone. See *Old Norwich*, comp. A.M. Cotman and F.W. Hawcroft
       (Norwich, 1961), 107–20.
[17]   The former main gatehouse into the Greyfriars may have been the property described in 1566 as a
       stable with a little chamber, then being used as a dovehouse, above it: P.A. Emery, *Norwich
       Greyfriars: Pre-Conquest Town and Medieval Friary* (East Anglian Archaeology, cxx, 2007), 56.

seen as the weak point in an opponent's defences, as in 1443, when the townsmen of Norwich attacked the cathedral priory by digging under the gates.[18] Once again, the practice of the religious institutions was mirrored by that of the public at large. Gates are not mentioned as often as some other features, but they come up occasionally in agreements and divisions of property: part of a messuage with a stone entry; a gate under the solar; free access through the back gate; free entrance and exit by the great gate of a messuage.[19] Private property was no more open to public access than monastic property.

A further and potentially more controversial use of gates was to block rights of way. Closure of rights of way was not a new phenomenon in the fifteenth century and is well-attested in the development of the precincts of all the major Norwich religious institutions.[20] As late as 1430–1 the Austin friars bought a lane adjoining their premises from the city for £20.[21] The same practice was adopted by private individuals anxious to enlarge, and the better to enclose, their holdings. One example comes from the eastern end of the present St. Andrew's Street, near the Blackfriars. The right to enclose the western part of this section of the street had been granted by the city to the owner of one of the adjoining properties in 1372, the dimensions given being 27½ yards long, 3¼ yards wide at the east end, and 3⅞ yards wide at the west. Permission to annex the remaining twenty-seven yards was given in 1495.[22] The civic authorities were obviously well-aware of the problems, for social control, as well as for health, likely to be caused by an unregulated cul-de-sac. The reason they gave in 1495 for allowing the rest of the lane to be enclosed with gates at the east end was 'because various unfortunate events and affrays had taken place in that lane, and it was filled to a considerable extent by dung and filth'. This was a formulaic response; similar wording had been used when permission was given to enclose another lane in 1414.[23]

It would also have been immediately apparent to the fifteenth-century inhabitants of Norwich that they lived in a city of running water and ponds (Fig. 3). This aspect of the local topography is mainly hidden from us today, when streams, sewers, and the main water supply alike have all been put underground, so that we are only aware of the river Wensum. The river was, and is, tidal to the mills on the western edge of the city, and still salt enough at times to support the occasional flounder.[24] In the fifteenth century it was also affected by pollution, both human

---

[18] Norman Tanner, 'The Cathedral and the City', in *Norwich Cathedral. Church, City and Diocese, 1096–1996*, ed. Ian Atherton, Eric Fernie, Christopher Harper-Bill and Hassell Smith (1996), 265.

[19] Examples from 1379 to 1426: Norfolk RO, MC 146/11, 624X2, cards for Norwich court roll 14 (NCR 1/14), rots. 5d, 25d, 35; NCR 1/18, rot. 8 (Nicholas Lomynour *et al.*).

[20] By archaeological and/or documentary evidence. For example: Gilchrist, *Norwich Cathedral Close*, 23–4; Margot Tillyard, 'The Acquisition by the Norwich Blackfriars of the Site for their Church c.1310–1325', in Serena Kelly, Elizabeth Rutledge and Margot Tillyard, *Men of Property. An Analysis of the Norwich Enrolled Deeds 1285–1311* (Norwich, 1983), 7; Emery, *Norwich Greyfriars*, 10, 26–7, 33.

[21] Norfolk RO, NCR 18A/1, f. 170v.

[22] The eastern end of St. Andrew's Street was reinstated at the end of the 19th century, when a tramway was put through: F.R. Beecheno, 'The Sucklings' House at Norwich', *Norfolk Archaeology*, xix (1917), 198.

[23] Norfolk RO, NCR 17B, Domesday Book, f. 29v; NCR 16D/1, f. 57v; Kirkpatrick, *Streets and Lanes*, 61.

[24] Mark Cocker, *Crow Country* (2008), 19.

and industrial. Industrial pollution came from the tanners, dyers and fullers who colonised the section of the Wensum separating the two halves of the city. In fact, in both respects the river was probably considerably less polluted than it had been in the early fourteenth century. Then the population had been three times the size, and the number of tanners and dyers considerably greater. By the fifteenth century weaving had become the major industry in Norwich, with dyers not even making the top ten occupations in terms of the numbers admitted to the freedom. Fullers (engaged in another anti-social craft) were initially more in evidence than before the Black Death, but numbers dropped after 1450.[25] The Wensum, however, must have remained throughout both insalubrious and dangerous. Drowning in it appears as a common cause of death in the coroners' inquests for the thirteenth and seventeenth centuries alike.[26] The city's (and the crown's)[27] main concern, however, was that by the end of the fourteenth century the river had become badly silted up. In 1467 the city assembly complained that at some times of year 'dry ground is observed in certain places in the same, and the flow of water prevented'.[28] This could have reduced the risk of drowning, but would have done nothing to curb the pollution.

Altogether, it may have been no bad thing that general access to the Wensum was limited. Most of the river bank not in the hands of religious institutions was taken up by privately-owned industrial premises or staithes. There were common quays, an original one near Fye Bridge, and two more in King Street acquired by the city in the late fourteenth century, but they were only 'common' in the sense that they belonged to the community. By the sixteenth century the common staithes along King Street were protected from casual access by stone walls and locked gates.[29] This is not to say that there was no public access, but the poor needing water from the river could only get it at particular points. From at least 1367–8 there was a common watering place for horses just upstream of the mills, above much of the pollution and where the water was most likely to be fresh as well as unpolluted. Further downriver another general watering place could be found on the north bank near Fye Bridge. In 1526 permission was given to close the lane leading down to the river here, on condition that the gate be left open during the day so that dwellers nearby could get down for water and to wash. There were also a number of points of access at the end of lanes along King Street, away from the worst of the industrial pollution, including a staithe built in 1422 specifically for the washing of linen cloths.[30]

[25]   Rutledge, 'Norwich before the Black Death: Economic Life', Table 2, 168–72, and Dunn, 'Trade', 215–17; Andrew King, 'The Merchant Class and Borough Finances in Later Medieval Norwich' (Univ. of Oxford D.Phil. thesis, 1989), Table 5.3.

[26]   Norfolk RO, NCR 6A/1; 8A/1, 2. Further details of cases of drowning, in ponds as well as in the river, are given in Carole Rawcliffe, 'Health and Safety at Work in Late Medieval East Anglia', in *Medieval East Anglia*, ed. Harper-Bill, 143–4.

[27]   The crown might be expected to have been concerned about the effect on shipping and trade, but in fact it ordered the cleansing of the river in connection with the city's defences: *CPR*, 1377–81, p. 121 (1378); 1381–5, p. 546 (1385); *The Records of the City of Norwich*, ed. William Hudson and J.C. Tingey (2 vols., Norwich, 1906–10), ii. 318 (1452).

[28]   *Records of Norwich*, ed. Hudson and Tingey, ii. 96.

[29]   Dunn, 'Financial Reform', 104–6; Mary Rodgers, *The River and Staithes of Tudor Norwich* (Norwich, 1996), 38.

[30]   Kirkpatrick, *Streets and Lanes*, 7–8, 73–4, 86.

Efforts to improve the state of the river predated 1400 and continued throughout the fifteenth century. The principal concern of the city authorities was to keep the river channel open, which led them to adopt a two-fold approach. The first was to deal with the situation as it existed. Strategies employed *inter alia* were to grant newly-formed islands near the banks, called 'bitmays', to neighbouring property owners who had an interest in their further consolidation, thus narrowing, and possibly deepening, the channel; and to order periodic cleansing of the river by the community.[31] The second approach was to limit the amount of rubbish and dung going into the river in the first place. In 1380 the private removal of muck by boat was prohibited (obviously because it was thought that too much ended up in the river) and a single contractor was appointed to do the job instead.[32] At the same time the authorities restricted the amount of dirt being brought down from higher ground along the water courses by installing cisterns at their junction with the river. It is not clear when these were first introduced, but they were certainly in operation by the end of the fifteenth century. The earliest may have been a cistern in Conesford (King Street) built in 1472–3. It was a substantial thatched structure, with a lockable door, whose construction required the services of a mason. For several years the costs of cleaning it out were borne directly by the city, but an assembly order in 1496 refers to financing the maintenance of a King Street cistern from the rent of a nearby property.[33] The building of what may have been a second cistern in the same area was mentioned in 1491, when the city granted Thomas Large a lane in King Street next to one of the common staithes.[34] Both of these cisterns would have dealt with muck coming down from the Ber Street ridge as well as along King Street. Further up the river a common cistern was recorded near Blackfriars bridge in 1505, when two masons and senior members of the civic governing body were ordered to inspect it.[35]

Quite apart from the river, however, few areas of Norwich were far from running water. A regular feature of the landscape was the small streams, known locally as cockeys, running down from the higher ground. The principal cockeys were probably spring-fed, although not all of them were accessible to the general public. Three, including the Dallingflete and the Fresflete, rose within the precinct of the Greyfriars and barely touched the margins of the city en route to the river Wensum. The remaining cockeys on the south side of the river, however, ran through the busiest part of Norwich and would have been far more visible. The larger of the two, known as the Great Cockey, rose just inside the walls and continued down the major valley between the castle and the great market place; the other, unnamed, flowed north from near the church of St. Giles, along a valley

---

[31] For example: Norfolk RO, NCR 17B, Domesday Book, f. 40; *Records of Norwich*, ed. Hudson and Tingey, i. 277; ii. 102.

[32] *Records of Norwich*, ed. Hudson and Tingey, ii. pp. cxxix, 84–5, 91.

[33] In 1474–5 its purpose was spelled out as 'receiving the muck from the streets lest it run into the royal river' (*recipient' putrida viarum ne currerent in regium flumen*): Norfolk RO, NCR 18A/2, ff. 48v, 73, 83, 93, 105v, 114v; Kirkpatrick, *Streets and Lanes*, 7.

[34] Norfolk RO, NCR 16D/1, f. 141v.

[35] *Ibid.*, NCR 16D/2, ff. 70–1. Later references to cisterns are given in Margaret Pelling, 'Health and Sanitation to 1750', in *Norwich since 1550*, ed. Carole Rawcliffe and Richard Wilson (2004), 130–1.

where willows grew in the sixteenth century.[36] North of the river the major stream was the Dalymond, the only watercourse (apart from the Wensum itself) that rose outside the city walls. Other possible spring-fed streams were the water of Muspol and an unnamed stream that ran west from near the Gildencroft. In addition, there were water courses fed by run-off from the higher ground. Properly channelled, run-off can produce a considerable stream over a remarkably short distance, and the more substantial of these watercourses were also sometimes referred to as cockeys. Water coming down from the Ber Street ridge, for example, approached the river along what was later known as Cockey Lane, while John Kirkpatrick refers to a cockey running down the north end of the market place to where it joined the Great Cockey.[37]

Run-off needed careful control in a hilly landscape such as that of Norwich, and there was a hierarchy of water courses for this purpose. Smaller channels, generally known as gutters, were used to lead waste water away in an efficient manner. The system is spelled out in a city assembly order of 1467, which required that the levelling of a street should begin at the higher end of the water course (*cursus aquatici*), so as not to impede the water flowing down to the great gutters (*magnos gurgites*) known as '*lez cokeys*'.[38] The upkeep of these public gutters or cockeys was accepted as the responsibility of the city; oak was bought for the repair of an un-located cockey in 1409–10 and bricks or tiles (*pro tegulis emptis*) for one near the Whitefriars in 1410–11.[39] Generally, the willingness to accept run-off on your land would, of course, depend on where you were in the city and how contaminated the water had become. Water from the Ber Street ridge, for example, might not have been welcome because of the butchers' premises along the street above.[40] Access to private gutters, on the other hand, was considered to be a definite asset as a means of draining waste water off your land, and was granted in the deeds from time to time. Also frequently mentioned is the right to eavesdrop (*aisiamentum severunde aque*), namely to have eaves which dripped onto a neighbour's property, sometimes within a measured distance.[41] Once again, the emphasis was on getting rid of the rain water, rather than considering it as a useful source.

River, and probably cockey, water was used for washing clothes, but the major religious institutions, and to a considerable extent the population at large, are likely to have got most of their cooking, brewing and (when required) drinking water from wells.[42] In an environment where most of the Norwich religious houses were

[36]   Kirkpatrick, *Streets and Lanes*, 50.
[37]   *Ibid.*, 7, 43. For a discussion of the use of the term 'cockey' see Pelling, 'Health and Sanitation', 126–30.
[38]   Norfolk RO, NCR 16D/1, f. 70.
[39]   Norfolk RO, NCR 7C, treasurers' rolls for 1409–10 and 1410–11 (also labelled 1411–12).
[40]   These almost certainly included slaughter houses. In 1586 the butchers were given permission to slaughter within the walls, despite a statute to the contrary, but only in Ber Street: Norfolk RO, NCR 16A/11 (10 Sept. 28 Elizabeth).
[41]   Norfolk RO, MC 146/11, 624X2, cards for Norwich court roll 14 (NCR 1/14). The water courses are described variously as gutters or cockeys. Eavesdrop was a common urban problem: for Winchester references see Derek Keene, *Survey of Medieval Winchester* (2 vols., Winchester Studies 2, Oxford, 1985), ii. 478, 481, 493, 557, 729, 737, 883, 899.
[42]   Carole Rawcliffe points out that the poor may have had little choice but to drink water, and that drinking water was sometimes recommended for health reasons: Rawcliffe, *Urban Bodies*, ch. 4.

close to the river or natural streams, they saw no need for elaborate works to bring in either drinking or washing water from a distance. Instead there is documentary and/or archaeological evidence for wells within the cathedral priory precinct and at the hospital of St. Giles. Similarly, excavations in the Greyfriars precinct have found at least eleven wells, about half of which were thought likely to date from before the Dissolution on the basis of their exclusively flint construction. One well in particular appears to have acted as a main water source, with lead pipes leading away from it to serve other buildings. The cathedral priory wells were also connected to pipes leading into the monastic domestic premises.[43]

There was no scheme to supply piped water for domestic use in Norwich until 1584, and no opportunity for the citizens to benefit from arrangements made by the religious houses, as occurred, for instance, at Bishop's Lynn in 1382.[44] Instead, many of the secular inhabitants of Norwich relied on private wells. Often described as draw wells (*fontes hauribiles*), these appear frequently enough in the title deeds to show that they were a regular feature of Norwich life, and a number of fifteenth-century and earlier wells (both lined and unlined) have been found in excavations.[45] It may be significant that a brief documentary search has uncovered none for the area south-east of St. Stephen's Street and along the Ber Street ridge. A well between the market place and the castle uncovered in 1888 was 50 ft. deep and lined with great stones at the bottom.[46] And this site was 20 ft., if not 30 ft., lower than the higher ground to the south and the south-east. The investment required in sinking so deep a well was considerable, and many of those living on the ridge may have contented themselves with a lined pit to collect rainwater instead. Neither the wells nor the pits should be denigrated as a source of water. Well water coming up through the chalk underlying Norwich would have been as pure as any, while low population and a lack of industry on the higher ground should have reduced the possible pollution of the rainwater pits.[47] For the poor with no private access to water, there was also a small group of perhaps seven common wells, one of which

---

[43] Gilchrist, *Norwich Cathedral Close*, 37; the stone culvert mentioned by Gilchrist appears to have been used for waste water and sewage disposal. Carole Rawcliffe, *Medicine for the Soul. The Life, Death and Resurrection of an English Medieval Hospital, St. Giles's, Norwich, c.1249–1550* (Stroud, 1999), 46; however, Rawcliffe suggests that the bakery, brewhouse and kitchen were later supplied from the river (*ibid.*, 56). Emery, *Norwich Greyfriars*, 75.

[44] For the 1584 Norwich scheme see *Records of Norwich*, ed. Hudson and Tingey, ii. pp. cxxviii, 392–4. In return for permission given to the Austin Friars to bring water pipes through Lynn, the townsmen there were allowed access to a conduit in Listergate from 6 a.m. to 7 p.m. between Easter and Michaelmas: *The Making of King's Lynn. A Documentary Survey*, ed. D.M. Owen (Records of Social and Economic History, new series, ix, 1984), 117–19. The delayed introduction of a public water supply at Norwich is likely to have been at least partly due to the considerable differences in level. The late 16th-century scheme involved pumping water up to the top of the tower of St. Lawrence's church before it could be conveyed to the market place.

[45] For example, for documentary references see Norfolk RO, MC 146/11, 624X2, cards for Norwich court roll 14 (NCR 1/14). For archaeological references see Malcolm Atkin, Alan Carter and D.H. Evans, *Excavations in Norwich 1971–78. Part II* (East Anglian Archaeology, xxvi, 1985), 95, 157; Atkin and Evans, *Excavations in Norwich 1971–78. Part III* (East Anglian Archaeology, c, 2002), 16, 83–4, 109, 126–7.

[46] Kirkpatrick, *Streets and Lanes*, 28, n. 9.

[47] As long as the slaughter houses were avoided. Most industry, and particularly polluting industry, was concentrated in the valley of the Wensum.

may have been the deep well mentioned above.[48] Drowning in wells, incidentally, seems to have been rare. The greater danger was of the earth falling in during their construction or of inhaling foul air.[49]

Only one of the known common wells (All Saints or All Hallows) lay north of the river, the rest being concentrated in central Norwich and the valley of the Great Cockey (Fig. 3). Furthermore, it is apparent that by the later fifteenth century, at least, not all the common wells were operative. An initial assembly order made in 1474, to repair two common wells in preparation for a royal visit, was followed soon after by a general requirement to open up and clean out all the wells that had become obstructed, the charge to fall on the parish.[50] Fortunately there were other supplies of drinkable water available to the poor in Norwich, namely the ponds or pits that marked the source of several of the major streams. That at the start of the Great Cockey was known by 1495–6 as Jakkes pit, possibly because there were pike in it.[51] This must have been a sizeable pond, as three women drowned there in the late thirteenth century. One drowned herself, but another was fetching water when the rope broke and she was pulled in by the weight of the jar.[52] There was also a pond called Lothmere at the source of the more westerly southern cockey, and together they must have provided an invaluable resource for the drier upper slopes of the city. Similar pits, one of which (Dalmund) involved another early drowning,[53] were connected with the three main cockeys north of the river.

The system of water courses and cockeys was not intended to deal with either industrial waste or human sewage. In 1390–1 Isabella Lucas stood charged with maintaining a noxious gutter and a barber was accused of throwing putrid blood into the street.[54] Information on sewage disposal systems in the city comes from both documentary and archaeological sources. From an early date, several of the Norwich religious houses are known to have operated sophisticated culverted

---

[48] Five of these are recorded before the Black Death: Tillyard, 'Acquisition', 8; Kirkpatrick, *Streets and Lanes*, 28; Norfolk RO, MC 146/52, plans 8 (All Saints), 68 (Thomas Bruman). The other two (in the parishes of St. Stephen and St. Michael at Plea) are first mentioned in 1474: Norfolk RO, NCR 16D/1, f. 97.

[49] Coroners' rolls, 1263–85 and 1669–90: Norfolk RO, NCR 6A/1; 8A/1, 2. For details see Rawcliffe, 'Health and Safety at Work', 144.

[50] Norfolk RO, NCR 16D/1, ff. 97–8. Only five of the seven wells appear in 16th-century surveys of Norwich: *Norwich Landgable Assessment 1568–70*, ed. Mary Rodgers and May Wallace (Norfolk Record Society, lxiii, 1999), 54, 84, 90, 111, 140.

[51] Kirkpatrick, *Streets and Lanes*, 17. The term 'Jack' was used for a young or small pike by 1587. The pond was apparently still in existence when Kirkpatrick was writing around 1700, and there is no evidence that the name derives from 'jakes', a term used for a privy from c.1530: *The Shorter Oxford English Dictionary*, ed. C.T. Onions (3rd edn. revised, Oxford, 1973).

[52] Described as the pit in the Old Swine Market: Norfolk RO, NCR 8A/2.

[53] *Ibid.*

[54] *Leet Jurisdiction in the City of Norwich during the Thirteenth and Fourteenth Centuries*, ed. William Hudson (Selden Society, v, 1892), 70, 72. Isabella was not the only person indicted for this offence in 1390–1: Norfolk RO, NCR 5B, leet roll. Both 1390 and 1391 were plague years in Norfolk: J.M.W. Bean, 'Plague, Population and Economic Decline in England in the Later Middle Ages', *EcHR*, new series, xv (1963), 428–9. While the civic authorities would undoubtedly have been influenced by the recurrent episodes of plague, and by the prevailing belief in foul air as a cause of disease (see below, n. 65), it is not clear that this led them to noticeably greater efforts in keeping the streets clean than are evident before the Black Death. Unfortunately, only two Norwich leet rolls survive between 1313 and 1542 (for 1375–6 and 1390–1), making it impossible to examine trends.

underground drainage systems for waste water, which included flushing out the garderobes.[55] Corporate and private provision was less elaborate. Private garderobes were known in Norwich before the Black Death, and a boy drowned in an uncovered cesspit in 1278–9.[56] Late fourteenth- and fifteenth-century deeds include occasional references to latrines – access to a latrine under the wall on the east end of a cottage; a room with a solar, two fireplaces and a latrine; a chimney and a latrine just built.[57] The city also maintained latrines on its corporate properties, but there is no clear evidence for the public latrines that were available in some other towns,[58] and the very poor may have had to make do as best they could. The records say nothing about how the tanners acquired the urine that they needed, and no doubt the lanes, and particularly the cul-de-sacs, were used for casual purposes. Archaeological evidence takes the form of cesspits, which were ubiquitous. In fifteenth-century Norwich these were generally positioned on the back wall of the house, often connected with chutes from an upper chamber, and sometimes with a soakaway.[59] Their proper cleaning seems to have become a recognised occupation. In 1411–12, for example, the city paid Master John, the cleaner of the latrines ('fower' *latrinarum*), 4s. 4d. for his work on one latrine at a property in the Fishmarket.[60] Paradoxically, the elaborate arrangements made by the religious houses were probably more polluting than the private cesspits, as their sewers ran into the river, while a properly maintained and regularly emptied cesspit will produce very little pollution.

An important element in the experience of life in Norwich in the fifteenth century would have been the condition of the streets. It is clear that, as in other major urban centres, the city authorities were in favour of the streets being paved, and that responsibility for their upkeep was placed on the neighbouring householders. However, a general order in 1467 for cleaning the streets included the requirement that every occupier level the street in front of his property 'with sand or stone pavement', as if both types of road were equally present in the city.[61] Quite what was meant by 'pavement' is another question, but it seems to have

---

[55] The Norwich cathedral priory system was in place by the 12th century, although, since the priory domestic buildings sat slightly above the flood plain, it seems unlikely that their drains were flushed out by water brought underground from the river, as Gilchrist suggests: Gilchrist, *Norwich Cathedral Close*, 37–8. It is possible, however, that the monks may have diverted water flowing down the gutter in the middle of Tombland for this purpose. For arrangements at St. Giles' hospital and the Greyfriars precinct, see Rawcliffe, *Medicine for the Soul*, 46, and Emery, *Norwich Greyfriars*, 75–9, 83.

[56] For instance, the ownership of a garderobe was conveyed by deed in 1319: Norfolk RO, NCR 1/9, rot. 4; NCR 8A/2. Archaeology has uncovered a garderobe turret in a 12th-century Norwich building: Ayers, 'Infrastructure of Norwich', 36.

[57] Examples from 1381–2 to 1402: Norfolk RO, MC 146/11, 624X2, cards for Norwich court roll 14 (NCR 1/14), rots. 12d, 22, 26d; NCR 1/16, rot. 21 (Thomas Dorham *et al.*).

[58] For example, repairs to a latrine at the guildhall, Norfolk RO, NCR 7C, treasurers' rolls 1411–12 (2). Common privies at Norwich are first mentioned in the 1650s: Pelling, 'Health and Sanitation', 137. For the availability of public latrines in other English towns and cities, see Rawcliffe, *Urban Bodies*, ch. 3.

[59] Atkin, Carter and Evans, *Excavations in Norwich. Part II*, 4, 12–13, 15, 21, 253–5; Atkin and Evans, *Excavations in Norwich. Part III*, 12, 16, 31–2, 47, 127, 163, 187, 242.

[60] Norfolk RO, NCR, 7C, treasurers' rolls 1411–12 (2).

[61] General orders for paving the streets had been passed in 1428–9: *Records of Norwich*, ed. Hudson and Tingey, ii. pp. cxxix, 96–7.

referred to a metalled surface of gravel, rammed chalk, or flint.[62] Even if the surface was good, there were other traps for the unwary. Presentments for leaving heaps of muck and dung in the streets were standard fare for the Norwich leet courts from the survival of the earliest records in the late thirteenth century, and lists of householders charged with doing so in 1375–6 make depressing reading.[63] As always, it is impossible to say whether the situation was particularly bad at the time, or whether this indicates a special campaign on the part of the civic authorities to stamp out the practice in the aftermath of a major epidemic.[64] Even here, however, it is clear that some muck was considered worse than less offensive waste – detritus from latrines, for instance, or horse manure.[65] Nonetheless, one can understand the temptation for the householder. By the fifteenth century it had become normal for domestic rubbish in Norwich not to be buried on site, which meant that residents almost certainly had to pay for it to be taken away.[66] It is also apparent that many of them did try to get rid of their waste by more acceptable methods, even if they ended up employing cowboys like John de Gyssyng, who took their money and piled all the muck on an island in the river.[67] And there were further hazards to avoid, such as the cattle and other animals being driven to the regular markets in the centre of the city.[68] The civic authorities were aware of this problem, and, after Norwich was granted two new fairs by the king in 1482, sought to minimise the potential disruption by controlling where within the walls the additional livestock should 'lie and walk'.[69] Other creatures to avoid were the domestic pigs, wandering the streets in contravention of assembly orders, and, surprisingly enough, ducks.[70] Then there were carts parked illegally, stones placed in the street, 'traves' (or posts) positioned in front of the gates of the wealthy (in return for an annual payment to the city), and even, in one case, a saw pit.[71] On the other hand, the topography of the city may have helped in cleaning the streets. John Kirkpatrick remarks on the foresight of those who laid out the market place on the steep western slope of the Great Cockey valley. While cleanliness would hardly have been the priority in the late eleventh century, the gradient undoubtedly, as Kirkpatrick says, helped to keep the area clean in rainy weather.[72] For twelve nights

---

[62] For examples of Norwich street surfaces see Ayers, 'Infrastructure of Norwich', 37–8.

[63] Norfolk RO, NCR 5B, leet roll 1375–6.

[64] There had been national outbreaks of plague in 1369 and in 1375: Bean, 'Economic Decline', 429. But see above, n. 54.

[65] The concern would have been to make the streets not only cleaner but also healthier. It was commonly accepted that diseases were spread by corrupt air: Carole Rawcliffe, *Medicine and Society in Later Medieval England* (Stroud, 1995), 42.

[66] Atkin, Carter and Evans, *Excavations in Norwich. Part II*, 255; Atkin and Evans, *Excavations in Norwich, Part III*, 12, 31, 50, 184.

[67] Norfolk RO, NCR 5B, leet roll 1375–6, m. 2.

[68] This situation did not change until 1960 when a new cattle market was established in the suburbs.

[69] *Records of Norwich*, ed. Hudson and Tingey, ii. 103.

[70] *Ibid.*, ii. 88. There had been a number of earlier orders to the same effect: Rawcliffe, 'Sickness and Health', 308. At least pigs were seen as a problem and not part of the system. In 19th-century Cincinnati the refuse was put in the middle of the street for the pigs to deal with: Fanny Trollope, *Domestic Manners of the Americans*, ed. Pamela Neville-Singleton (1997), 34–5.

[71] *Leet Jurisdiction*, ed. Hudson, 66, 68, 76; Norfolk RO, NCR 17B, Domesday Book, f. 40.

[72] Kirkpatrick, *Streets and Lanes*, 24.

at Christmas time there was even street lighting, when every householder was required to place a lantern or tallow candle outside his door or window.[73]

All the efforts of the civic community to keep the streets clean, however, must have been frustrated by yet another aspect of fifteenth-century Norwich – namely that so much of it was a building site. As part of their campaign to kick-start the local economy, the city authorities began a sustained programme of civic building in the late fourteenth century. Projects included the Cow Tower, part of the defences on the corner of the river near the hospital of St. Giles, in 1398–9; new water mills on the Wensum near the western boundary of the city, from 1401 to 1430; the sumptuous guildhall on the site of the old tollhouse in the market place, in 1407–12; a new market cross in 1411; and a freestone quay for one of the common staithes in King Street in 1432.[74]

Nor were the major religious institutions totally immune from this process. At the cathedral the fifteenth century saw both the completion of the cloister, and the construction of the magnificent stone vault over the nave and of the present 315 ft. spire on the top of the tower. The Erpingham gate into the cathedral priory precinct, one of the most splendid of cathedral gateways, was built between 1416 and 1425, and the gate to the bishop's palace shortly before 1436. At the hospital of St. Giles the chancel of the church had been erected in about 1380, but the rest of the church was refashioned 100 years later, and the cloister in about 1450. Further work took place at the Blackfriars' southern site, where the immense church (265 ft. long) and cloister were completely rebuilt during the period 1440–70, after a fire in 1413.[75] And then there were the churches. Medieval parishioners as a whole must have been more or less resigned to worshipping for much of the time in the middle of a building site, but in a multi-parish city like Norwich the effects would have been multiplied and the noise, dirt and disruption spread far into the surrounding streets. Because much church rebuilding is undocumented, and its dating depends entirely on the adoption of the perpendicular style, we have to consider the evidence from the point of view of the long fifteenth century, lasting from the late fourteenth century to the early sixteenth century. Fig. 4 shows the Norwich churches that underwent major reconstruction during this period – at the very least investing in a new aisle or a rebuilt tower and often much more. Bishop Goldwell visited forty-three Norwich parishes in 1492 and the churches of twenty-nine of them appear on this plan.[76] The time taken to complete these alterations varied from church to church. Barely had the market place recovered from the disruption caused by the construction of the new guildhall and the market cross when work started on the complete rebuilding of the great market church of St. Peter Mancroft. This was a fairly short campaign, beginning in 1430, with the

---

[73] *Records of Norwich*, ed. Hudson and Tingey, ii. 90–1.

[74] Ayers, *Norwich*: '*A Fine City*', 111–13.

[75] Pevsner and Wilson, *Norfolk I*, 192, 198, 226, 265–6, 269, 276, 278.

[76] N.P. Tanner, *The Church in Late Medieval Norwich, 1370–1532* (Toronto, 1984), 179–88. It has been suggested that only eight churches missed out altogether on this building boom. However, fig. 4 does not include those churches where the rebuilding was limited to new windows or porches, disruptive as the work must have been. See C.P. Graves, *The Form and Fabric of Belief. An Archaeology of the Lay Experience of Religion in Medieval Norfolk and Devon* (British Archaeological Reports, British Series, cccxi, 2000), 60; and Jonathan Finch, 'The Churches', in *Medieval Norwich*, ed. Rawcliffe and Wilson, 62, 354, n. 58.

new church being consecrated in 1455. In contrast, the rebuilding of the church of St. Lawrence, 'perpendicular and all of a piece', as Pevsner says, was begun in about 1449, but they were still finishing off the tower six decades later. Not all building campaigns were continuous. At St. Michael Coslany the tower was rebuilt in the 1420s, but most of the sumptuous flint flush-work for which it is best known actually dates from the early sixteenth century.[77]

Finally, there was private development. The few standing medieval houses that we have in Norwich are exceptional survivals and a far better idea of the extent of domestic rebuilding can be gained from the number of fifteenth-century under-crofts (Fig. 5). Over sixty under-crofts still exist in Norwich, almost all of them dating from the fifteenth century, and the sites of over thirty others are known.[78] Not surprisingly, they were clustered on the heavily-developed north-facing slope down from the market place, and were often cut back into the hill to provide a platform for the building above. As a result, anyone living in this area would have had to contend not only with the major remodelling of many of the churches, but also with the excavation and building work connected with the new under-crofts and the houses above them.

One area might seem to have escaped the worst of the building frenzy – namely King Street in the south-eastern corner of the city. But this was to be affected by a related environmental hazard. All the rebuilding work led to a considerable demand for flint, lime and mortar. There is no indication in the late thirteenth and early fourteenth centuries that quarrying for chalk and flint was actually taking place within Norwich, but by the beginning of the fifteenth century the situation had changed, with the exploitation of the steep slope up to the Ber Street ridge above King Street by a series of chalk and lime workings. The earliest known lay a short way up from the wall and is recorded from 1400, when the city acquired an interest in it.[79] Two further kilns on the slope behind King Street are mentioned in an account of 1488–9.[80] Lime-working was definitely an anti-social activity, and in 1561 there was a complaint about the lime causing damage to clothes being washed at two staithes in the area.[81]

So what conclusions can be drawn about the environment of fifteenth-century Norwich? In 1400 the civic authorities inherited an infrastructure little changed, and almost certainly run-down, since the Black Death. Also apparently little changed since the late thirteenth century despite the onset of plague, either qualitatively or in quantity, was the nature of the urban government's response to problems of cleanliness and sanitation.[82] On the other hand, both the city and

---

[77] Pevsner and Wilson, *Norfolk I*, 230–53.
[78] Ayers, *Norwich: 'A Fine City'*, 113–18, 122.
[79] Norfolk RO, NCR 17A, Liber Albus, f. 13.
[80] Norfolk RO, NCR 18A/2, f. 128–8v.
[81] *Records of Norwich*, ed. Hudson and Tingey, ii. 135.
[82] But see below, pp. 113–14. An exception is the establishment of the cisterns at the mouths of the cockeys. Municipal muck carts to clear the streets were not introduced until the beginning of the 16th century: *ibid.*, ii. 109–10. An assembly order of 1496 mentioned by Jørgensen, which named two men in each aldermanry in connection with street cleaning, appears to have been setting up a sub-committee rather than appointing new employees. The two men chosen for the aldermanry of Conesford, Thomas Large and William Heyward, were both councillors and were to become aldermen in due course. Large was also currently acting as one of the chamberlains, the city's main financial officers. Jørgensen, 'Cooperative Sanitation', 564; *Records of Norwich*, ed. Hudson and

private individuals made a considerable investment in building during the period and in some areas changed the cityscape completely, while a smaller population and a less polluting industrial base probably made fifteenth-century Norwich a generally cleaner city to live in than it had been in the early fourteenth century. The real failure related to the river, which became a matter of increasing concern. It was not to be until the middle of the sixteenth century that the newly-confident post-Dissolution city took the bull by the horns, established the river and streets committee and made the maintenance of the Wensum a wholly civic responsibility.[83]

How its inhabitants considered Norwich is yet another matter, for the quality of the urban environment that you experienced depended to a large extent on who you were. The hilly landscape, the streams, the stench and pollution of the river and the streets disrupted by building works would have been common to all.[84] But the reality of life for an inhabitant of fifteenth-century Norwich was crucially determined by access – access to a clean water supply, access to a private latrine, access, even, to the river – and above all on access to the gardens, orchards and open spaces for which Norwich was renowned by the seventeenth century.

Tingey, i. 288; Timothy Hawes, *An Index to Norwich City Officers 1453–1835* (Norfolk Record Society, lii, 1986), 82, 94.

[83] Jørgensen, "'All Good Rule of the Citee'", 309–10; *Norwich's River and Street Accounts*, ed. Fay.

[84] Dirty streets are mentioned in the 15th-century doggerel verse quoted in n. 15, above, although this reference may be to a specific lane notorious for prostitution, rather than to the Norwich streets in general: see Rutledge, 'Norwich before the Black Death: Economic Life', 182.

Elizabeth Rutledge

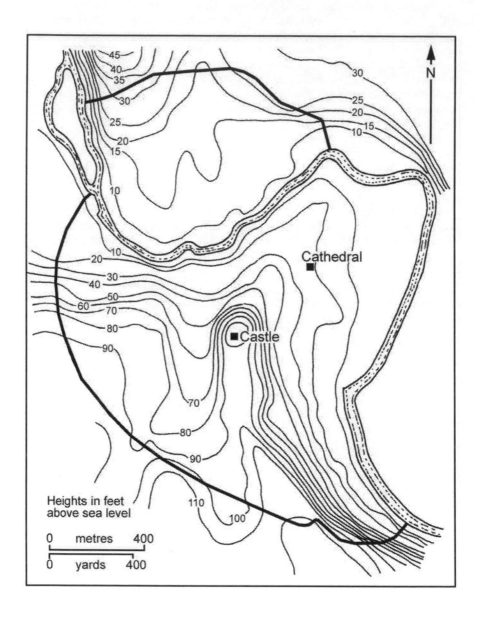

Fig. 1: Norwich contours in 1884 (Phillip Judge, after Dan Jones).

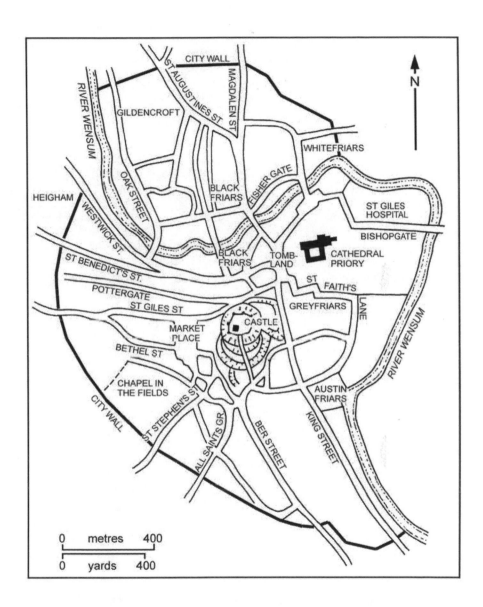

Fig. 2: Medieval Norwich (Phillip Judge).

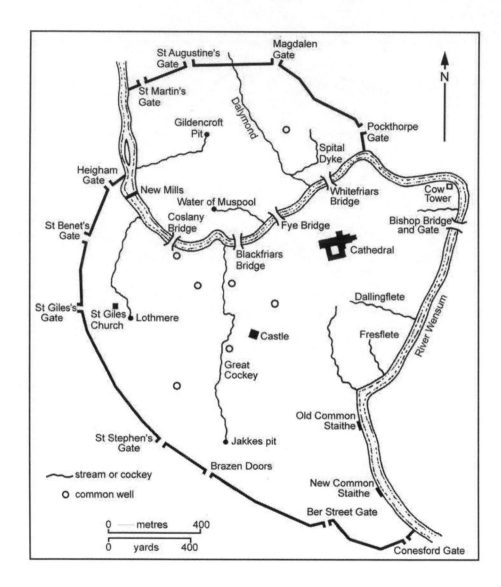

Fig. 3: Ponds and streams of medieval Norwich (Phillip Judge).

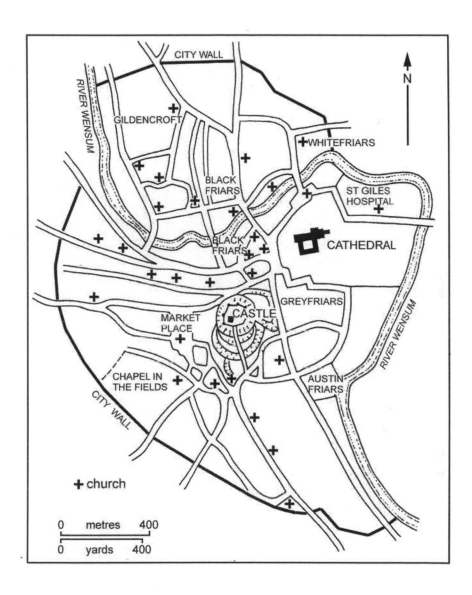

Fig. 4: Norwich churches remodelled in the long fifteenth century (Phillip Judge).

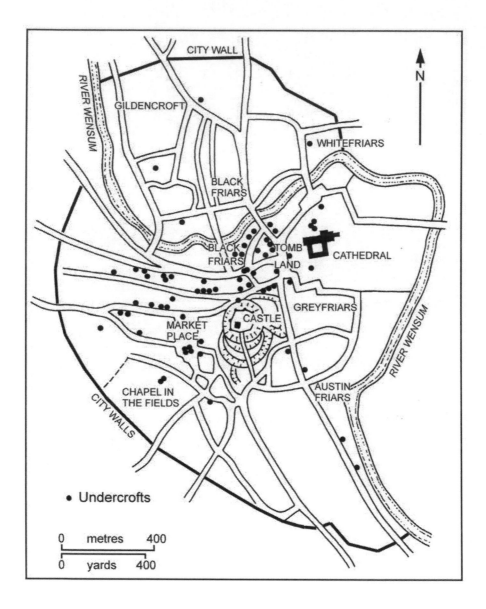

Fig. 5: Norwich undercrofts (Phillip Judge, after Ayers, *Norwich*: '*A Fine City*', 124).

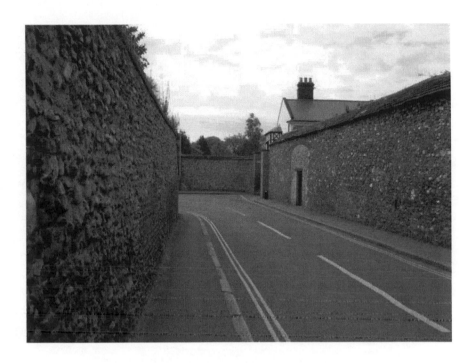

Plate 1: Bishopsgate, Norwich, showing the walls of the bishop's palace, left, and of the Great Hospital (formerly the hospital of St. Giles), right. Photograph: Carole Rawcliffe.

MID-LEVEL OFFICIALS IN FIFTEENTH-CENTURY NORWICH

Samantha Sagui

John Clement, a brewer, entered the Norwich franchise in 1447. Over the next decade he was a constable nine times and a tax collector once, but he never discharged any other civic office.[1] In spite of their important role in administering and maintaining order in English cities, men like Clement have been neglected as a result of English urban historians' tendency to focus on the better-documented and wealthier mercantile elite. Prosopographical analyses of urban political, economic, and social groups have directed some attention towards middling artisans and retailers because of their focus on collective biography, but the relative dearth of information about these groups has made even this approach more effective for understanding the senior officials.[2] Moreover, although these studies have revealed much about civic hierarchies, they have perhaps encouraged the perception that a mercantile elite dominated all aspects of urban political life. Although no one would deny the virtual monopoly of high office by a privileged few, there is

[1] Norfolk RO, NCR 16D/1, ff. 21v, 24v, 27, 31, 38v, 43.

[2] Lawrence Stone, *The Past and Present Revisited* (New York, 1989), 57–8. Prosopographical studies of medieval English towns include: Sylvia Thrupp, *The Merchant Class of Medieval London* (Ann Arbor, Mich., 1989), 65, 80–5; D.G. Shaw, *The Creation of a Community: The City of Wells in the Middle Ages* (Oxford, 1993), 166–7; Maryanne Kowaleski, *Local Markets and Regional Trade in Medieval Exeter* (Cambridge, 1995), 101–19; R.H. Frost, 'The Aldermen of Norwich, 1461–1509: A Study of a Civic Elite' (Cambridge Univ. Ph.D. thesis, 1996), 40–1; *eadem*, 'The Urban Elite', in *Medieval Norwich*, ed. Carole Rawcliffe and Richard Wilson (2004), 243; Jenny Kermode, *Medieval Merchants: York, Beverley and Hull in the Later Middle Ages* (Cambridge, 1998), 26–68; Charlotte Carpenter, 'The Formation of Urban Élites: Civic Officials in Late-Medieval York 1476–1515' (Univ. of York Ph.D. thesis, 2000), 58–67, 109; Lorraine Attreed, *The King's Towns: Identity and Survival in Late Medieval English Boroughs* (New York, 2001), 5–6; Caroline Barron, *London in the Later Middle Ages: Government and People, 1200–1500* (Oxford, 2004), 356–74; Christian Liddy, *Politics and Finance in Late Medieval English Towns: Bristol, York and the Crown, 1350–1400* (Woodbridge, 2005), 101–10, 217–19; Nicholas Amor, *Late Medieval Ipswich: Trade and Industry* (Woodbridge, 2011), 17–18, 236–68. Those that analyze mid- and lower-level urban political groups include: Kowaleski, *Local Markets*, 101–19; Carpenter, 'Formation of Urban Élites', 58–67, 109; Shaw, *Creation of a Community*, 166–7; Kermode, *Medieval Merchants*, 39–40. For comparable studies of continental cities see, for example, Hilde de Ridder-Symoens, 'Prosopographical Research in the Low Countries Concerning the Middle Ages and the Sixteenth Century', *Medieval Prosopography*, xiv (1993), 38–41; F.J.W. van Kan, 'Elite and Government in Medieval Leiden', *Journal of Medieval History*, xxi (1995), 51–75; David Nicholas, 'The Governance of Fourteenth-Century Ghent: The Theory and Practice of Public Administration', in *Law, Custom and the Social Fabric in Medieval Europe*, ed. Bernard Bachrach and David Nicholas (Kalamazoo, Mich., 1990), 235–60.

considerable evidence that mercantile control was not so comprehensive in the lower levels of civic government.[3]

Non-elite urban officials have received little sustained analysis.[4] Indeed, on the few occasions that mid-level offices have been examined they have generally been cast as part of the *cursus honorum* or as unwelcome chores rather than as potentially valuable positions.[5] By focusing on a group of non-elite personnel, namely, constables, assessors, collectors, supervisors and searchers in Norwich between 1414 and 1473, this paper demonstrates the essential role played by such individuals and postulates that not all urban office-holders nursed greater ambitions.[6] In doing so it suggests that historians need further to examine the likelihood that mid-level offices were desirable in their own right rather than simply being regarded as stepping stones to higher things, and provides a useful corrective to the prevailing tendency to emphasize the increasingly powerful reach of urban oligarchies.[7]

Norwich was among England's largest cities: in 1334, it ranked as the fifth wealthiest and, according to the 1377 poll tax, it was by then also the fifth largest city in the country. By 1525 Norwich occupied an even stronger position as the second largest and wealthiest city in England. This development suggests that it was becoming comparatively richer and more populous during the later Middle Ages.[8] Although many towns show evidence of decline in the fifteenth century, Norwich experienced a period of sustained prosperity fostered by an influx of immigrants and a rise in the manufacture of worsted cloth.[9] Yet, in spite of its

---

[3] Carpenter, 'Formation of Urban Élites', 58–67, 109; Shaw, *Creation of a Community*, 166–7; Kermode, *Medieval Merchants*, 39–40.

[4] Carpenter ('Formation of Urban Élites', 52–3) includes bridge wardens, who were mid-level York officials, in her study. Yet, although she notes that such appointments may have been attractive in their own right, and were more than just a launching pad to higher things, she treats mid-level offices as part of the *cursus honorum* and thus does not fully investigate the individuals who never achieved higher political status. Also see: Maryanne Kowaleski, 'The Commercial Dominance of a Medieval Provincial Oligarchy: Exeter in the Late Fourteenth Century', in *The English Medieval Town: A Reader in English Urban History, 1200–1540*, ed. Richard Holt and Gervase Rosser (New York, 1990), 184.

[5] See, for example, Carpenter, 'Formation of Urban Élites', 52–3; Frost, 'Aldermen', 15–17; Charles Phythian-Adams, *Desolation of a City: Coventry and the Urban Crisis of the Late Middle Ages* (Cambridge, 1979), 125; Barbara Hanawalt, '"Good Governance" in the Medieval and Early Modern Context', *Journal of British Studies*, xxxvii (1998), 255; Stephen Rigby and Elizabeth Ewan, 'Government, Power, and Authority, 1300–1540', in *The Cambridge Urban History, Vol. 1, c.600–c.1540*, ed. D.M. Palliser (Cambridge, 2000), 312.

[6] This study begins with the first surviving 15th-century Norwich assembly records and ends in 1473, which allows a 20-year study of constables whose names are only consistently recorded after 1453. These particular offices have been chosen because they are the only mid-level positions for which it is possible to identify a significant number of occupants, at least 50 in the extant documents.

[7] See, for example, Steven Rigby, 'Urban "Oligarchy" in Late Medieval England', in *Towns and Townspeople in the Fifteenth Century*, ed. J.A.F. Thomson (Gloucester, 1988), 76; Phythian-Adams, *Desolation of a City*, 272; Kowaleski, *Local Markets*, 108; Kermode, *Medieval Merchants*, 30; Frost, 'Urban Elite', 243.

[8] Alan Dyer, 'Ranking Lists of English Medieval Towns', in *The Cambridge Urban History, Vol. 1*, ed. Palliser, 752–65; James Campbell, 'Norwich before 1300', in *Medieval Norwich*, ed. Rawcliffe and Wilson, 29; John Pound, *Tudor and Stuart Norwich* (Chichester, 1998), 55.

[9] Penelope Dunn, 'Trade', in *Medieval Norwich*, ed. Rawcliffe and Wilson, 212–16; Elizabeth Rutledge, 'Economic Life', in *ibid.*, 160, 188; John Pound, 'The Social and Trade Structure of Norwich, 1525–1575', *Past and Present*, xxxiv (1966), 60.

relative wealth, Norwich went through a period of turbulence at the beginning of the fifteenth century, caused, in part, by the acquisition of a new royal charter that transformed the city into a county and granted its citizens the right to elect a mayor.[10] Although the new charter augmented the status and privileges of the city, it required an overhaul of the upper echelons of civic government, as a mayor and two sheriffs replaced the four bailiffs who had previously headed the official hierarchy. According to Ben McRee, the conflicts that erupted in the following years stemmed from a competition for authority between the top two tiers of the ruling elite.[11] Even though this conflict was sufficiently alarming for the king to assume control of the city on two separate occasions, both McRee and Phillipa Maddern have argued that Norwich does not deserve its reputation for being a particularly disorderly city. Instead, conflict may have been confined to the emerging aldermanic elite and members of the common council who sought to consolidate their position.[12]

Notwithstanding the turmoil that surrounded the adoption of its new constitution, Norwich retained aspects of its older administrative structure. Civic governance continued to revolve around a system of four great leets – later called wards in deference to London – which were responsible for presenting breaches of customary law to the local courts (see Map 1). As the city developed, these wards also became the locus for the election of aldermen, who formed a council of twenty-four that effectively ruled the city. These powerful individuals and the mayor constituted the highest level of the ruling elite, here called Rank A.[13] Below them was a common council of sixty men, also chosen by ward, who participated in elections of officials and approved new legislation; they comprise Rank B.[14] The wards were subdivided into three separate aldermanries (or small wards), each of which had its own constables and taxation officials by the mid fifteenth century. These mid-level office-holders, along with men appointed as supervisors or

---

[10] Although Norwich made a remarkable economic recovery, its population may have declined by as much as 68% between the 1330s and the 1370s. It is possible that this heavy death toll created administrative problems as office-holders died and it became increasingly difficult to find suitable replacements. See Carole Rawcliffe, 'Sickness and Health', in *Medieval Norwich*, ed. Rawcliffe and Wilson, 317–18; Richard Britnell, 'The Black Death in English Towns', *Urban History*, xxi (1994), 205, 208.

[11] Ben McRee, 'Peacemaking and its Limits in Late Medieval Norwich', *EHR*, cix (1994), 831–66; Brian Ayers, *Norwich: Archaeology of a Fine City* (Stroud, 2009), 116. In this respect Norwich was by no means unique; many other historians have speculated that tensions within the civic elite must have played a significant role in exacerbating urban disorder. See, for example, R.B. Dobson, 'The Risings in York, Beverley and Scarborough, 1380–1', in *The English Rising of 1381*, ed. R.H. Hilton and T.H. Aston (Cambridge, 1984), 139–42; Christian Liddy, 'Urban Conflict in Late Fourteenth-Century England: The Case of York in 1380–1', *EHR*, cxviii (2003), 1–16; Kermode, *Medieval Merchants*, 56; Pamela Nightingale, 'Capitalists, Crafts and Constitutional Change in Late Fourteenth-Century London', *Past and Present*, cxxiv (1989), 33.

[12] McRee, 'Peacemaking', 831–66; P.C. Maddern, *Violence and Social Order: East Anglia 1422–1442* (Oxford, 1992), 173–92. It is possible that the arbitrators charged with effecting a compromise shared this assumption, and attempted to ameliorate the situation in 1415 by allowing the aldermen and councillors to share responsibility for appointing constables. See Rigby, 'Urban "Oligarchy"', 68; Kowaleski, *Local Markets*, 103.

[13] This ranking system is adapted from Kowaleski, *Local Markets*, 103.

[14] For a full discussion of the Norwich jurisdictions see *The Records of the City of Norwich*, ed. William Hudson and J.C. Tingey (2 vols., Norwich, 1906–10), i. pp. cii–iv.

searchers, have been assigned to Rank C.[15] Although in some cases members of these groups differed from others only in terms of securety of tenure, as a general rule more significant factors separated them.[16] In addition to being wealthier than their compatriots, the aldermen of Norwich exercised far greater control over elections and the passage and enforcement of legislation.[17] Moreover, aldermen were elected for life, whereas councillors and lesser officials often retained their positions for only a few years. Thus, while an aldermen's place in the urban hierarchy was secure, a councillor's could prove short-lived, and therefore these two groups should be regarded as correspondingly unequal in status.[18]

An additional measure of political participation may be found in membership of the freedom of the city, which provided access to civic power.[19] The 'Old Free Book' of Norwich, which contains a register of admissions, is, however, notoriously incomplete and has proved of limited value in this study.[20] Candidates for office in Norwich had to join the freedom before becoming aldermen, yet 27 per cent of the aldermen considered here are not even mentioned in the 'Old Free Book'. Similarly, councillors were required to enroll in the city's franchise, yet roughly 45 per cent of them cannot be identified from the surviving records. Indeed, Penelope Dunn maintains that barely half (53 per cent) of the men described as citizens elsewhere can be traced in the freedom registers.[21] Nevertheless, although these lists are incomplete, they help us to determine the occupations of some city officials and to investigate the political connections of Norwich constables.[22]

The surviving archives contain references to 651 named individuals who held the mid-level offices of constable, assessor, collector, supervisor or searcher between 1414 and 1473. Although there were other officials of similar rank in Norwich, they are not consistently noted in these sources; and, because too few of them can be identified for meaningful analysis, they have been excluded from this

---

[15] Norwich's bureaucracy, including aldermen, councillors and upper- and mid-level officials, called upon the services of at least 155 individuals each year. Approximately one in twelve male householders might have participated directly in local government at some point in their lives. See P.C. Maddern, 'Order and Disorder', in *Medieval Norwich*, ed. Rawcliffe and Wilson, 192–30.

[16] Frost, 'Urban Elite', 239.

[17] Frost, 'Aldermen', 87–105; Kowaleski, *Local Markets*, 103; Shaw, *Creation of a Community*, 167; Carpenter, 'Formation of Urban Élites', 72–4.

[18] McRee, 'Peacemaking', 835; Frost, 'Aldermen', 18. For more detail on the role of urban councils see, for example, Carpenter, 'Formation of Urban Élites', 218; Derek Keene, *Survey of Medieval Winchester* (2 vols., Winchester Studies 2, Oxford, 1985), i. 70–9.

[19] Kowaleski, *Local Markets*, 96; Frost, 'Aldermen', 7; Catherine Patterson, 'Town and City Government', in *A Companion to Tudor Britain*, ed. Robert Tittler and Norman Johns (Malden, Mass., 2004), 119.

[20] Frost, 'Urban Elite', 239; R.B. Dobson, 'Admissions to the Freedom of the City of York in the Later Middle Ages', *EcHR*, new series, xxvi (1973), 1–22; J.F. Pound, 'The Validity of Freemen's Lists: Some Norwich Evidence', *ibid.*, xxxiv (1981), 48–59; *Records of Norwich*, ed. Hudson and Tingey, ii. pp. xxx–xxxii.

[21] Penelope Dunn, 'After the Black Death: Society and Economy in Late Fourteenth-Century Norwich' (Univ. of East Anglia Ph.D. thesis, 2003), 77.

[22] Membership in the freedom cannot, however, be regarded as an indicator of prosperity. While some men did not join the freedom because they lacked the means to do so, others elected to pay fines in the leet courts rather than enroll in the city franchise, despite their sometimes considerable wealth. See Dunn 'Trade', 233.

study.[23] The earliest Norwich sources regularly to list such office-holders are the assembly rolls, which survive from 1365 and include two rolls from the period under discussion.[24] In addition to recording the proceedings of the city assembly, including the promulgation of ordinances and admissions to the freedom, the rolls name the aldermen and certain city officials. In total these rolls contain 134 references to the five civic offices analyzed here. The sequence ends in 1426, after which there are no surviving records from the city assembly until 1434, when the first assembly book begins. Although the early part of this book only sporadically lists office-holders, it consistently names the ward constables after 1453.[25] The end date for this study (1473) has been selected in order to provide a twenty-year sample from the better-documented period. In total, the first ninety-five folios of the assembly book provide 591 references to the officials in this study. A third source, the mayor's court book, begins in 1424 and covers a wider range of business, which gave rise to an almost random organisation.[26] Its eighty-six folios (written front and dorse) record recognizances for debt, occasional lists of fines, a few admissions to the freedom, extensive lists of pledges for keeping the peace, and lists of searchers. In total they identify 236 mid-level office-holders. Together, these sources furnish the names of all of the Norwich constables after 1453 and probably of all of the collectors, assessors and supervisors after that date as well. The sample of searchers is somewhat more limited, as is that of other officials prior to 1453.[27]

By far the best-documented mid-level officials in fifteenth-century Norwich are the constables, whose wide-ranging responsibilities were largely concerned with maintaining order. According to the constables' oath, their primary role was keeping the peace within their wards, suppressing insurrections, and arresting any rebels found within the city. They also undertook to detain nightwalkers, miscreants, and players of dice and other games of chance.[28] In addition to organizing the watch in his own ward, each constable swore to 'execute all commandementes and precepts geven by [the mayor]'.[29] The assembly records reveal that, besides their other responsibilities, constables occasionally took charge of collecting taxes and assisted with the supervision of public works.[30]

Norwich had employed constables with peace-keeping functions from at least 1288, but they assumed a much more significant role in governing the city during

---

[23] Other mid-level offices include key-bearers, bellmen, serjeants of the chamber, mayor's serjeants, keepers of the dike and beadles. See, for example, Norfolk RO, NCR 16D/1, ff. 7v, 16v, 39v, 78, 91; Pound, *Tudor and Stuart Norwich*, 109.

[24] Norfolk RO, NCR 8D/1414; 8D/1420–6; selections printed in *Records of Norwich*, ed. Hudson and Tingey, i. 273–80.

[25] Norfolk RO, NCR 16D/1, ff. 1–95; selections printed in *Records of Norwich*, ed. Hudson and Tingey, i. 281–6.

[26] Norfolk RO, NCR 16A/1; selections printed in *Records of Norwich*, ed. Hudson and Tingey, i. 305–6.

[27] These officials have been examined with the aid of a Policing Officials Database, which stores data derived from 2,832 references to Norwich officials culled from records of the city assembly, mayor's court, leet courts and sessions of gaol delivery.

[28] The Norwich constables seem to have played a similar role to that of their London counterparts. Moreover, in both cities these officials were assigned to specific wards. See Barron, *London in the Later Middle Ages*, 125.

[29] *Records of Norwich*, ed. Hudson and Tingey, i. 124–5.

[30] Norfolk RO, NCR 16D/1, f. 54v; 8D/1420–6, m. 2.

the fifteenth century.[31] The 'Composition' of 1415 (a document intended to settle conflicts over the balance of power in Norwich) decreed that there should be sixteen constables, eight elected each year by the aldermen and eight by the common councillors. Although this number had been increased to twenty-four by 1453, so that there might be two constables in each lesser ward, the manner of election remained the same. The 'Composition' also granted constables the right to participate in the common assembly, a privilege they retained at least until 1462.[32] The selection procedure established by the 'Composition' and the constables' right to sit in the assembly were new developments, which suggested to William Hudson that these lower status officials were 'being put forth as a counterpoise to the rising power of the Aldermen'.[33] While it is certainly possible that a multi-tiered ruling elite would have contained political strife by giving substantial artisans a role in decision-making,[34] we should also bear in mind that these changes fostered closer relationships between different governing groups.[35]

An analysis of the constables who took office between 1453 and 1473 demonstrates that men from all political ranks occupied the post; the constabulary was not just an effective springboard for launching one's career as an alderman.[36] Ruth Frost's assertion that 60 per cent of aldermen between 1461 and 1509 had previously served as constables encourages scholars to examine the position through the lens of an ambitious civic elite. Yet, as Table 1 shows, most constables never went on to scale such heights.[37] Although nearly half of the constables belong to Rank B, about 43 per cent were never elected to either of the city's legislative bodies.[38] Indeed, although evidence about the city franchise is limited, the pattern of admission strongly suggests that constables were not always freemen. All of the aldermen who can be identified had joined the freedom prior to becoming a constable, with the possible exception of Edmund Colman, who served during the year that he became a freeman.[39] For most future aldermen there was a two- to six-year gap between joining the freedom and becoming a constable. Some of the other constables, however, entered the city's franchise up to four years *after* holding office.[40] Although roughly 40 per cent of constables who never rose higher up the civic hierarchy can be identified in the 'Old Free Book', it seems likely that a small

---

[31] Norfolk RO, NCR 5B/1, mm. 1, 2.

[32] *Records of Norwich*, ed. Hudson and Tingey, i. p. ciii; Norfolk RO, NCR 16D/1, f. 53v.

[33] *Records of Norwich*, ed. Hudson and Tingey, i. p. cii.

[34] Kowaleski, *Local Markets*, 103; McRee, 'Peacemaking', 853.

[35] Phythian-Adams, *Desolation of a City*, 72.

[36] This analysis of constables is limited to the period after 1453. Although it is possible to identify 39 constables from the preceding period, the inconsistent approach to listing before this date makes it impossible to assess patterns of service or the political status of most constables.

[37] Frost, 'Aldermen', 16.

[38] Although all of the constables, councillors and aldermen can be identified after 1453, it is possible that a few men who had served as common councillors prior to 1453 went on to become constables; even so, it is unlikely that many followed this pattern, considering that only six men in the known sample first became constables after ascending to Rank B.

[39] Norfolk RO, NCR 16D/1, f. 22.

[40] One of the men from Rank C became a freeman four years after his only term in office, while six councillors joined between one and three years after serving as constables. None of these men held the office more than twice.

portion of them remained un-enfranchised throughout their lives, as was the case with many low-level office-holders in Exeter.[41]

Not surprisingly, political status had a significant impact on constables' future careers. All but a single individual in Rank A held additional civic offices, as did just over 60 per cent of the men in Rank B, but only about a quarter of those in Rank C. Because lower-level office-holders are not named in the assembly records, it is possible that those in Rank C served in other capacities or participated in the leet court system, but they did not generally ascend to higher offices or other mid-level positions. When men in Rank C took up other posts they were most likely to become tax collectors or assessors. Some individuals also served as coroner, sergeant-at-mace, custodian of the worstead weavers or keeper of the dike. Men in Rank B likewise resurface most often as collectors and assessors, though several became key bearers, supervisors, sheriffs, coroners, chamberlains and auditors. There were no obstacles to the heights reached by men in Rank A, seven of whom went on to become mayors of Norwich.

Similar considerations determined how often an individual might serve as constable.[42] The majority of Rank A constables held office for two years, and only one person, John Swayn, was a constable more than four times.[43] The term spent in office varied far more within Ranks B and C. Although these men were much more likely to serve for only one year, six individuals remained in post for a remarkable ten or more years.[44] Among them only John Mundeford and William Norfolk became city councillors.[45] One man, Robert Jolsy, a shoemaker who joined the freedom in 1465, was constable eighteen times between 1469 and 1490, before being appointed the dike-keeper of the city in 1494, 1496 and 1498.[46] Richard Wesell and Robert Wrong, who were constables for eleven and twelve years respectively, were also tax collectors, but none of the other men who notched up such long periods of service held other documented civic offices.[47] Neither Robert Everard nor Robert Salle (who were both constables for fifteen years in Holme Street and Spitelond) can be found among the freemen of the city – although it is possible that their names are simply missing from the records, these two men might further demonstrate that service to the city was not contingent upon membership of the freedom.[48]

---

[41] In Exeter, as few as 26% of men in Rank C were members of the freedom: see Kowaleski, *Local Markets*, 103. The percentage in Norwich was undoubtedly higher, but there is no reason to assume, as Maddern ('Order and Disorder', 192) does, that all office-holders were freemen.

[42] See Table 2.

[43] Swayn was one of the few constables in Rank A not to belong to one of the distributive trades. There was also at least a 25-year gap between his admission to the freedom and his election as alderman. These facts suggest that he may not initially have been a strong candidate for Rank A and may have used his time as constable to help his ascent to higher office. Norfolk RO, NCR 16D/1, ff. 52, 56, 63, 64, 66, 69, 74, 78, 82, 95, 130v.

[44] A similar pattern is evident in Exeter, where men who were not in the aldermanry tended to hold office much less often: see Kowaleski, 'Commercial Dominance', 192.

[45] Norfolk RO, NCR 16D/1, ff. 43v, 47, 52, 56, 59, 63, 66, 70, 74, 78, 82, 88.

[46] *Ibid.*, ff. 82, 91, 95v; *An Index to Norwich City Officers: 1453–1835*, ed. Timothy Hawes (Norfolk Record Society, lii, 1989), 90.

[47] Norfolk RO, NCR 16D/1, ff. 31, 35v, 38, 52, 56, 59, 63, 66, 70, 74v, 78, 82, 91, 95v.

[48] It may be that these men were not eligible to join the freedom, since they lived in parts of Norwich that were under monastic jurisdiction. The city began to elect constables for these districts in 1460,

This divergent pattern of office-holding suggests that the motives of men in Rank A may have differed substantially from those in Ranks B and C. For high achievers who were likely to become aldermen, the constabulary offered valuable administrative experience. For others, however, the office provided different benefits. Perhaps those who repeatedly served as constables simply wanted 'to be at the centre of things and to savour the consequent respect and status'.[49] But there were also financial incentives. The participation of constables in elections before 1462 may have allowed them to protect their economic interests.[50] Even after the constables lost their right to attend council meetings, there would still have been many opportunities to cultivate potentially useful relationships with the future rulers of the city. Office-holding also conferred prestige and authority at ward level, albeit at the risk of provoking resentment. Moreover, although being a constable consumed significant time and energy, some financial support was available. From at least 1422, constables were empowered to collect fines of 6*d.* from repeat offenders, half of which was paid into the community chest, while half could be retained by the constable himself.[51] Finally, it is possible that some of these men were driven by a sense of civic responsibility.

The high portion of men who held office only once, particularly in Rank C, might suggest that these incentives were not always sufficient to compensate for the burdens of office, or that individuals might not be selected a second time if they were incompetent or corrupt. Although no one specifically sought a dispensation from discharging the office of constable (in marked contrast to the multiple applications to be excused from becoming sheriff) there are other indications that Norwich may have experienced some difficulty in filling mid-level positions.[52] For example, there were several years during which no constables were elected for Trowse, Holme Street or Spitelond. Although such lacunae might well be explained by the conflict between the civic and ecclesiastical authorities for control of these exempt jurisdictions, there is no analogous reason why the post of bellman should occasionally have been left vacant.[53] Moreover, there are a few instances in which the name of one constable has been crossed out and replaced by another. Except in 1461, when five replacements were made (perhaps because of the fraught political situation), there were never more than two such substitutions in a single year, and there is no indication that any fines for refusal to serve were collected.[54] These cases may have been the result of clerical errors, or they may reveal some problem in finding suitable candidates.[55]

---

but in the following decade only appointed them sporadically. See Norfolk RO, NCR 16D/1, ff. 59, 63, 78, 82, 88, 91, 95v; Maddern, 'Order and Disorder', 199–201.

[49]   Kermode, *Medieval Merchants*, 68.

[50]   See, for example, Frost, 'Aldermen', 108; *eadem*, 'Urban Elite', 243; Kowaleski, 'Commercial Dominance', 185, 193–4.

[51]   Norfolk RO, NCR 8D/1420–6, m. 4.

[52]   See, for example, Norfolk RO, NCR 16D/1, f. 47v.

[53]   See, for example, *ibid.*, ff. 47, 52, 63, 70.

[54]   See, for example, *ibid.*, ff. 27, 52.

[55]   Although this evidence may suggest that some posts were hard to fill, it does not support an argument for flight from office, see: Frost, 'Urban Elite', 253; *eadem*, 'Aldermen', 36; J.I. Kermode, 'Urban Decline? The Flight from Office in Late Medieval York', *EcHR*, new series, xxxv (1982), 180–2; Shaw, *Creation of a Community*, 172; Phythian-Adams, *Desolation of a City*, 249–51.

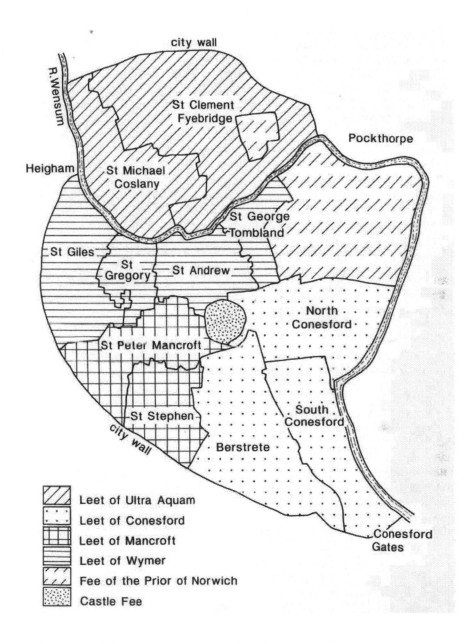

Map 1: The leets of late medieval Norwich (Phillip Judge).

These contrasting patterns of office-holding are in part a reflection of individual goals and aspirations, but an analysis of constables by occupation suggests that other factors distinguished one rank from another and, perhaps, stood in the way of any realistic expectation of achieving aldermanic office. We know the occupations of 53 per cent of the constables in this study, but since many of them have been identified through the freemen's registers, this sample is biased in favour of the wealthier officers. The findings summarized in Table 3 confirm that men from the distributive trades dominated Rank A and that certain occupations (notably inn-keeping and butchery) precluded the exercise of power. This pattern may reflect an attempt among the elite to project an image of wisdom, authority and good order.[56] Some of the individuals from Rank B were also engaged in the distributive trades, but they were slightly more likely than those from either of the other groups to be victuallers of one kind or another, a discrepancy that might be due to the exclusion of butchers from Rank A. The occupational profile of Rank C constables is slightly closer to that of the residents at large; although they were, if anything, disproportionately likely to be employed in cloth production – particularly worstead weaving – they were also heavily involved in making clothing, victualling and distribution.[57] On the whole, a third of Rank B constables and half of Rank C constables were not engaged in any of the eighteen trades that Frost has identified as being appropriate for aldermen.[58] If medieval townsmen recognized and accepted these implied limitations, it is probable that many of the men who served as constables did not expect to ascend further up the civic ladder.[59] Nevertheless, the exclusion of certain occupational groups, notably hostellers, from the constabulary may indicate that the office still commanded a certain amount of prestige, which would have been undermined by the appointment of men who so often attracted public censure.[60]

Although the distributive trades were favoured most by aldermen, Susan Reynolds has argued that wealth was a more critical factor than occupation in determining one's qualifications for membership of the civic elite.[61] Unfortunately, it is difficult to assess individual wealth in this period, as the lay subsidies of the early fourteenth century and early sixteenth century are too far removed in time to be of value, and too few of the wills left by Rank B and C constables have survived for comparative analysis. The only way to measure the relative prosperity of constables is through the tax assessments of 1451 and 1472. The 1451 tax return names 163 people in Norwich with annual landed incomes from £2 to £200, including several members of the local gentry who resided in the countryside for most of the year. The list is confined to no more than the wealthiest 2 per cent of

---

[56] Frost, 'Aldermen', 57–61; Kermode, *Medieval Merchants*, 65; Maddern, 'Order and Disorder', 179; Carpenter, 'Formation of Urban Élites', 62–7; Kowaleski, *Local Markets*, 103.

[57] Dunn, 'After the Black Death', 130; *eadem*, 'Trade', 216; Rutledge, 'Economic Life', 168–72.

[58] Frost, 'Aldermen', 59.

[59] See Kowaleski, 'Commercial Dominance', 214.

[60] See Carpenter, 'Formation of Urban Élites', 67; Frost, 'Aldermen', 57. For more on the prestige of urban officials, see Rigby and Ewan, 'Government, Power and Authority', 305–9; Susan Reynolds, 'Medieval Urban History and the History of Political Thought', *Urban History Yearbook*, ix (1982), 15.

[61] Reynolds, 'Medieval Urban History', 20; D.M. Palliser, 'Urban Society', in *Fifteenth-Century Attitudes: Perceptions of Society in Late Medieval England*, ed. Rosemary Horrox (Cambridge, 1994), 141; Shaw, *Creation of a Community*, 167; Carpenter, 'Formation of Urban Élites', 72.

Norwich inhabitants, among whom were twenty aldermen and twenty-six of the common councillors who served in 1453. It also includes three constables from Rank C and ten from Rank B. Although far from comprehensive, the 1451 tax return indicates that some constables could be quite prosperous, even if they were not destined to become aldermen, but on the whole they were less well off than members of the elite.[62] The 1472 tax, which was also based on landed wealth, but did not impose a minimum threshold for liability, could potentially help to delineate patterns of wealth more accurately, in spite of the fact that half of the assessment is missing.[63] Because the surviving rolls itemised each property separately, rather than listing all of an individual's holdings together, we cannot necessarily assume that the information available for each contributor is complete. Nonetheless, the 1472 tax return definitively shows that at least twelve Rank A constables, thirty-six Rank B constables, and twenty-two Rank C constables owned property in Norwich. Once again, it confirms that those in Rank A were significantly wealthier than the others.[64] Moreover, the average property value for Rank C was approximately three-quarters that of Rank B: at least if Thomas Storme, a particularly elusive individual who appears as both sheriff and constable in 1472, but is not mentioned anywhere else in the assembly records, is excluded.[65] Not surprisingly, constables in Rank C appear to have been less likely to own property than those in Rank B. Though this evidence is not conclusive, it suggests that there might have been a greater differential in wealth between these two groups than is apparent from their respective patterns of office-holding or occupations. Less affluent individuals in Rank C might not have had the resources to join either civic council and might, therefore, have nursed limited political aspirations from the outset.[66]

Another group of mid-level officials in Norwich, tax collectors and assessors, may have enjoyed a higher social status than is generally assumed.[67] In Norwich, collectors and assessors seem to have been appointed as needed to raise specific taxes, while searchers and constables shared responsibility for routine collection at other times.[68] When they are recorded in the assembly books, collectors and assessors are almost always listed together; although they are usually

---

[62] Roger Virgoe, 'A Norwich Taxation List of 1451', *Norfolk Archaeology*, xl (1988), 145–54.

[63] Maureen Jurkowski, 'Income Tax Assessments of Norwich, 1472 and 1489', in *Poverty and Wealth: Sheep, Taxation and Charity in Late Medieval Norfolk*, ed. Mark Bailey, Maureen Jurkowski and Carole Rawcliffe (Norfolk Record Society, lxxi, 2007), 99–138.

[64] Properties held by Rank A constables were valued at 61s. on average, whereas the average valuation for properties held by Ranks B and C constables was 35s. and 31s. respectively.

[65] Norfolk RO, NCR 16D/1, f. 95v.

[66] Six individuals in Rank B served as constables only after being elected to the common council. Others undertook a second or third term while they were councilmen. Thus, it seems that, while acting as constable might have helped individuals to become aldermen, it was hardly a prerequisite for membership of the council. Shaw (*Creation of a Community*, 158) has demonstrated that in Wells men never took a step backwards down the civic ladder. The activities of the Rank B constables might, then, suggest that there was some difficulty in finding people to be constables. Alternatively, the *cursus honorum* in Norwich may have been more flexible than in Wells, or the post of constable more prestigious.

[67] See, for example, Attreed, *The King's Towns*, 151; Shaw, *Creation of a Community*, 159.

[68] See, for example, Norfolk RO, NCR 16D/1, ff. 53–4v. Also Attreed, *The King's Towns*, 151; *The English Government at Work, Vol. 2, 1327–1336: Fiscal Administration*, ed. W.A. Morris and J.R. Strayer (Cambridge, Mass., 1947), 36.

distinguishable from one another, there are a few instances in which it is not clear who was responsible for the collection as opposed to the assessment of taxes.[69] The assembly records list the tax officials charged with nineteen separate collections between 1414 and 1473. In 1440 and every previous year, between two and four collectors and/or assessors were nominated for each of the city's four great leets. In 1442, however, there were two or three assessors assigned to each of Norwich's twelve small wards, presumably to improve efficiency. Although the number of officials employed in each ward varied considerably thereafter (with an especially high number being involved in levying the 1453 tax), they were always appointed by ward. There seems to have been an administrative change between 1440 and 1442, whereby these smaller units became the preferred locus for assessment and collection.[70]

The records of the civic assembly furnish the names of 206 collectors and 131 assessors – a total of 308 individuals, thirty-one of whom served in both capacities.[71] Because collectors were not appointed annually, it is hardly surprising that no one occupied the same position on a regular basis. Yet many taxation officials were actively involved in other aspects of civic administration – nearly half of them held other offices in the city. Collectors were most likely to serve as constables, while assessors were slightly more inclined to seek positions in the upper echelons of the civic hierarchy. Each group, however, supplied Norwich with two mayors. Assessors were significantly more likely to reach Rank A than collectors, who were more comparable to constables in terms of status. Even so, nearly half of the collectors and approximately 40 per cent of assessors fall into Rank C.

Although any analysis of the occupations pursued by taxation officials must remain speculative, it seems that they were drawn from the same socio-economic group as constables. Assessors and constables alike tended to be involved in cloth production, the making of clothing and accessories, victualling and the distributive trades.[72] Collectors were broadly similar, but were slightly more likely to be victuallers and were correspondingly less often found in the distributive trades. Given the dominance of mercantile groups at the pinnacle of the urban elite,[73] this analysis of occupations suggests that collectors were drawn from a marginally less prestigious circle, but such an assumption remains tentative, given the limited sample available for study and its probable bias in favour of wealthier men.

The tax records also point to the existence of a financial hierarchy in which the assessors were wealthier than the constables who, in turn, amassed more landed wealth than the collectors. In order to make viable comparisons, only men who held office between 1440 and 1460 have been included in the following analysis of the 1451 tax returns. Within this group 18 per cent of assessors, 11.5 per cent of constables, and just short of 9 per cent of collectors appear in the surviving tax

---

[69]   See, for example, Norfolk RO, NCR 16D/1, f. 60.

[70]   *Ibid.*, ff. 15, 15v, 20v.

[71]   The sporadic nature of appointments complicates any evaluation of these offices. It is possible that some elections of taxation officials have been omitted, although there are no obvious lacunae, and the data that survive cover complete years.

[72]   See Table 4.

[73]   Frost, 'Aldermen', 239–43; Kermode, *Medieval Merchants*, 39; Palliser, 'Urban Society', 141.

list.[74] Since only the most prosperous residents were enumerated, these percentages may be regarded as a reliable indicator of relative wealth. The 1472 tax return covered a wider range of people, but, being incomplete, includes less than a third of office-holders. On the basis of this narrow sample, the assessors' property was valued at 46*s*. on average – somewhat more than the 38*s*. 6*d*. average for both collectors and constables.[75] On the whole, the taxation lists suggest that, although the assessors were slightly wealthier than collectors and constables, all three groups were more affluent than the majority of people living in Norwich.

Whereas collectors, assessors and constables came from a broadly similar socio-economic spectrum, the supervisors charged with oversight of particular tasks were more likely to be drawn from the ranks of the ruling elite. The Norwich records furnish the names of fifty-seven supervisors, who were responsible for civic projects often involving sanitation (most commonly cleansing the river or streets) or maintenance of the city wall.[76] In the wake of the plague, hygiene became a high priority as civic authorities, who believed that pollution posed a risk to public health, sought to prevent another outbreak.[77] Supervisors were normally appointed in teams of two, for the length of the project, which could last for many weeks or even a year. The fact that several of them could be chosen over the course of any one year suggests that multiple sets of supervisors may have functioned at the same time and that terms of service were negotiated on an *ad hoc* basis.[78] Perhaps because of the time and expenditure involved, as well as the perceived importance of their tasks, these men were often generously remunerated for services rendered. For example, the assembly roll for 1367 notes that, when William Staloun and John de Gnateshale were elected to supervise the cleansing of the river, each of them was to be paid half a mark per week for his labours.[79] In 1401 John Swanton received 46*s*. 8*d*. in return for overseeing a similar project for thirty-five weeks.[80] Although there is some evidence to suggest that the city levied taxes in order to hire specialist equipment,[81] it is not clear whether the supervisors retained all their pay or used a portion of it to engage workers.

Because these assignments could be both lucrative and extremely onerous, they were usually undertaken by members of the elite. Over half of our fifty-seven supervisors were drawn from Rank A, while a further quarter belonged to Rank B. Indeed, no fewer than eight of them became mayor of Norwich. John Gilbert even

---

[74] Virgoe, 'Norwich Taxation', 149–51.

[75] Jurkowski, 'Income Tax', 118–38.

[76] As with the taxation officials, the sporadic appointment of supervisors complicates the task of determining how many of them were actually recorded. Although it seems likely that the sources after 1453 are fairly complete, it is possible that members of the elite were more likely to be noted, particularly in the early period. Also see Isla Fay, 'Health and Disease in Medieval and Tudor Norwich' (University of East Anglia Ph.D. thesis, 2007), 293–306; Dolly Jørgensen, '"All Good Rule of the Citee": Sanitation and Civic Government in England, 1400–1600', *Journal of Urban History*, xxxvi (2010), 300–15; Norfolk RO, NCR 16D/1, f. 38v.

[77] Barron, *London in the Middle Ages*, 241; Ernest Sabine, 'City Cleaning in Mediaeval London', *Speculum*, xii (1937), 28. Several subsequent attempts to clean the city were inspired by epidemics. The outbreak of plague in 1365, for example, caused the city authorities to order that the river be cleansed in that year and again two years later. See Fay, 'Health and Disease', 293.

[78] See, for example, Norfolk RO, NCR 16D/1, ff. 20v, 60v, 61.

[79] Norfolk RO, NCR 8D/1, m. 6d.

[80] *Records of Norwich*, ed. Hudson and Tingey, ii. 54.

[81] See, for example, *ibid.*, 110.

accepted responsibility for a major cleansing programme three years after he had first served as mayor and immediately before his second term in office, such was its importance to the city.[82] This is similar to the pattern observed in Exeter and London, where men of high status often supervised public works.[83] In total, about three-quarters of Norwich supervisors occupied other civic offices at some point in their lives. This striking level of participation could indicate that supervisory duties involved an element of reward for loyal service, although it is also a reflection of the seriousness with which the civic authorities approached campaigns for environmental health during a period notable for several serious outbreaks of plague.[84]

Although many prominent figures were appointed as supervisors, they did not exercise a monopoly of these positions; nearly a quarter of overseers came from Rank C. On the other hand, supervisors were more likely to be associated with the distributive trades than constables or either type of taxation official, and were only marginally less involved in mercantile pursuits than aldermen.[85] They were about as likely as constables and assessors to be victuallers, but were slightly less prominent in the fields of cloth production and the manufacture of clothing and accessories. The varied social and occupational status of supervisors reflects the fact that not all tasks were equal in terms of the time and effort required, the importance of the work, or the level of remuneration on offer. On occasion, constables also assumed supervisory duties, which may indicate that the civic authorities sometimes had difficulty in filling these positions. The constables were ideally qualified for the overseeing of certain projects. For example, in 1422 the assembly mandated that all residents of Norwich should assist in cleansing the River Wensum and assigned a stretch of it to each great ward. It was the constables who were charged with ensuring that every person who was able to do so either contributed his labour or paid 4*d.* for a workman to take his place.[86] In this case, the constables were undoubtedly chosen because their local knowledge made it far easier for them to implement these orders, and, if necessary, to use their official powers to overcome resistance.

Regardless of their personal standing or the task in hand, it is clear that, although supervisors did not undertake manual labour, they were expected to visit worksites regularly in order to ensure that projects were completed properly. Their personal involvement in the physical wellbeing of the urban body supports

---

[82] Norfolk RO, NCR 16D/1, f. 61. In this particular instance cleansing the river seems to have been one of Gilbert's personal goals: in addition to championing and supervising the work involved, he left a generous bequest to be spent on public sanitation in his testament. See Carole Rawcliffe, *Medicine for the Soul: The Life, Death and Resurrection of an English Medieval Hospital, St. Giles's, Norwich, c. 1249–1550* (Stroud, 1999), 36.

[83] Kowaleski, *Local Markets*, 104–5; Sabine, 'City Cleaning', 22.

[84] Frequent presentments for environmental offences in the leet courts also reflect a widespread effort to prevent epidemics by cleansing the urban environment. This concern may have grown in the 15th century as the city increased expenditure to ensure the cleanliness of its waterways. See Fay, 'Health and Disease', 292, 298–300.

[85] Frost ('Aldermen', 59) demonstrates that, between 1461 and 1509, 53.3% of aldermen were mercers, grocers or drapers.

[86] Norfolk RO, NCR 8D/1420–6, m. 2.

Lorraine Attreed's hypothesis that, far from being despotic oligarchs, urban officials sought to protect the community and promote public welfare.[87]

A final group of mid-level officials, the searchers, was significantly less involved in other aspects of civic governance than the supervisors, tax officials or constables. Each craft or trade elected its own searchers (sometimes the masters or wardens of the guild in question), who, according to their respective oaths, were to 'make good and trewe serche' of the membership each year in order to ensure that the bylaws of the city were being observed.[88] They swore to report forestallers, dubious activities and defective merchandise to the mayor, and to ensure that all practitioners of their trades and crafts who had lived in the city for a year and a day were made known to the authorities.[89] Should they fail in any of these requirements they were liable to a fine. The bailiffs of Norwich are known to have appointed searchers for various trades and crafts from the mid fourteenth century onwards.[90] After the 'Composition' of 1415, the guilds and fraternities were allowed to select their own searchers, although the latter continued to be sworn in by the mayor and remained subservient to him, being still obliged to report offences to his court. Furthermore, should any craft fail to choose two acceptable candidates, the mayor was entitled to make the selection himself.[91] He was also empowered to review the fines levied by the searchers, half of which were allocated to the community chest.[92] It is worth noting that on at least one occasion the searchers were charged with assessing and collecting taxes.[93] Such evidence suggests that the craft guilds, although not particularly powerful in Norwich, played an auxiliary political role as agents of the civic authorities.[94]

Because the searchers were subordinate to the mayor, their names ought properly to have been inscribed in his court book, which, unfortunately, only lists them for a period of six years in the 1440s, when the city was largely under the stewardship of a royally-appointed governor. The number of different trades and crafts mentioned at this time ranged from nine, in 1446, to twenty-six in 1447. Although most craft guilds retained two searchers, the worsted weavers always

---

[87] Attreed, *The King's Towns*, 44–5. London aldermen and lesser officials also played a direct role in providing for the cleanliness of the streets. See, for example, Barron, *London in the Middle Ages*, 261; Carole Rawcliffe, 'Sources for the Study of Public Health in the Medieval City', in *Understanding Medieval Primary Sources*, ed. Joel Rosenthal (New York and London, 2012), 182–91.

[88] *Records of Norwich*, ed. Hudson and Tingey, ii. 315. In addition to regulating trade, the searchers' activities were likely intended to preserve health by preventing the sale of putrid meat, which was thought to cause disease. See Fay, 'Health and Disease', 351; Carole Rawcliffe, *Leprosy in Medieval England* (Woodbridge, 2006), 79.

[89] *Records of Norwich*, ed. Hudson and Tingey, ii. 287.

[90] *Ibid.*, p. xliii.

[91] *Ibid.*, p. lxv.

[92] *Ibid.*, 284.

[93] *Ibid.*, 289; Norfolk RO, NCR 16D/1, f. 53v.

[94] Heather Swanson, 'The Illusion of Economic Structure: Craft Guilds in Late Medieval English Towns', *Past and Present*, cxxi (1988), 29–48; Kermode, *Medieval Merchants*, 56; Matthew Davies, 'Artisans, Guilds and Government in London', in *Daily Life in the Late Middle Ages*, ed. Richard Britnell (Stroud, 1998), 133–7; Barbara Green and Rachel Young, *Norwich: The Growth of a City* (Norwich, 1972), 17–18; Phythian-Adams, *Desolation of a City*, 117; Gervase Rosser, 'Crafts, Guilds and the Negotiation of Work in the Medieval Town', *Past and Present*, cliv (1997), 3–31.

elected six or eight, whereas in 1445 a few crafts had only one.[95] It seems that some crafts did not choose a searcher every year – perhaps because they were too small and unimportant. Since the 'Composition' of 1415 had decreed that each of the London mysteries was to have a counterpart in Norwich, some of the more specialist crafts would hardly have needed, or been able to appoint, one.[96] It was not until 1456 that the number of guilds formally required to make a return was set at twenty-four, after a period of flux in the 1440s. The irregular listing of searchers in the mayor's court book may reflect a disagreement on this score, although it seems likely that some crafts encountered a dearth of volunteers. Nor do we know how systematically such matters were recorded by the mayor's clerk.[97]

The surviving lists furnish references to 145 individuals elected as searchers.[98] During this short period under review, it is apparent that over 30 per cent of them acted in the same capacity more than once. This tendency suggests that specialised knowledge or skills were necessary to fulfil the duties involved. Alternatively, it may be that office-holding was reserved for the wealthiest men, who could occupy these powerful positions for extended periods of time.[99] The 1451 tax return indicates that at least seventeen of the searchers were among the most prosperous landholders in Norwich.[100] These men, however, were no more likely than the other searchers to serve more than once; about one quarter did so altogether. Only two served for each of the six years, however, indicating that the position was not a permanent one. Significantly, they both also became constables at other points in their careers. In total, thirty searchers held other civic offices, and they were disproportionately more likely to be a searcher at least twice. Although, on the whole, searchers were less inclined than constables to move up the civic hierarchy, their readiness to serve repeatedly within the context of their guilds presupposes some sense of obligation, even if it was directed towards their fellow craftsmen rather than the city.[101]

Although the high level of repeated service among searchers suggests either that the wealthy clung to these positions or that a specialised skill set was required, the post did not necessarily demand expert knowledge of a particular craft. It is possible to identify the occupations of thirty-two searchers. Most of them were elected by the guild to which they belonged at the time of their admission to the freedom of the city, but 22 per cent were not. Although some of them may have changed their principal occupation afterwards, eight men in this study served as the searcher for more than one craft.[102] Was there a dearth of individuals with the

---

95 See Norfolk RO, NCR 16A/1, f. 43; Dunn, 'Trade', 216.
96 *Records of Norwich*, ed. Hudson and Tingey, ii. p. xlv.
97 *Ibid.*, 92.
98 These individuals represent 70% of the maximum number of searchers who could potentially have served over the six years; given the likelihood of inconsistencies discussed above, they may represent all of the searchers appointed in those years.
99 Kowaleski, *Local Markets*, 101.
100 At least 12% of the searchers may be found among the wealthiest 2% of Norwich residents; this percentage could have been higher, since some searchers may have died or left the city before the assessment of the tax. See Virgoe, 'Norwich Taxation', 149–51.
101 Although it is not possible to establish the official status of most searchers because so few aldermen and councillors can be identified before 1453, we know that at least three searchers became aldermen and 20 became councillors.
102 Frost, 'Aldermen', 58.

administrative proficiency, experience, social status, and willingness to take up some of these posts? Or had some of the men who were associated with multiple crafts been appointed by the mayor? In the latter case, these positions may have been highly desirable and a certain level of wealth and prestige, or a personal relationship with the mayor, may have been the most important prerequisites for office.[103] In either event, it seems likely that Norwich's searchers were perceived to play a vital role in regulating local commerce, because when the liberties of the city were taken into the king's hands in 1442 Sir John Clifton, the royal governor, immediately appointed new searchers for twenty-three crafts.[104]

By examining five mid-level civic offices, this paper has demonstrated that the rulers of Norwich consistently relied upon the assistance of men outside the upper echelons of the governing elite to maintain order, and that participation in these offices may have afforded artisans and retailers access to political power. There is some evidence to suggest that the lower incomes and status of those in Rank C prevented them from aspiring to membership of the two legislative bodies of the city. Urban historians would certainly profit from viewing mid-level positions as desirable in their own right, and re-examining the motives that led people to become involved in peace-keeping and the daily administrative tasks that were so essential to a city's well-being. The men who occupied these positions in fifteenth-century Norwich were influenced by a variety of considerations. Some may have been inspired by a sense of communal obligation, or even have relished the opportunity to take responsibility for preserving local order, while others may have sought the prestige of civic employment. Mid-level offices often promised financial benefits, opportunities to cultivate potentially lucrative relationships with the future rulers of the city, and some (albeit limited) involvement in the processes of legislation and election, especially before 1462. This pattern of recruitment from outside the elite may have smoothed over social differences between the rulers and the ruled and encouraged residents to accept the authority of what remained a fairly narrow oligarchy.

---

[103] Norfolk RO, NCR 16A/1, ff. 2, 40; *Records of Norwich*, ed. Hudson and Tingey, ii. p. xxii.
[104] Norfolk RO, NCR 16A/1, f. 39. Clifton may have sought to spread his own patronage or simply to remove incompetent or potentially troublesome men from office.

TABLES

Table 1: Political Rank of Mid-Level Officials in Norwich, 1453–73

Political Rank	Constables (no.)	%	Collectors (no.)	%	Assessors (no.)	%	Supervisors (no.)	%
A	(22)	9.2	(9)	7.7	(12)	25.5	(12)	52.2
B	(115)	48.1	(51)	43.6	(16)	34.0	(6)	26.1
C	(102)	42.7	(57)	48.7	(19)	40.4	(5)	21.7
Total	(239)	100	(117)	100	(47)	99.9	(23)	100

Source: Data taken from the Policing Officials Database, constructed from references to service in a wide variety of civic offices in Norwich and other medieval English towns, particularly offices concerned with policing or other supervisory functions. The main Norwich sources used in this table are the assembly book (1434–73), and mayor's court book (1424–49). Also see nn. 24–7, above.

Note: Individuals who held multiple offices are listed once in each category.

Table 2: Number of Years Served as Constable in Norwich

No. of years	Rank A (no.)	%	Rank B (no.)	%	Rank C (no.)	%	Total (no.)	%
1	(5)	22.7	(46)	40.0	(61)	59.8	(112)	46.8
2	(12)	54.5	(27)	23.5	(16)	15.7	(55)	23.0
3	(3)	13.6	(14)	12.2	(10)	9.8	(27)	11.3
4	(1)	4.6	(8)	6.9	(5)	4.9	(14)	5.9
5	(0)	0.0	(9)	7.8	(0)	0.0	(9)	3.8
6	(0)	0.0	(3)	2.6	(1)	1.0	(4)	1.7
7	(0)	0.0	(1)	0.9	(2)	1.9	(3)	1.3
8	(1)	4.6	(4)	3.5	(1)	1.0	(6)	2.5
9	(0)	0.0	(1)	0.9	(1)	1.0	(2)	0.8
10+	(0)	0.0	(2)	1.7	(5)	4.9	(7)	2.9
Total	(22)	100	(115)	100	(102)	100	(239)	100

Source: Policing Officials Database.
Note: This table includes all of the men who became constables between 1453 and 1473; when necessary their careers have been traced into the subsequent period.

Samantha Sagui

Table 3: Occupations of Norwich Constables, 1453–73

Occupation	Rank A (no.)	%	Rank B (no.)	%	Rank C (no.)	%	Total (no.)	%
Artists	(0)	0.0	(2)	3.1	(0)	0.0	(2)	1.6
Building	(0)	0.0	(1)	1.5	(2)	4.8	(3)	2.3
Clerical and legal	(0)	0.0	(0)	0.0	(4)	9.5	(4)	3.1
Cloth production	(2)	9.5	(9)	13.8	(11)	26.2	(22)	17.1
Clothing and accessories	(3)	14.3	(10)	15.4	(7)	16.7	(20)	15.6
Distribution	(14)	66.7	(12)	18.4	(5)	11.9	(31)	24.2
Leather production	(0)	0.0	(1)	1.5	(1)	2.4	(2)	1.6
Metal work	(0)	0.0						5.4
Miscellaneous services	(0)	0.0	(0)	0.0	(3)	7.1	(3)	2.3
Provisions/ victualling	(2)	9.5	(18)	27.7	(5)	11.9	(25)	19.5
Transport	(0)	0.0	(4)	6.1	(1)	2.4	(5)	3.9
Wood, horn and bone	(0)	0.0	(2)	3.1	(2)	4.8	(4)	3.1
Total	(21)	100	(65)	100	(42)	100	(128)	100

Source: Policing Officials Database.
Note: In order to facilitate comparison with other studies of Norwich, the occupational categories in this table have been adopted from Rutledge, 'Economic Life', 168–72. This scheme is rather unusual in a couple of respects: most importantly, Rutledge includes retailers in the distribution category; however, the only tradesmen in this category who held office were drapers, mercers, merchants and grocers.
This table includes all constables in Norwich between 1453 and 1473 for whom occupations can be identified, including 95.5% of the men in Rank A, 55.7% of those in Rank B, and 41.2% of the individuals in Rank C. As a result, this table underestimates the less easily identified and less remunerative occupations.

Table 4: Occupations of Norwich Tax Officials, Constables and Supervisors, 1414–73

Occupation	Collectors (no.)	%	Assessors (no.)	%	Constables (no.)	%	Supervisors (no.)	%
Artists	(1)	1.2	(0)	0.0	(2)	1.6	(0)	0.0
Building	(7)	98.6	(3)	7.9	(3)	2.3	(1)	5.3
Clerical and legal	(0)	0.0	(0)	0.0	(4)	3.1	(0)	0.0
Cloth production	(11)	13.6	(8)	21.1	(22)	17.1	(2)	10.5
Clothing and accessories	(12)	14.8	(7)	18.4	(20)	15.6	(1)	5.3
Distribution	(12)	14.8	(8)	21.1	(31)	24.2	(9)	47.4
Hosteller	(1)	1.2	(2)	5.3	(0)	0.0	(1)	5.2
Leather production	(1)	1.2	(1)	2.6	(2)	1.6	(0)	0.0
Metal work	(6)	7.4	(0)	0.0	(7)	5.4	(2)	10.5
Miscellaneous services	(0)	0.0	(0)	0.0	(3)	2.3	(0)	0.0
Provisions/ victualling	(20)	24.7	(7)	18.4	(25)	19.5	(3)	15.8
Transport	(6)	7.4	(2)	5.3	(5)	3.9	(0)	0.0
Wood, horn and bone	(4)	4.9	(0)	0.0	(4)	3.1	(0)	0.0
Total	(81)	100	(38)	100	(128)	100	(19)	100

Source: Policing Officials Database.
Note: In order to facilitate comparison with other studies of Norwich, the occupational categories in this table have also been adopted from Rutledge, 'Economic Life', 168–72; see the caveat for Table 3. This data must be treated with caution because occupations could only be ascertained for 40% of collectors, 29% of assessors, 53% of constables, and 33% of supervisors. As a result, this table once again underestimates the less easily identified, less remunerative occupations.

LEPROSY AND PUBLIC HEALTH IN LATE MEDIEVAL ROUEN[*]

Elma Brenner

In Rouen, as in many other major European cities, following the Black Death (1347–50) there was increased anxiety about environmental health, and it was thought necessary to protect the urban population from the spread of disease through corrupt, or miasmatic, air. These preoccupations were linked to growing concerns about cleanliness, stench, 'infection' and the elimination of 'pollution', as a result of which certain features of civic life appeared particularly dangerous, including vagrant pigs and poultry, open latrines, the slaughter of animals in public places, rotten food, rubbish and contaminated water.[1] Such anxieties were closely linked to the Galenic model of human health and physiology as disseminated in *regimina sanitatis*, the health manuals that were becoming increasingly popular in the later Middle Ages.[2] In theory at least, these *regimina* were addressed to the upper echelons of society, as reflected, for example, by their advice regarding the consumption of expensive foodstuffs.[3] While Galen maintained that good health resulted from the internal balance of the four bodily humours, he also devoted considerable attention to the non-naturals, which were external phenomena and psychological states that could either prevent or cause illness. They included the quality of the environment, food and drink, exercise, sleep, the purgation of bodily fluids and emotional wellbeing.[4]

Late medieval concerns about such hazards as fly-blown meat, the presence of human and animal waste, and the attendant corruption of the air were clearly

[*]   I am very grateful to Professor Carole Rawcliffe for her invaluable comments and suggestions.

[1]   On pollution and public health measures in late medieval and early modern Rouen, see Philippe Lardin, 'Les Rouennais et la pollution à la fin du Moyen Âge', in *Des châteaux et des sources*: *archéologie et histoire dans la Normandie médiévale. Mélanges en l'honneur d'Anne-Marie Flambard Héricher*, ed. Élisabeth Lalou, Bruno Lepeuple and Jean-Louis Roch (Mont-Saint-Aignan, 2008), 399–427; Louis Porquet, *La peste en Normandie du XIVe au XVIIe siècle* (Vire, 1898), 123–8. On such measures in 15th-century Brittany and Savoy, see Jean-Pierre Leguay, 'Esquisse d'une politique sanitaire médiévale: les mesures sociales et médicales prises dans les villes bretonnes et savoyardes au XVe siècle', in *Médecine et société de l'antiquité à nos jours*, ed. Anne-Marie Flambard Héricher and Yannick Marec ([Rouen], 2005), 90.

[2]   On the *regimina sanitatis* and their origins, see Pedro Gil Sotres, 'The Regimens of Health', in *Western Medical Thought from Antiquity to the Middle Ages*, ed. M.D. Grmek and trans. Antony Shugaar (Cambridge, Mass., 1998), 291–318.

[3]   *Ibid.*, 300, 309.

[4]   *Medieval Medicine: A Reader*, ed. Faith Wallis (Readings in Medieval Civilizations and Cultures, xv, Toronto, 2010), 485–6, 548; C.A. Bonfield, 'The *Regimen Sanitatis* and its Dissemination in England, c. 1348–1550' (Univ. of East Anglia Ph.D. thesis, 2006), 1–6.

connected to Galenic ideas about the preservation of health. They also reflect the significant influence, by the fourteenth century, of Latin translations of Arabic medical texts made in the twelfth and thirteenth centuries.[5] These translated texts, above all Avicenna's *Canon*, explored theories of infection and contagion, as well as the effects of environmental pollution, poor diet and contact with, or proximity to, the sick, in their discussions of the causation of disease.[6] As a result, *regimina* warn repeatedly against the adverse effects of the noxious air that could result from pungent smells (associated with animals such as cows and pigs and birds such as pigeons, and, significantly, with lepers, whose breath and sores emitted unpleasant odours) and from the putrefaction of organic waste.[7] At the same time, an analogy could be drawn between the human and the urban body, one of the most obvious parallels being the healthy flow of blood inside the body and the availability of clean water within the city.[8] From this perspective, civic welfare depended on the elimination of pollution and similar threats to survival.

This article will investigate how attitudes towards lepers and leprosy in late medieval Rouen, France's second largest city in this period, changed in the context of contemporary ideas about the transmission of disease and a growing awareness of the need to maintain public health, which evolved against the violent backdrop of the Hundred Years' War (1337–1453). It will also consider how central leprosy, a notorious source of toxic vapours, may have been in generating anxieties about the spread of epidemics, and whether it sometimes became symbolic of disease in general. Although it has often been assumed that, historically, 'progress' in medical thought has been marked by a shift from concepts of infection by miasmatic air to more 'advanced' notions of contagion, Annemarie Kinzelbach underlines the fact that transmission both by corrupt air and by contagion (in the sense of epidemics being 'spread by direct or indirect contact with the sick or deceased') *together* formed part of the understanding of disease in the late medieval and early modern periods.[9] Indeed, the need for pre-modern measures aimed at ensuring public health and hygiene to be approached 'on their own terms', rather than from a teleological perspective, predicated upon the concept of progress towards modern-day biomedicine, has recently been emphasised by Guy Geltner.[10] He argues that such measures should be studied comparatively, in different locations and over time, and in their broader social and religious contexts. Even though late medieval societies may not have used the term 'public health', and

---

[5]   Gil Sotres, 'Regimens', 296–300.
[6]   For Arabic medical texts on the causation of leprosy, see François-Olivier Touati, 'Historiciser la notion de contagion: l'exemple de la lèpre dans les sociétés médiévales', in *Air, miasmes et contagion: les épidémies dans l'antiquité et au Moyen Âge*, ed. Sylvie Bazin-Tacchella, Danielle Quéruel and Évelyne Samama (Langres, 2001), 175–81.
[7]   Gil Sotres, 'Regimens', 303.
[8]   Bonfield, 'Regimen Sanitatis', 8–9, 139–40 and, more generally, chs. 4 and 5.
[9]   Annemarie Kinzelbach, 'Infection, Contagion, and Public Health in Late Medieval and Early Modern German Imperial Towns', *Journal of the History of Medicine and Allied Sciences*, lxi (3) (2006), 369–89, especially 369–71, 373–7, 385–6, 388. On the coexistence of concepts of miasma and contagion at this time, also see the article by John Henderson, below, pp. 175–9.
[10] Guy Geltner, 'Public Health and the Pre-Modern City: A Research Agenda', *History Compass*, x (3) (2012), 231–2. See also Carole Rawcliffe, 'Sources for the Study of Public Health in the Medieval City', in *Understanding Medieval Primary Sources*, ed. J.T. Rosenthal (London and New York, 2012), 177–8.

undoubtedly advanced ideas about the causation of disease and what constituted a salubrious environment that were very different to our own, Geltner makes the interesting point that an awareness of pre-modern sanitary legislation can still be relevant to today's public health workers.[11]

The so-called 1321 'Lepers' Plot', as a result of which lepers and Jews were accused of poisoning the water supply of the kingdom of France so that people would die or become leprous (an accusation indicative of concerns about communal health prior to the Black Death), is widely viewed as heralding an increasingly negative response to presumed lepers.[12] Nevertheless, there appears to be no direct evidence that Rouen's lepers were persecuted at this time.[13] Chronicles originating in Rouen record the event, but simply refer in general terms to the fact that 'all the lepers as it were throughout the kingdom ... were burnt', observing that 'all the lepers throughout the kingdom of France were captured, and condemned by the pope, and many in various places were burnt by fire, and those who remained were shut up in their houses'.[14] Whereas these accounts create a vivid picture of widespread violence against lepers in France, and the confinement of suspects in its aftermath, they do not explicitly describe any such persecution in Rouen. Although there was a striking decline in the number of charitable gifts received by the city's *leprosaria* in the fourteenth and fifteenth centuries, this may have been due as much to the fact that the disease itself was in retreat as it was to any residual hostility towards its victims.[15]

Did leprosy, therefore, cease to play much part in late medieval thinking about disease, or did it remain among those threats that seemed to present a particular danger to the health of urban populations? This article will address both questions through an examination of royal ordinances and municipal records from the fifteenth century. While the former, as prescriptive sources, do not necessarily reveal which measures were put into practice and how successful they were, the latter may be more indicative of actual responses to disease.[16] We will also assess

---

[11] Geltner, 'Public Health', 234–5, 238. See also C.E. Rosenberg, 'Epilogue: *Airs, Waters, Places*. A Status Report', *Bulletin of the History of Medicine*, lxxxvi (4) (2012), 661–70.

[12] On this 'plot', see Malcolm Barber, 'Lepers, Jews and Moslems: The Plot to Overthrow Christendom in 1321', *History*, lxvi (1981), 1–17; David Nirenberg, *Communities of Violence: Persecution of Minorities in the Middle Ages* (Princeton, N.J., 1996), 93–124 (focusing on the spread of the accusation to the Crown of Aragon).

[13] For a study of a locality in Switzerland where evidence for the persecution of lepers in 1321 does exist, see Piera Borradori, *Mourir au monde: les lépreux dans le Pays de Vaud (XIIIe–XVIIe siècle)* (Cahiers lausannois d'histoire médiévale, vii, Lausanne, 1992), 84–90.

[14] '*omnes leprosi quasi per totum regnum ... combusti sunt*': 'E Chronici Rotomagensis continuatione', in *Recueil des historiens des Gaules et de la France, XXIII*, ed. J.N. de Wailly, L.V. Delisle and C.M.G.B. Jourdain (Paris, 1876), 349; '*Capti fuerunt omnes leprosi per totum regnum Franciæ, et a domino papa condemnati, multique in diversis locis igne combusti; et qui remanserunt in domibus suis inclusi sunt*': 'E Chronico sanctæ Catharinæ de Monte Rothomagi', in *ibid.*, 409. Also see *Normanniae nova chronica ab anno Christi CCCCLXXIII ad annum MCCCLXXVIII. E tribus chronicis mss. Sancti Laudi, Sanctae Catharinae et Majoris Ecclesiae Rotomagensium collecta*, ed. Adolphe Chéruel (Caen, 1850), 31.

[15] On the numerous gifts received by the *leprosarium* of Mont-aux-Malades, Rouen, in the 12th and 13th centuries, see Elma Brenner, 'Charity in Rouen in the Twelfth and Thirteenth Centuries (with Special Reference to Mont-aux-Malades)' (Cambridge Univ. Ph.D. thesis, 2007), especially chs. 1 and 2.

[16] Geltner, 'Public Health', 234–6. For attempts to restrict the participation of lepers in communal rituals at Amiens, see below, p. 156.

the institutional status of Rouen's *leprosaria* in this period, especially that of Mont-aux-Malades, its principal leper house, an Augustinian priory, which catered for male and female lepers, and that of Salle-aux-Puelles, a house for leprous women, which was granted by King Charles V of France (1364–80) to the city's hospital for the sick poor, La Madeleine, in 1366. Although Charles's transfer of Salle-aux-Puelles could suggest that responding to the social and medical problems caused by plague and the Hundred Years' War appeared to be more urgent than addressing those associated with leprosy at this time, careful provision was made for it to continue functioning as a *leprosarium*. Carole Rawcliffe has noted that the decline of leper houses in the later Middle Ages 'sits oddly with the obvious – and in some cases growing – concern leprosy still provoked'.[17] The discussion below will evaluate how prominently leprosy and its sufferers featured both in anxieties and theories regarding civic health in late medieval Rouen, and in the lived environment of the city and its hinterland.

The fourteenth and fifteenth centuries marked a turbulent period in Rouen's history, characterised by plague epidemics, famine, flooding, popular uprisings and the protracted impact of the Hundred Years' War.[18] In the eyes of the citizenry, who had previously supported Rouen's *leprosaria* through their charity, the needs of the leprous may well have paled in comparison with these troubles.[19] According to the *Normanniae nova chronica* (documenting the years 473 to 1378), the plague arrived in the Rouen countryside and in the city itself around the feast of St. John the Baptist (24 June) 1348, although the city had probably been infected in late April.[20] Both the *Nova chronica* and the chronicle of Pierre Cochon (ending in 1430) describe a great mortality in 1348: the former claims that between the last week of August and Christmas 1348 more than 100,000 people died in the city of Rouen alone.[21] Further outbreaks of plague occurred there in 1362, 1369, 1379, 1387, 1390, 1417, 1457, 1483–4, 1499, 1503, 1505, 1511, 1518, 1520, 1521–2 and 1523.[22] Three urban cemeteries, those of the parishes of Saint-Martin-du-Pont, Saint-Martin-sur-Renelle and Saint-Godard, were enlarged during this period, reflecting the mass mortality caused by pestilence.[23] In addition, a new cemetery was established to serve the heavily populated parish of Saint-Maclou soon after the Black Death: blessed in May 1357, it replaced an earlier, but now inadequate,

[17] Carole Rawcliffe, *Leprosy in Medieval England* (Woodbridge, 2006), 8.
[18] Alain Sadourny, 'Des débuts de la guerre de cent ans à la Harelle', in *Histoire de Rouen*, ed. Michel Mollat (Univers de la France et des pays francophones, xliii, Toulouse, 1979), 99–100, 116–21.
[19] On earlier charity for Rouen's lepers, see Brenner, 'Charity in Rouen'.
[20] *Normanniae nova chronica*, ed. Chéruel, 33; O.J. Benedictow, *The Black Death 1346–1353: The Complete History* (Woodbridge, 2004), 102; Sadourny, 'Débuts', 100.
[21] *Normanniae nova chronica*, ed. Chéruel, 33; *Chronique normande de Pierre Cochon, notaire apostolique à Rouen*, ed. Charles de Robillard de Beaurepaire (Rouen, 1870), 73–4; Sadourny, 'Débuts', 100.
[22] Jean Fournée, 'Les normands face à la peste', *Le pays bas-normand*, cxlix (1) (1978), 35, 36; Sadourny, 'Débuts', 100; Porquet, *La peste en Normandie*, 124, 128. For the plague outbreak of 1499, see Rouen, Archives départementales de Seine-Maritime [henceforth Rouen, AdSM], Archives Municipales de Rouen [henceforth AMR], Délibérations, Registre A 9, f. 318; Lardin, 'Rouennais et pollution', 418; Porquet, *La peste en Normandie*, 124–5 (dating the relevant document to 1498).
[23] Sadourny, 'Débuts', 100.

parochial graveyard.[24] It was subsequently enlarged several times, most notably in 1432 and during the plague-ridden 1520s. Between 1526 and about 1533, wooden galleries were erected to serve as a charnel house, which is one of very few buildings of this type still remaining in Europe today.[25] The charnel house is famous for its wooden, and originally painted, carvings of skulls, bones, gravediggers' spades and picks, the Dance of Death and other macabre images (plate 1),[26] reflecting the preoccupation with death apparent throughout Europe in an age of plague.[27] There were many more such epidemics in Rouen in the sixteenth and seventeenth centuries, with what appears to have been the last occurring in 1668–70.[28]

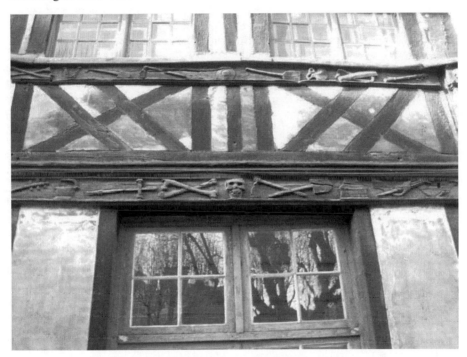

Plate 1: Wooden carvings in the Aître Saint-Maclou, Rouen. Photograph: Elma Brenner.

[24] Sabine Delanes, 'L'aître Saint-Maclou', in Christiane Decaëns, Henry Decaëns, Jérôme Decoux and Sabine Delanes, *L'église et l'aître Saint-Maclou, Rouen, Haute-Normandie* (Patrimoine et Territoire, vii, [Rouen], 2012), 54; *Chronique normande de Pierre Cochon*, ed. de Beaurepaire, 73.

[25] In Normandy, another 16th-century charnel house still stands, the *aître* of Brisgaret in the town of Montivilliers: Delanes, 'L'aître', 56–9.

[26] Nicétas Periaux, *Dictionnaire indicateur et historique des rues et places de Rouen* (Rouen, 1870; repr. Saint-Aubin-les-Elbeuf, 1997), 574; Delanes, 'L'aître', 59.

[27] On the macabre art and literature of the 14th to 16th centuries, which actually began to appear before the Black Death, see Paul Binski, *Medieval Death: Ritual and Representation* (1996), 126–34, and Karen Smyth's article, above, pp. 42–5.

[28] Fournée, 'Les normands', 36; Porquet, *La peste en Normandie*, 128–33.

Public Health Measures

Measures put in place by the kings of France and the civic government of Rouen in the fifteenth century testify to tangible concerns about communal welfare and the prevention of disease at this time, as well as about the visual appearance of the city.[29] These anxieties focused upon matters of general cleanliness, with particular and predictable reference to butchery and the supply of wholesome meat. Certain parts of the city were undoubtedly heavily polluted: for example, the Aubette and Robec rivers, tributaries of the Seine running through the eastern districts of Rouen, were contaminated by both human waste (latrines were located on their banks) and the chemical by-products of the dyeing and fulling of cloth. The sewage that overflowed from another public latrine, in an alleyway leading from the rue des Certains in the parish of Saint-Maclou, led to the temporary closure of the alleyway in the latter part of the fifteenth century.[30]

A set of statutes regulating the activities of butchers selling meat in two new butcheries, in the halles of the Vieux-Marché, Rouen's main market square, and at the Porte Beauvoisine, on the city's northern edge, was issued by the *bailli* of Rouen and Gisors on 28 June 1432 and confirmed by Charles VIII (1483–98) many years later in November 1487.[31] The Vieux-Marché was the place where Joan of Arc was burnt as a heretic in 1431; another public space at Rouen, the Mare-du-Parc in the suburb of Saint-Sever, had previously witnessed the burning of heretics in the third quarter of the thirteenth century.[32] Significantly, rotten or corrupt meat was also often burnt in public markets. Such meat was believed to contaminate the physical environment, while heresy was associated with the spread of spiritual pollution.

The statutes first promulgated in June 1432 reveal the existence of a concept of the '*bien commun de la chose publique*', and an awareness of the need to protect this 'common public good' from disease. This phrase was used from at least the early fifteenth century: for example, the importance of serving '*la chose publique*' is stressed in a confirmation of the statutes of Rouen's surgeons issued by Charles VII (1422–61) in April 1453.[33] In keeping with the ideas expressed so forcefully in

---

[29] On public health measures implemented by Rouen's magistrates to combat plague between c.1450 and c.1560, see also Neil Murphy's article, below, pp. 142–6, 148, 149, 151, 154, 155–6, 157, 158.

[30] Periaux, *Dictionnaire*, 155 and n. 5; Jean-Pierre Leguay, *La pollution au Moyen Âge* (Paris, 1999), 17, 18.

[31] 'Statuts des bouchers vendant dans les halles du Vieux-Marché et de la Porte Beauvoisine, à Rouen', in *Ordonnances des rois de France de la troisième race*, *XX*, ed. Claude de Pastoret (Paris, 1840), 39–45. On the butcheries at the Porte Beauvoisine and the Vieux-Marché, see Periaux, *Dictionnaire*, 35–6, 61, 147, 658.

[32] On 22 June 1253, Jean Marel was condemned as a heretic at the Mare-du-Parc; on 18 Apr. 1266, a lapsed Jewish convert was declared a heretic and an apostate at a public gathering near the Mare-du-Parc and burnt: *Regestrum visitationum archiepiscopi Rothomagensis: journal des visites pastorales d'Eude Rigaud, archevêque de Rouen. MCCXLVIII–MCCLXIX*, ed. Théodose Bonnin (Rouen, 1852), 160, 541; *The Register of Eudes of Rouen*, ed. J.F. O'Sullivan and trans. S.M. Brown (Records of Civilization, Sources and Studies, lxxii, New York, 1964), 175, 618. On the Mare-du-Parc, see Periaux, *Dictionnaire*, 364.

[33] Lardin, 'Rouennais et pollution', 401; 'Lettres de Charles VII, par laquelle il confirme les statuts des chirurgiens de Rouen et ordonne de s'y conformer, données à Tours en avril, avant Pâques 1453', in François Hue, *La communauté des chirurgiens de Rouen: Chirurgiens – Barbiers-Chirurgiens – Collège de Chirurgie, 1407–1791* (Rouen, 1913), 28.

contemporary *regimina*, the document regulating practice at Rouen's new butcheries also warned that bad meat could be 'of very great danger and prejudice to human creatures'.[34] Consequently, its authors sought to ensure that no pork, beef or lamb 'infected with any diseases' went on sale there.[35] The list of prohibitions was both detailed and comprehensive. For example, '*porc fresq seursemé*' (pork bearing signs of corruption) might only be sold if it was salted; otherwise it would be confiscated and given to 'poor prisoners'.[36] No butcher was to deal in beef infected with '*fy*' (understood to be a type of bovine leprosy) or any other sickness, or lamb contaminated by '*clavelée*' (a disease causing spots, akin to smallpox) or '*bouquet*' (a sore usually affecting the sheep's muzzle). Nor was he to market the flesh of any 'beast whatever it is that comes from a leper house'.[37] Any rotten meat found on the butchers' stalls would henceforth be seized by the wardens of their guild and thrown in the river Seine.[38]

These prescriptions indicate that there was considerable anxiety about potential health hazards in fifteenth-century Rouen, no doubt primarily with respect to plague, but also regarding leprosy and other communicable diseases. It was clearly believed that once animals fell sick humans might become infected too, through the consumption of their flesh. A diet of substandard meat would, in any event, destabilise the humours, rendering an individual especially vulnerable to miasmatic air.[39] The statutes may also reflect a more general suspicion of butchers and concern to regulate their trade: in the first half of the fifteenth century, during the social dislocation and food shortages caused by the Hundred Years' War, they had prospered by exploiting the market and charging unacceptably high prices.[40] Even so, the prohibition placed on the sale of meat from animals reared at *leprosaria* is emphatic, encompassing all livestock without exception. This suggests that it may then have been difficult for leper house communities in Normandy to sell their agricultural produce, and that the disease was still feared, even if fewer cases were actually being confirmed. Another document, an ordinance of Charles VIII authorizing the location of butcheries in the suburbs of Rouen, issued in December 1487, also testifies to continuing anxieties about the consumption of infected meat. Butchers trading there were forbidden to sell 'pork or [the flesh of any] other beast nourished at the house of a lord, a marshal or a leper'.[41] Pork was particularly associated with leprosy, as it could manifest spots and tubercules very similar to those of the leprous.[42] Interestingly, the reference here to the house of a single

---

[34] '*très-grant dangier et prejudice des creatures humaines*': 'Statuts des bouchers', ed. de Pastoret, 39.

[35] '*entechiez d'aucunes maladies*': *ibid.*, 41.

[36] '*povres prisonniers*': *ibid.*, 41–2. For the word '*seursemé*', or 'susmy', which means 'corrupted with blood or matter', see D.R. Carr, 'Controlling the Butchers in Late Medieval English Towns', *The Historian*, lxx (2008), 458, n. 43.

[37] '*beste quelle qu'elle soit qui vienne de maladerie*': 'Statuts des bouchers', ed. de Pastoret, 42.

[38] *Ibid.*, 42.

[39] Carole Rawcliffe, *Urban Bodies: Communal Health in Late Medieval English Towns and Cities* (Woodbridge, 2013), ch. 4.

[40] Lucien-René Delsalle, *Rouen et les Rouennais au temps de Jeanne d'Arc, 1400–1470* (Rouen, 1982), 71–2.

[41] '*porc ne austre beste nourrie de l'ostel d'un saigneur, d'un mareschal ou d'un ladre*': 'Création de boucheries dans les faubourgs de Rouen', in *Ordonnances des rois de France, XX*, ed. de Pastoret, 50.

[42] Rawcliffe, *Leprosy*, 80.

'*ladre*' indicates that some lepers, probably those of high status or members of the priesthood, remained in their private residences after developing the disease, rather than entering *leprosaria* (or, indeed, taking to the road as beggars). It is unclear why animals belonging to lords or marshals posed a problem, other, perhaps, than being intended for the royal army. However, the restriction placed upon pigs and other beasts reared by lepers was almost certainly prompted by beliefs about the transmission of the disease from humans to animals and *vice versa*.

On the face of it, certain aspects of these two sets of prescriptions from June 1432 (confirmed in November 1487) and December 1487 appear inconsistent with concerns about the medical risks arising from the sale of contaminated meat. In 1432, for example, it was considered acceptable for poor prisoners to eat diseased pork. It is likely that these individuals were believed to be impervious to the ill effects of such food because of the immunity bestowed over the years by their own unwholesome diets.[43] Nonetheless, according to contemporary notions of disease transmission, both by miasmatic air and through physical contact, their consumption of infected meat might still result in the spread of disease among the wider urban population. The city's prisons, such as that of the official of Rouen close to the cathedral, and the gaol of the *bailliage* in the rue Bouvreuil, were located within the walls; and, as is the case today, not all of the inmates were incarcerated on a permanent basis.[44] Indeed, since medieval prisons were accessible, permeable institutions, they represented a recognised source of airborne pollution, especially as so many inmates came into contact with members of mainstream society, both within and outside the gates.[45] In December 1487 Charles VIII ordered that any corrupt or diseased pork confiscated from the butcheries outside Rouen should henceforward be given to the poor in general, whose own digestions were, once again, deemed to be more robust and whose health, perhaps, was of secondary importance.[46] Yet poor people could similarly spread disease to others with ease, particularly since they so often lived in cramped, insanitary conditions.

It is also perplexing to discover that in both 1432 and 1487 bad meat was to be thrown in the river Seine, despite late medieval concerns about the pollution of water supplies, as manifested in the 1321 'Lepers' Plot'.[47] Admittedly, the inhabitants of Rouen may not have obtained their drinking water from the Seine, instead using the fountains located throughout the city.[48] This type of waste disposal may also have been acceptable because it was believed that offensive

---

[43] Some canon lawyers maintained that simple, inexpensive, even substandard, food was appropriate for the poor, while rich, high quality fare might damage their health: Brian Tierney, 'The Decretists and the "Deserving Poor"', *Comparative Studies in Society and History*, i (1958–9), 366.

[44] On Rouen's prisons, see Periaux, *Dictionnaire*, 23, 501, 587, 663. On the relative freedom of prisoners in late medieval Italian prisons, see Guy Geltner, *The Medieval Prison: A Social History* (Princeton, N.J., 2008), 77–80.

[45] On the permeability of medieval prisons, see Geltner, *Medieval Prison*, 72–3.

[46] 'Création de boucheries', ed. de Pastoret, 50.

[47] 'Statuts des bouchers', ed. de Pastoret, 42; 'Création de boucheries', ed. *idem*, 50.

[48] Rouen's water supply was described in detail in Jacques Le Lieur's famous *Livre des fontaines* (1525): Rouen, Bibliothèque Municipale [henceforth Rouen, BM], MS G3; Jacques Le Lieur, *Le livre des fontaines*, ed. Lucien-René Delsalle, Benoît Eliot and Stéphane Rioland (facsimile edition, Bonsecours, 2005).

matter would soon be carried away on the tide.[49] Nonetheless, there had been a ban upon the disposal of rubbish in the river Robec, one of the Seine's tributaries, since 1407. Later, in 1518 (a plague year), it was decided to clean the river Renelle, in the western part of the city.[50] Such initiatives testify to a continuing awareness of the need to keep Rouen's water courses unpolluted and free from blockages, which would cause stagnant water and thus disease.

Royal and municipal provisions regarding the activities of butchers were not confined to Rouen: for instance, many such ordinances were promulgated in the towns and cities of England in the fourteenth and fifteenth centuries.[51] David Carr argues that these measures resulted from the stench and mess generated by the butchers' trade. The best way to provide fresh meat was to slaughter animals within the walls, which inevitably gave rise to unpleasant smells, blood and offal in public places.[52] Regulations for the removal of rubbish from the streets of late medieval cities often focused upon the offensive matter resulting from butchery, not least because magistrates were so concerned about the respectability and proper appearance of their cities, as well as preventing the spread of disease through contaminated food and miasmatic air. In towns such as Bristol, Coventry and Northampton, as in Rouen, they were determined that butchers should not harm the community and its reputation by selling spoiled, corrupt meat. Whereas in Rouen substandard pork was given to prisoners and the poor, in Northampton in 1460 it was assigned to the 'sick men' at the *leprosarium* of St. Leonard, reflecting a widespread assumption that lepers could also eat 'susmy' meat with impunity, since they were already infected.[53]

In October 1499, a group of *conseillers* (councillors) of Rouen's civic government met to discuss the preventative measures needed to contain a recent outbreak of plague. They may well have been made responsible for protecting the city from pestilence, and thus have possessed a specialised knowledge of matters concerning public health.[54] On Sunday 13 October 1499, following deaths 'from the black plague' in the parishes of Saint-Jean-sur-Renelle and Saint-Maclou, 'and other places', they drew up a set of '*Reglements pour le fait de la Contagion*'.[55] The account of their deliberations reflects entrenched beliefs about the need for cleanliness in the city, and about the role of livestock, as well as carcasses and offal, in the transmission of disease. One councillor, Monsieur de Longpaon, asserted that 'the matter and sickness would cease if pigs and fowl were removed',

---

[49] Similarly, in 1343, the rulers of London accorded butchers the right to dispose of offal from a wharf on the Fleet, apparently believing that the power of the stream would flush the waste into the tidal Thames: E.L. Sabine, 'Butchering in Mediaeval London', *Speculum*, viii (1933), 343–4; Carr, 'Controlling the Butchers', 452–3.

[50] Fournée, 'Les normands', 43, 44.

[51] For London, see Sabine, 'Butchering', 335–53.

[52] Carr, 'Controlling the Butchers', 450, 452, 461; see also Lardin, 'Rouennais et pollution', 418.

[53] Carr, 'Controlling the Butchers', 450–1, 458–9, 460–1. On the gift of bad food to leper communities, see also Rawcliffe, *Leprosy*, 79–80.

[54] See Kinzelbach, 'Infection', 380, on the 'experts' in southern German municipal governments who dealt with pestilence between c.1450 and c.1550.

[55] '*de la peste noire … et autres lieux*': Rouen, AdSM, AMR, Registre A 9, f. 318; Lardin, 'Rouennais et pollution', 418, 419; Porquet, *La peste en Normandie*, 124–5.

and that rubbish should not be deposited in the streets.[56] Another, identified as Master Guillaume, agreed that vagrant pigs and other beasts should be rounded up and the streets kept clean. He also urged prayer to God, underscoring the value placed upon spiritual remedies in combating plague. Monsieur de Ponicer argued that the civic abattoirs should be reactivated, and the butchers compelled to use them. His proposal testifies to continuing concern about the slaughter of animals in public places and the mess thereby created, as well as to the by now unshakeable conviction that such noxious waste helped to transmit disease. Pierre de Quevremont appears to have had a clear understanding of person-to-person contagion, maintaining that 'with regard to … the poor sick, one must forbid them from communication among the people'.[57] On the other hand, he also observed that pigs and fowl 'engender infections'.[58]

Pigs were regarded as an insanitary nuisance in European cities from at least the early fourteenth century. The association of swine and fowl with infection stemmed in part from the fact that these animals consumed waste material, itself linked to the spread of disease.[59] Pigs also left dung in public places, constituted a notorious threat to small children and were, moreover, associated with wider problems of disorder and vagrancy. However, the suggestions made by officers of Rouen's municipal government in 1499 were wide-ranging, addressing not only the unwelcome presence of livestock, but also the cleanliness of the streets, the use of slaughterhouses and the risks of contagion from human to human. An outbreak of the plague was clearly the occasion for urgent debate among the ruling elite about how best to preserve the health of the city. Philippe Lardin argues that the word 'infection' in late medieval documents generally signifies a bad smell which appeared damaging to human health, although sometimes, particularly with regard to the clothing and houses of plague victims, air was judged to be dangerous without carrying any obvious stench.[60] This account of deliberations in 1499, therefore, reveals an awareness both of the risks posed by miasmas, and, apparently, of theories concerning the transmission of disease between people through touch and other types of close personal contact.

Institutional Change: Rouen's Leprosaria in the Later Middle Ages

Although anxiety about leprosy clearly helped to shape measures for safeguarding communal health in late medieval Rouen, the city's *leprosaria* were themselves in decline at this time, as was the disease itself across most of Western Europe. While it is clear that leprosy did recede in the later Middle Ages, as a result of the adoption of tighter diagnostic criteria, the spread of better living conditions and the development of higher levels of immunity, as well as, perhaps, climatic change, it is important to recognise that the disease only ever affected a relatively small

---

[56] '*cessera la chose et malladie en brief si des porcs et oysons les s'oster*': Rouen, AdSM, AMR, Registre A 9, f. 318.
[57] '*en regard de ceulx que les pauvres mallades on leur doit deffendre la communication parmi le peuple*': *ibid.*
[58] '*engendrent infections*': *ibid.*
[59] See Lardin, 'Rouennais et pollution', 417–18.
[60] *Ibid.*, 419–22.

number of people, even during its apparent peak in the twelfth and thirteenth centuries.[61] In short, it aroused a mixed response of fear and compassion that was out of all proportion to the percentage of the population at risk. Charity for lepers and *leprosaria* became less fashionable after 1300, in tandem with increasingly negative responses to the leprous (or at least those of low status) and growing concerns about contagion.[62] By 1586, the small *leprosarium* of Saint-Léger-du-Bourg-Denis, east of Rouen, which had served the parishes of Saint-Paul, Saint-Maclou and Saint-Cande-le-Vieux, was described as being 'ruined and destroyed'.[63] It is likely that many, if not all, of the other smaller *leprosaria* around the city, at Répainville (immediately north-east of Rouen), Darnétal (further eastwards), Bois-Guillaume (north of Rouen), Saint-Sever (immediately south of the river Seine), and Sotteville-lès-Rouen (south of Rouen), had also fallen into disuse or disappeared completely by the later sixteenth century, if not one or two hundred years earlier.[64]

As we have seen, on 31 August 1366, the *leprosarium* of Salle-aux-Puelles at Petit-Quevilly, south-west of Rouen, with all its rights and possessions, was awarded to La Madeleine, Rouen's hospital for the sick poor, by Charles V.[65] The king made his gift at the behest of Thomas Le Tourneur, a royal clerk and canon of Rouen cathedral from 1357 to 1384.[66] Le Tourneur exercised considerable influence in court circles: he served as master of accounts and first secretary to Charles V, and was one of the king's executors on his death in 1380.[67] As a cathedral canon, his support for La Madeleine is hardly surprising, since from its foundation, in the eleventh century or earlier, the hospital had been closely associated with Rouen cathedral. La Madeleine's memorial book, first compiled in the 1460s, but apparently containing entries from an earlier volume, reveals that Thomas also made substantial gifts to the hospital himself.[68]

The context for the unification of Salle-aux-Puelles with La Madeleine was the great financial need of the latter institution in the 1360s, following the Black Death (and the more recent plague outbreak of 1362) and the first decades of the Hundred

---

[61] Rawcliffe, *Leprosy*, 345, 346.

[62] *Ibid.*, 347–8. On the development of the idea that leprosy might be contracted through proximity to, or physical contact with, its victims, as well as other external hazards, see Touati, 'Historiciser', 175–83.

[63] '*ruinée et desmollye*': Rouen, AdSM, G6897, ff. 90–1; Charles de Robillard de Beaurepaire, *Inventaire-sommaire des Archives Départementales antérieures à 1790: Seine-Inférieure, archives ecclésiastiques – Série G*, v (nos. 6221–7370) (Rouen, 1892), 287–8; Jean Fournée, 'Les maladreries et les vocables de leurs chapelles', *Lèpre et lépreux en Normandie, Cahiers Léopold Delisle*, xlvi (1997), 111.

[64] On Rouen's *leprosaria*, see Philippe Deschamps, 'Léproseries et maladreries rouennaises: le prieuré du Mont-aux-Malades et ses rapports avec Thomas Becket', *Revue des sociétés savantes de Haute-Normandie*, xlviii (1967), 31–2. The majority of English leper houses declined, changed their function or disappeared in the 14th century (Rawcliffe, *Leprosy*, 348–50); Rouen's *leprosaria* could well have followed a similar pattern.

[65] Rouen, BM, MS Y42 (15th-century memorial book of La Madeleine hospital), f. 50v.

[66] *Ibid.*, f. 31.

[67] Vincent Tabbagh, *Fasti ecclesiae gallicanae: répertoire prosopographique des évêques, dignitaires et chanoines de France de 1200 à 1500. Tome II: diocèse de Rouen* (Turnhout, 1998), 378–9; Catherine Dubois, 'Les Rouennais face à la mort au XVe siècle, d'après l'obituaire du prieuré de la Madeleine' (Rouen Univ. Master's thesis, 1990), 47.

[68] Rouen, BM, MS Y42, f. 31; Dubois, 'Les Rouennais', 10–11, 47.

Years' War. In October 1359, the future Charles V, then duke of Normandy, had already taken steps to assist La Madeleine by exempting it from taxes (*octrois*), specifically because of the losses sustained through the destruction wrought by the English. His grant observed that, at the same time, 'the good people of the countryside' were taking refuge there in growing numbers, including the sick and women made pregnant by the enemy.[69] It was necessary to accommodate the latter until after they had given birth and, in due course, to feed their infants.[70] Besides caring for the acutely sick, La Madeleine customarily provided assistance to women in childbirth, as we can see from the appearance in its memorial book of an *obstetrix*, Agnes La Gorelle, who worked as a midwife there for twenty-five years.[71] It also took responsibility for abandoned infants, often sending them to wet nurses in the countryside around Rouen.[72] These obligations help to explain why the hospital's resources were so stretched during a period of warfare and social and economic turmoil.

Salle-aux-Puelles is traditionally believed to have catered for aristocratic women suffering from leprosy, and was a wealthy institution. Its earliest endowment dated from between 1185 and 1188, when Henry II, king of England (1154–89) and duke of Normandy (1150–89), donated a manor house and other property from his estates at Petit-Quevilly, together with an annual income of 200 *livres* of Anjou from the *vicomté* of Rouen, 'to the leprous women of Quevilly'.[73] The English king's patronage probably explains why, following the annexation of Normandy to France in 1204, it seemed appropriate for a French monarch to donate the *leprosarium* to another religious house. Henry II had also granted the women a meadow at Quevilly, and the right to put their animals to pasture in the nearby forest of Rouvray, where they could commandeer wood to heat and repair their buildings.[74] Salle-aux-Puelles thus possessed valuable agricultural resources, as confirmed by an account of the visit of Eudes Rigaud, archbishop of Rouen (1248–75), in 1258, which mentions 'lands before the gate', a grange at Quevilly, and 'meadows that suffice well for the pasture of their animals for the use of the house'.[75] In addition, Salle-aux-Puelles exercised the patronage of two local churches, Saint-Martin of Grand-Couronne and Saint-Jacques of Moulineaux, which yielded tithes and other emoluments.[76] Its annexation to La Madeleine thus conferred significant revenues, lands and property on Rouen's principal hospital.

---

[69] '*des bonnes gens du pais*': *Documents concernant les pauvres de Rouen: extraits des archives de l'hôtel-de-ville*, ed. Gustave Panel (3 vols., Rouen, 1917–19), i. pp. xxviii, 3. On refugees flocking to Rouen later in the Hundred Years' War, in 1417 and 1423, see Delsalle, *Rouen*, 71.

[70] *Documents*, ed. Panel, i. pp. xxviii, 3.

[71] Rouen, BM, MS Y42, f. 6.

[72] *Documents*, ed. Panel, i. pp. xxviii–ix.

[73] '*feminis leprosis de Keuilli*': charter of Henry II in favour of the leprous women of Salle-aux-Puelles, Cherbourg, undated (April 1185/January 1188): Rouen, AdSM, 27HP95 (14th-century? copy made under the seal of the *mairie* of Rouen); *The Letters and Charters of King Henry II (1154–1189)*, ed. Nicholas Vincent *et al.* (Oxford, forthcoming); *Recueil des actes de Henri II, roi d'Angleterre et duc de Normandie*, ed. Léopold Delisle and Élie Berger (4 vols., Paris, 1909–27), ii. 296–7.

[74] Charter of Henry II in favour of Salle-aux-Puelles (April 1185/January 1188).

[75] '*terras ante portam … prata que eis sufficient bene pro suis animalibus pascendum ad usum domus*': *Regestrum*, ed. Bonnin, 325; *Register*, ed. O'Sullivan, 372.

[76] *The Letters and Charters of King Richard I (1189–1199)*, ed. Judith Everard and Nicholas Vincent (Oxford, forthcoming) (donation of the church of Grand-Couronne to the leprous women of

In the context of plague and war, which affected large numbers of people in Rouen and the surrounding area, the needs of the leprous women of Salle-aux-Puelles must have seemed less compelling. There might also have been fewer of them at the house by 1366 than there had been in the late twelfth and thirteenth centuries, due to both the impact of pestilence and enemy action (Salle-aux-Puelles was located in the vulnerable countryside) and the decline of leprosy itself. When discussing events in the 1330s, the chronicler Pierre Cochon describes, in passing, a deserted scene outside Salle-aux-Puelles, where the only person to be found was a mad woman begging at the edge of the woods.[77] The Black Death alone could well have destroyed the entire community, as it did, for example, at the female *leprosarium* of St. James, Westminster.[78] Since the establishment at Salle-aux-Puelles was small even in the mid thirteenth century – in 1258 there were just ten leprous sisters there and one who was 'healthy' – these factors alone would have justified the diversion of its revenues to La Madeleine.[79]

Yet the arrangements regarding the royal donation of Salle-aux-Puelles to La Madeleine in 1366 were predicated on the assumption that the *leprosarium* would still continue to function, in terms of both the spiritual and the physical care of the sick, and suggest that the merger may, in fact, have been prompted by a desire to improve falling standards there. Charles V's award, as recorded in La Madeleine's memorial book, specified that Mass was to be celebrated in the church of Saint-Julien at Salle-aux-Puelles every Sunday, and on solemn days and feasts.[80] His donation charter of November 1366 (a document distinct from the entry in the memorial book) expressed hope that the spiritual health of 'the miserable persons infected with the disease of leprosy' would be tended 'more devotedly and more carefully', and stipulated that the residents were in future to have 'a sufficiency of victuals'.[81] The existing situation at Salle-aux-Puelles clearly left much to be desired. The king instructed the archbishop of Rouen to annex the church of Saint-Julien to La Madeleine in such a way that, when the living fell vacant, the prior of La Madeleine or a nominee would take responsibility for it and ensure that the divine office was regularly celebrated and the sacraments were administered to the inmates, 'as has been the custom there thus far'.[82] Tellingly, he ordered that temporal affairs were to be managed in such a way that 'there should not be a lack of humanity and physical support for the miserable persons staying there and who

Quevilly by Richard I, king of England, 4 Apr. 1195); François Farin, *Histoire de la ville de Rouen* (2 vols., Rouen, 1731), ii (5), 122; Pierre Duchemin, *Petit-Quevilly et le prieuré de Saint-Julien* (Pont-Audemer, 1890; repr. Saint-Étienne-du-Rouvray, 1987), 231 (on the donation of the tithes of Grand-Couronne to Salle-aux-Puelles by Roger Deshays, his wife Jeanne, his brother Étienne and his son Guillaume); Fournée, 'Les maladreries', 106 (on Henry II's donation of the church of Moulineaux to Salle-aux-Puelles, for which I have not found original documentation, although 13th-century documents confirm the *leprosarium*'s possession of the church by this time).

[77] *Chronique normande de Pierre Cochon*, ed. de Beaurepaire, 67.

[78] Rawcliffe, *Leprosy*, 349.

[79] *Regestrum*, ed. Bonnin, 325; *Register*, ed. O'Sullivan, 371.

[80] Rouen, BM, MS Y42, f. 50v.

[81] '*miserabilibus personis morbo lepræ infectis ... devotius et curiosius ... sufficientiam victualium*': Rouen, AdSM, H-Dépôt 1, A39 (from a 17th-century? printed copy, 1–2).

[82] '*sicut est inibi hactenus consuetum*': *ibid.* (printed copy, 2).

will live there in the future'.[83] He further emphasised this point by insisting that 'all the necessities should be administered to every single one of these persons, so that they should not have to scavenge for supplies through need of victuals'.[84]

These provisions indicate that, by the ruling authorities at least, the leprous women of Salle-aux-Puelles were viewed with compassion: they were 'miserable persons' who had evidently been neglected and were henceforward to be treated more humanely. Such solicitude challenges the view that attitudes towards the leprous became uniformly less positive in the fourteenth century, particularly following the Black Death.[85] Here, in 1366, the king of France appears to have been genuinely concerned about the suffering and needs of the sick, albeit those from reputable families. Similarly, Thomas Le Tourneur's initiative for the annexation of Salle-aux-Puelles could have arisen as much from an awareness of poor conditions at the *leprosarium* as from a desire to meet the urgent needs of La Madeleine. It was clearly expected that there would be leprous women at Salle-aux-Puelles in the future, and recognised that they should be supported in a decent fashion, according to established practices which had been allowed to lapse. In July 1377, Pope Gregory XI (1370–8) confirmed the donation, instructing the bishop of Paris to annex the church of Saint-Julien and the house of Salle-aux-Puelles to La Madeleine. Like Charles V's charter, the papal confirmation provided for the continuation of spiritual and bodily care at Salle-aux-Puelles, ordering the bishop to ensure 'that in the said church and house there are as many chaplains and ministers as there are now and is the custom, and that in the church divine offices are served, and that the sick in the house are received and nourished as previously'.[86] Thus, although the resources of Salle-aux-Puelles were centralised in order to benefit other categories of the sick and needy, the institution itself was still to provide for lepers, in a more effective and sympathetic manner. In light of the reference to scavenging, we might, perhaps, also conclude that steps were being taken to dissuade the inmates from begging in public places and thus posing a threat to the healthy.

By the mid fifteenth century, the *leprosarium* of Mont-aux-Malades, like many other monastic houses in the Rouen area, was also feeling the effects of the Hundred Years' War.[87] In March 1443, the religious of Mont-aux-Malades appealed to Pope Eugenius IV (1431–47) for assistance, since their income had fallen 'because of the upheavals of the wars in those parts and especially in the

---

[83] '*ne quid in miserabilibus personis inibi morantibus et quæ ibi degent imposterum humanitatis et temporalitatis desit*': *ibid*.

[84] '*quinimo unicuique ipsarum personarum ita sufficienter ministretur in temporalibus, quod super victualium penuriâ non habeant materiam conquirendi*': *ibid*.

[85] On historians' views about changing responses to leprosy in the 14th century, see Elma Brenner, 'Recent Perspectives on Leprosy in Medieval Western Europe', *History Compass*, viii (5) (2010), 390–2.

[86] '*quod in ecclesia et domo predictis sint tot capellani et ministri sicut nunc sunt et esse consueuerunt ac in ecclesia in diuinis deseruiatur et infirmi in dicta domo recipiantur et alimententur sicut prius*': Rouen, AdSM, H-Dépôt 1, A39.

[87] For the difficulties faced by other religious houses in Rouen and the surrounding area between 1417 and 1451, including the abbey of Saint-Ouen, the hospital of La Madeleine and the priories of Saint-Lô and Notre-Dame-du-Pré, see *La désolation des églises, monastères, hôpitaux en France vers le milieu du XVe siècle*, ed. Henri Denifle (3 vols., Mâcon and Paris, 1897–9), i. nos. 177–86, pp. 66–70.

Pays de Caux, in which such revenues were for the most part founded'.[88] Mont-aux-Malades had received land in this fertile area, west of Rouen, from Henry II in the 1170s, and the devastation of so much rich agricultural territory during the ongoing hostilities had serious financial implications for the community.[89] At least according to the petition of 1443, which may have resorted to special pleading, the hospital was still actively providing for lepers at this time. It accommodated patients of both sexes from twenty-one of Rouen's parishes, as well as offering bed and board to passing lepers, thereby discharging obligations which were 'not without great expenses'.[90] In the fourteenth and fifteenth centuries, therefore, it seems that Rouen's two major *leprosaria* still sheltered the leprous, fulfilling a vital public health function by separating individuals believed to be a major source of miasmatic air and infection from mainstream society. The service performed by Mont-aux-Malades in lodging itinerant lepers, who were associated with vagrancy and the spread of disease, must have seemed particularly important.

Conclusion: *Leprosy and Public Health in Sixteenth-Century Rouen*

Although leprosy in Western Europe was undoubtedly in decline by the sixteenth century, contemporary sources indicate that cases of the disease were still being confirmed in Rouen, and that lepers still resided at Mont-aux-Malades. In the early modern period there was 'an increasing elasticity in the identification of leprosy', which may have led to a number of mistaken diagnoses, as had previously happened in the twelfth and thirteenth centuries.[91] On 19 February 1524, three civic *conseillers*, Jean Le Roux, Guillaume Auber and Jean du Hamel, reported to royal officers on their inspection of Mont-aux-Malades. They had found that the church, refectory, kitchen, dormitory and other buildings were in good repair, but were being used by religious members of the community rather than by the sick, which suggests that the care of lepers was no longer the primary focus there.[92] Nonetheless, three lepers from Rouen (two men from the parish of Saint-Lô and a woman from that of Notre-Dame-de-la-Ronde) were living there in separate lodgings. The *conseillers* noted that the woman, 'who was in her bed, extremely sick', occupied a room without a fire, which implies a degree of neglect, as it must then have been very cold.[93] Mont-aux-Malades also still catered for itinerant lepers

---

[88] '*causantibus tamen guerrarum turbinibus in partibus illis et potissime in patria Caleti, in qua hujusmodi introitus pro majori parte fundati sunt*': *ibid.*, i. no. 186, p. 70.

[89] Charter of Henry II granting various privileges, rights and lands to Mont-aux-Malades, including an area of land in the Pays de Caux between Nointot and the valley road from Bolbec to Mirville, undated (May 1172/July 1178 or perhaps between May 1172 and May 1175): Rouen, AdSM, 25HP1, folder 1, document i; *Letters and Charters of Henry II*, ed. Vincent *et al.*; *Désolation*, ed. Denifle, i. no. 186, p. 70.

[90] '*non sine magnis expensis*': *Désolation*, ed. Denifle, i. no. 186, p. 70.

[91] Luke Demaitre, *Leprosy in Premodern Medicine: A Malady of the Whole Body* (Baltimore, Md., 2007), 155.

[92] AN, S4889B, dossier 13, last document, ff. 1, 2v.

[93] '*La quelle estoit en son lit bien fort mallade*': *ibid.*, f. 1–1v.

at this time, since the *conseillers* visited 'the hospital for the poor passing sick', which was probably located well away from the main priory buildings.[94]

The content and tone of the councillors' account of their inspection confirm that they were inquiring into conditions of care at Mont-aux-Malades, and were displeased by the indifference shown by the canons to the needs of the lepers, particularly since, as they argued, the original intention of the foundation had been for the sick to be treated in the same way as the religious themselves.[95] It certainly appears that, by the sixteenth century and probably far earlier, civic health concerns regarding leprosy encompassed the needs and wellbeing of the leprous themselves. While the urban community as a whole had to be protected from infection, those within it who succumbed to the disease were to be properly supported, since their spiritual and physical welfare, like that of other citizens, still remained paramount.

In October 1536, Jean du Tremblé, 'suspected of the disease of leprosy', was taken to Mont-aux-Malades, where he was examined by the leprous brothers and sisters (evidently still being accommodated there twelve years after the municipal inspection), who confirmed the diagnosis.[96] Almost half a century later, in September 1586, residents of the parish of Saint-Maclou paid two physicians and a surgeon 6 *livres* for examining Madeleine Morin, the wife of Jehan Prévost, and their daughter Robine to ascertain whether the two women had been infected. Another positive verdict was accompanied by the customary warning that they would have to live apart from the healthy. The parochial authorities duly arranged for the ruined *leprosarium* of Saint-Léger-du-Bourg-Denis, to which they traditionally sent confirmed lepers, to be rebuilt to accommodate them.[97]

These careful examinations and the subsequent arrangements for segregating the sick indicate that there was still appreciable fear of leprosy in early modern Rouen. Following the Black Death, and in the light of recurrent outbreaks of plague in the fifteenth and sixteenth centuries, anxiety about the interconnected threat of leprosy and miasmatic air was manifested in regulations concerning the sale of meat, efforts to diagnose and isolate those perceived to be leprous, and the revival of at least one *leprosarium*, as well as the continuity of care provided by Mont-aux-Malades and perhaps also Salle-aux-Puelles. Social and economic factors, particularly the impact of epidemic disease and of the Hundred Years' War, together with shifting patterns in lay piety, undoubtedly affected the status and prosperity of *leprosaria* and their residents. Although leprosy retained much of the spiritual symbolism that had surrounded it in earlier centuries, its transformation into a perceived health hazard in late medieval Rouen should be understood in the context of changing ideas about the spread of disease, shaped above all by *regimina sanitatis*, and a new awareness of the 'common public good' of the city and the importance of protecting it.

---

[94]   '*l'hospital ordonne pour les povres mallades*'. This hospital was situated near the parish church of Saint-Jacques at Mont-aux-Malades, 'within the enclosure' ('*dedens l'enclos*'), meaning that, although it lay inside the confines of the priory grounds, it was probably some distance from the central complex of buildings: *ibid.*, f. 1v.

[95]   *Ibid.*, f. 2–2v.

[96]   '*de morbo lepre suspectus*': Rouen, AdSM, G6606.

[97]   Rouen, AdSM, G6897, ff. 89–90v. *Leprosaria* were also sometimes rebuilt in England: see, for example, the case of Beverley, Yorkshire, discussed in Rawcliffe, *Leprosy*, 319.

PLAGUE ORDINANCES AND THE MANAGEMENT OF INFECTIOUS DISEASES IN NORTHERN FRENCH TOWNS, c.1450–c.1560[*]

Neil Murphy

During the first half of the sixteenth century, municipal councils across northern France issued ordinances designed to combat outbreaks of plague. The measures contained in these ordinances were extensive and formed the core of urban responses to plague throughout the early modern period. These ordinances did not appear out of a vacuum; rather, they represented the codification of stratagems adopted during the second half of the fifteenth century. This article will describe and account for the growth of the public health system developed by the magistrates of towns lying in the urban belt of northern and north-eastern France from the 1450s to the 1550s. It will concentrate on the towns and cities of Abbeville, Amiens, Beauvais, Paris, Rouen and Tournai, all of which possess good administrative records for the period.[1] In addition to the texts of plague ordinances, the most valuable documents for this study are the registers of municipal deliberations, which allow us to follow the decision-making process that lay behind the development of plague legislation.

Many of the more celebrated measures against pestilence originated in fourteenth- and fifteenth-century Italy, and the bulk of our knowledge regarding

[*] I wish to thank Professors Samuel Cohn and Carole Rawcliffe for their insightful comments on this article.

[1] Registers of deliberations were kept at Amiens from 1406 (Archives Municipales Amiens [henceforth AMA], BB 1); at Paris from 1499 – *Registres des délibérations du Bureau de la ville de Paris. Tome premier, 1499–1526*, ed. François Bonnardot (Paris, 1883) – and at Rouen from 1389 (Archives Municipales Rouen [henceforth AMR], A 1). Although the municipal archives of Abbeville, Beauvais and Tournai were largely destroyed in 1940, extensive extracts from them were published in the late 19th and early 20th centuries, while manuscript copies of the registers for Abbeville and Beauvais were made in the 18th and 19th centuries. For Abbeville: Bibliothèque Municipale Abbeville [henceforth BMA], 347, 371; A.A. Ledieu, *Ville d'Abbeville. Inventaire sommaire des archives municipales antérieures à 1790* (Abbeville, 1902). For Beauvais: Bibliothèque Municipale Beauvais [henceforth BMB], Collection Bucquet-aux-Cousteaux, 55, 57; Renaud Rose, *Ville de Beauvais. Inventaire sommaire des archives communales antérieures à 1790* (Beauvais, 1887). For Tournai: A.L. de La Grange, 'Extraits analytiques des registres des consaulx de la ville de Tournai, 1431–1476', *Mémoires de la société historique et littéraire de Tournai*, xxiii (1983), 1–396; Henri Vandenbroeck, 'Extraits analytiques des anciens registres des consaux de la ville de Tournai, 1388–1422', *Société historique et littéraire de Tournai. Mémoires*, vii (1861), 1–302. For registers of municipal deliberations in France generally, see Graeme Small, 'Municipal registers of deliberations in the fourteenth and fifteenth centuries: Cross-Channel Observations', in *Les idées passent-elles la Manche. Savoirs, Représentations, Pratiques (France-Angleterre, Xe–XXe siècles)*, ed. J.-P. Genet and F.-J. Ruggiu (Paris, 2007), 27–66.

the ways in which urban administrations reacted to these outbreaks is based on studies of northern Italian cities, such as Florence and Venice.[2] Although historians have expanded the geographical scope of such studies to consider municipal responses to plague in England, Spain, Switzerland, Germany and the Low Countries, little research has been done on France during the fifteenth and sixteenth centuries.[3] Most studies examining the impact of plague in France concentrate on the devastating outbreaks of the fourteenth, seventeenth and early eighteenth centuries. As a result, scant attention has been paid to the development of municipal plague legislation during the years between 1400 and 1600.[4] This is a significant oversight, as the methods devised by municipal councils to cope with plague during this period laid the foundations of urban responses to the disease right through to the end of Louis XIV's reign. Although it appeared almost forty

[2]   Among the numerous studies on this topic, see especially W.M. Bowsky, 'The Impact of the Black Death upon Sienese Government and Society', *Speculum*, xxxix (1964), 1–34; Ann Carmichael, *Plague and the Poor in Renaissance Florence* (Cambridge, 1986); *eadem*, 'Plague Legislation in the Italian Renaissance', *Bulletin of the History of Medicine*, lvii (1983), 508–25; Élisabeth Charpentier, *Une ville devant la peste: Orvieto et la peste noire de 1348* (Paris, 1962); Giala Calvi, *Histories of a Plague Year: The Social and the Imaginary in Baroque Florence* (Berkeley, Calif., 1989); C.M. Cipolla, *Cristofano and the Plague* (1973); *idem*, *Fighting the Plague in Seventeenth-Century Italy* (1981); S.K. Cohn, Jr., *Cultures of Plague: Medical Thinking at the End of the Renaissance* (Oxford, 2010); J.L. Stevens Crawshaw, *Plague Hospitals: Public Health for the City in Early Modern Venice* (Aldershot, 2012); John Henderson, 'Plague in Renaissance Florence: Medical Theory and Government Response', in *Maladies et sociétiés (XIIe–XVIIIe siècles)*, ed. Neithard Bulst and Robert Delort (Paris, 1989), 165–86; *idem*, 'The Black Death in Florence: Medical and Communal Responses', in *Death in Towns: Urban Responses to the Dying and the Dead, 100–1600*, ed. Steven Bassett (Leicester, 1992), 139–41; R.J. Palmer, 'The Control of Plague in Venice and Northern Italy, 1348–1600' (Univ. of Kent Ph.D. thesis, 1978).

[3]   Bartolomé Bennassar, *Recherches sur les grands épidémies dans le nord de l'Espagne à la fin du XVIe siècle* (Paris, 1969); J.L. Betrán, *La peste en la Barcelona de los Austrias* (Lleida, 1996); W.P. Blockmans, 'The Social and Economic Effects of Plague in the Low Countries', *Revue belge de philologie et d'histoire*, lviii (1980), 833–63; J.G. Carmona García, *La peste en Seville* (Seville, 2004); A.P. Cook and N.D. Cook, *The Plague Files: Crisis Management in Sixteenth-Century Seville* (Baton Rouge, La., 2009); M.L. Hammond, 'Contagion, Honour and Urban Life in Early Modern Germany', in *Imagining Contagion in Early Modern Europe*, ed. C.L. Carlin (Basingstoke, 2005), 179–201; Paul Slack, *The Impact of Plague in Tudor and Stuart England* (1985); W.G. Naphy, *Plagues, Poisons and Potions: Plague-Spreading Conspiracies in the Western Alps c.1530–1640* (Manchester, 2002).

[4]   For works on France, see Jean Canard, *Les pestes en Beaujolais, Forez, Jarez, Lyonnais du XIVème au XVIIIème siècle* (Régny, 1979); M.P. Chase, 'Fevers, Poisons, and Apostemes: Authority and Experience in Montpellier Plague Treatises', in *Science and Technology in the Middle Ages*, ed. P.O. Long (New York, 1985), 153–70; Jean Delumeau and Yves Lequin, *Les Malheurs des temps. Histoire des fléaux et des calamités en France* (Paris, 1987); Jean Delumeau, *La Peur en occident (XIIe–XVIIIe siècles)* (Paris, 1978); R.W. Emery, 'The Black Death of 1348 in Perpignan', *Speculum*, xlii (1967), 611–23; Colin Jones, 'Plague and its Metaphors in Early Modern France', *Representations*, liii (1996), 97–127; Monique Lucenet, *Les Grandes Pestes en France* (Paris, 1985); Daniel Gordon, 'The City and Plague in the Age of Enlightenment', *Yale French Studies*, xcii (1997), 67–87; Françoise Hildesheimer, *Le Bureau de santé de Marseille* (Marseilles, 1980); *eadem*, *La Terreur et la pitié: l'ancien régime à l'epreuve de la peste* (Paris, 1990); François Lebrun, *Les Hommes et la mort en Anjou* (Paris, 1971); Ferreol Rebuffat, *Marseille: ville morte* (Paris, 1968); Jacques Revel, 'Autour d'une peste ancienne: la peste de 1666–70', *Revue d'histoire moderne et contemporaine*, xvii (1970), 583–93; D.L. Smail, 'Accommodating Plague in Medieval Marseille', *Continuity and Change*, xi (1996), 11–41; J.K. Takeda, *Between Crown and Commerce: Marseille and the Early Modern Mediterranean* (Baltimore, Md., 2011), 106–30; A.P. Trout, 'The Municipality of Paris Confronts the Plague of 1668', *Medical History*, xvii (1973), 418–23.

years ago, J.-N. Biraben's *Les hommes et la peste dans les pays européens et méditerranéens* remains the principal study of plague in France.[5] Yet, while still valuable, this book looks more generally at responses to plague across the entire country from the fourteenth to the eighteenth centuries. With the exception of Sylvette Guilbert's pioneering 1963 article on Châlons-sur-Marne, historians have not specifically focused on the measures developed by French local authorities to combat plague during the more neglected fifteenth and sixteenth centuries.[6]

While some plague legislation was introduced in response to the Black Death of 1348–9, the ruling elites of northern French towns failed to develop a comprehensive set of institutional responses to subsequent outbreaks of plague before the 1450s.[7] The lack of any coherent attempt by these elites to manage outbreaks of plague during the first half of the fifteenth century can be attributed to the dire conditions arising in the north as a result of the campaigns of the Hundred Years' War. Indeed, the administration of Amiens collapsed for three months in late summer 1433 because of the combined pressures of war and plague.[8] Towns and cities in the south-east of the kingdom, such as Lyon, which were located far from the principal zones of persistent conflict in later medieval France, led the way in developing a comprehensive system to contain epidemics.[9] In contrast to these southern towns, the vast majority of the official business of northern French municipal councils was concerned with warfare during this period. It was only with the drawing to an end of the Hundred Years' War, and the return of relative stability to the northern parts of the kingdom, that urban administrations could feasibly seek to curb the impact of plague. The first concerted and wide-ranging attempts came in response to the devastating outbreak that struck the region in 1457–9.

Hygiene, Sanitation and Health

One of the first measures taken by municipal councils in their efforts to prevent the spread of plague was to organise the cleansing of the urban fabric; indeed, French towns were often at their most hygienic during outbreaks of epidemic disease.[10] The impetus to remove refuse and expel animals, such as pigs, from public places derived from a fear of miasmatic air, which was believed to be an agent of plague. Disease entered the body when contaminated air was inhaled, which the infected then spread to others on their polluted breath.[11] The cleaning of city streets for the

---

[5]   J.-M. Biraben, *Les hommes et la peste en France et dans les pays européens et méditerranéens* (2 vols., Paris, 1975).
[6]   Sylvette Guilbert, 'A Châlons-sur-Marne au XVe siècle: un conseil municipal face aux épidémies', *Annales. Histoire, Sciences Sociales*, vi (1968), 1283–1300.
[7]   See, for example, the sanitary measures adopted in Paris in response to plague by the ministers of John II in 1353: *Ordonnances des roys de France de la troisième race*, ed. E.J. de Laurière *et al.* (21 vols., Paris, 1723–1849), ii. 383.
[8]   AMA, BB 4, ff. 40–2.
[9]   For plague at Lyon, see Monique Lucenet, *Lyon malade de la peste* (Paris, 1981).
[10] For the fear of filth, see Alain Corbin, *Le miasme et la jonquille* (Paris, 1982).
[11] Carole Rawcliffe, *Urban Bodies: Communal Health in Late Medieval English Towns and Cities* (Woodbridge, 2013), ch. 3. I wish to thank Professor Rawcliffe for allowing me to consult the manuscript in advance of publication.

purposes of communal health was not an innovation of the fifteenth century; such measures can be found in European towns long before the Black Death.[12] However, it was not until the pestilence of 1457–9 that northern French towns systematically employed this method of combating infection. The exception is to be found at Tournai, where street cleaning in response to plague occurred from the outbreak of 1438 onwards.[13] Tournai's distinct geo-political situation may explain its early adoption of these sanitary precautions. By the fifteenth century it formed a French enclave in the county of Hainault, deep within the Burgundian Low Countries, where towns had developed institutional responses to plague far in advance of their French neighbours. Although street cleaning is documented in Paris during the plague outbreak of 1353 (following an ordinance of John II), towns lying on the north-eastern frontier of the kingdom drew their inspiration from the Low Countries.[14] Indeed, the rulers of Amiens actually noted that their attempts to improve the environment during times of plague derived from knowledge of developments in Tournai, Valenciennes, Saint-Omer and Lille.[15]

Refuse removal was initially organised on a parish level, with municipal councils directing their sergeants to ensure that townspeople cleaned both the front of their houses and the street outside.[16] Especially polluted areas, such as market-places and rivers, were targeted for vigorous cleaning by specially-appointed teams of workmen. Sanitary practices originally developed in response to plague soon became standard. Urination in public was first prohibited at Abbeville during the plague outbreak of 1457–9, and the legislation remained in place thereafter.[17] Concern to eliminate human waste from busy thoroughfares became increasingly apparent during the early decades of the sixteenth century; and, while northern towns lagged behind their southern counterparts in implementing plague legislation, they took the lead in initiating sanitary measures designed for this purpose. In contrast to southern towns, such as Grenoble (where public conveniences were not introduced until the pestilence of 1582), when a severe outbreak of plague hit Amiens in 1538 the council both orchestrated a city-wide inspection to ensure that all houses possessed latrines and constructed the first public privies.[18] Similar measures had been taken two decades earlier in Rouen: during the plague of 1518, the council had ruled that any house without a latrine now had to acquire one.[19]

Once municipal councils had attempted to eliminate human waste, they turned their attention to the animals with which they shared the urban space. In contrast to other parts of Europe, cats and dogs were not routinely killed in northern French

---

[12] Carmichael, *Plague and the Poor*, 96; Cohn, *Cultures of Plague*, 204–5; E.L. Sabine, 'Butchering in Mediaeval London', *Speculum*, viii (1933), 335–53; *idem*, 'Latrines and Cesspools of Mediaeval London', *ibid.*, ix (1934), 303–21; Lynn Thorndike, 'Sanitation, Baths, and Street-Cleaning in the Middle Ages and Renaissance', *ibid.*, iii (1928), 192–203.
[13] La Grange, 'Registres des consaulx, 1431–1476', 56.
[14] *Ordonnances des roys de France*, ed. de Laurière, ii. 383. See also Delumeau and Lequin, *Les Malheurs des temps*, 186.
[15] AMA, BB 9, f. 124.
[16] *Ibid.*, f. 19v.
[17] Ledieu, *Inventaire sommaire, Abbeville*, 91.
[18] Lucenet, *Grandes pestes*, 115; AMA, BB 23, f. 61v. For the construction of public latrines during times of plague, see also AMA, BB 24, f. 131.
[19] AMR, A 11, f. 17v.

towns during outbreaks of plague.[20] The only example that I have found of the culling of dogs came in response to the plague of 1564 in Amiens. On this occasion, the authorities ordered the executioner to round up and kill in public all the stray dogs found within the walls.[21] This epidemic was especially severe and had entered the town from an unknown source. By having the dogs executed in public, like common criminals, magistrates could use them as a scapegoat for spreading disease and show the townspeople that they were taking steps to deal with the crisis. It is also significant that only strays were targeted, in a move that replicates the harsh measures which were currently being introduced against vagrants aross Europe during times of plague. Like stray dogs, such people were homeless and masterless, and they, too, were prohibited from circulating in city streets.[22]

The animal identified as the principal vector of disease in many European towns was the pig. Where possible, intra-mural meat markets were closed down and moved to designated areas safely outside the city walls. However, the ubiquity of warfare in the north-east meant that it was not always possible to rear animals beyond the security of urban fortifications. Since the plague outbreak of 1467 coincided with heavy fighting in the region between Louis XI and Charles the Bold, Amiens' civic council reluctantly permitted pigs to be brought within the walls, where they were kept in designated areas that were subject to especially vigorous cleaning.[23] Anxious to avoid the risks posed by miasmatic air, magistrates also regulated the slaughter of animals and sale of meat during epidemics. In response to the arrival of plague in Amiens in 1520, a new market was constructed specifically to keep butchers and their meat away from places where corn and other victuals were sold. Municipal elites made full use of their extensive powers during times of crisis, and this important step led to a major reconfiguration of urban space in Amiens, including the destruction of private residences.[24] Although Rouen's butchers were permitted to exercise their craft inside the walls at such times, their activities were confined to specially constructed slaughterhouses.[25] Nervousness on this score was clearly growing. When plague struck Abbeville in 1488, the municipal council had the pens that were previously used to keep pigs inside the town demolished and moved the animals into the suburbs. These measures threatened the livelihood of the town's butchers and, when their appeal to have the pens reinstated was rejected by the authorities in March 1490, for fear of plague, they proposed to take their case to the parlement of Paris.[26] As an added, but even more controversial, precaution, the flesh of animals slaughtered in Amiens during epidemics could only be purchased from butchers who had

[20] For the killing of dogs and cats, see Delumeau, *La Peur en occident*, 112; Mark Jenner, 'The Great Dog Massacre', in *Fear in Early Modern Society*, ed. W.G. Naphy and Penny Roberts (Manchester, 1997), 44–61; Keith Thomas, *Man and the Natural World: Changing Attitudes in England, 1500–1800* (Oxford, 1983), 105.

[21] AMA, BB 36, f. 166. Dogs were again targeted in Amiens in 1596, during another serious outbreak of plague: AMA, AA 17, f. 166; BB 46, f. 104.

[22] Jenner, 'Great Dog Massacre', 56.

[23] AMA, BB 9, f. 176.

[24] AMA, BB 21, f. 31v.

[25] AMA, BB 16, ff. 90–1. See also Elma Brenner's article, above, pp. 127–31.

[26] Ledieu, *Inventaire sommaire, Abbeville*, 128.

successfully petitioned the council for a special licence. This led to the growth of a black market in illegal meat, with hucksters coming into towns to sell their wares.[27]

Magistrates did not deliberately seek to cause economic hardship to their fellow townspeople as a result of such measures. Where possible, they balanced their efforts to stop the spread of disease by restricting the movement of people and goods with attempts to alleviate the negative economic effects of plague on residents.[28] In 1493, for example, one Quentin Vecquart was excused the rent of his stall in the fish market of Amiens by the civic council because one of his children had died of plague that year.[29] The decline in trade which accompanied outbreaks of plague was a source of utmost concern to urban communities, which were reliant on the import of food for survival. During the plague of 1457, for instance, Rouen's council abolished the taxes which farmers from the surrounding countryside paid when bringing goods into the city for sale, in order to encourage them to continue supplying the market.[30] Prices inevitably rose during times of epidemic disease, even though magistrates constrained victuallers, such as bakers and butchers, to sell their produce at reasonable prices.[31] It was crucial that the food supply should be maintained, as a poor diet also made people more vulnerable to infection; and any serious interruption to the market during pestilences increased the risk of starvation for the poorer classes.[32] Should this happen, the financial burden of providing relief would fall on the ruling elite.[33]

The conditions resulting from a combination of war, plague and famine were frequently harsh, and town councils did what they could to lessen their severity. In 1523 the duke of Suffolk's forces ravaged Picardy at the same time as an outbreak of plague struck the region.[34] Hundreds of refugees flocked into Amiens, where the authorities had to levy additional taxes in order to meet the cost of feeding them.[35] It was also necessary to prevent the hoarding of foodstuffs and the export of grain during times of plague. In 1512 Rouen's council successfully blocked moves made by the seneschal to requisition grain for consumption by the royal army.[36] During the second half of the fifteenth century, the initiatives taken by urban elites against plague included measures to cushion the economic impact of the disease on the labouring poor. The desire to protect the working classes also derived from a concern to maintain social stability. In October 1435, a revolt of artisans had erupted in Amiens, partly in response to the local government's failure to alleviate

---

[27] AMR, A 10, f. 83.
[28] K.W. Bowers, 'Balancing Industrial and Communal Needs: Plague and Public Health in Early Modern Seville', *Bulletin of the History of Medicine*, lxxxi (2007), 335–58.
[29] AMA, BB 16, f. 260v.
[30] AMR, A 8, f. 27. For similar measures introduced at Amiens, see AMA, BB 16, f. 265; BB 22, f. 22.
[31] AMA, AA 12, f. 13. Ledieu, *Inventaire sommaire, Abbeville*, 97, 155. For price rises in the north during times of plague, see Delumeau and Lequin, *Les Malheurs des temps*, 202.
[32] For links between epidemic diseases and famine, see A.M. Appleby, 'Epidemics and Famine in the Little Ice Age', *Journal of Interdisciplinary History*, x (1980), 643–63; and Rawcliffe, *Urban Bodies*, ch. 5, for late medieval beliefs about malnourishment and the spread of plague.
[33] AMA, AA 12, f. 22; BB 17, f. 265; BB 22, f. 24v.
[34] AMA, BB 22, ff. 79, 83, 85. For the campaign, see S.J. Gunn, 'The Duke of Suffolk's March on Paris in 1523', *EHR*, ci (1986), 595–634.
[35] AMA, BB 22, f. 83.
[36] AMR, A 10, f. 16.

the financial hardships caused by a combination of plague and warfare, which had placed the bulk of the tax burden on those least able to pay.[37]

A Plague Industry

The creation of a range of official positions specifically to cope with the impact of epidemics during the second half the fifteenth century led to the development of what might be termed a 'plague industry'. Among the first official appointees were those individuals hired to dispose of the bodies of the dead in plague cemeteries.[38] In contrast to Italian cities such as Venice, where porters and gravediggers were employed on permanent contracts, in northern French towns such posts were seasonal, and were filled only during times of plague, with the rate of pay rising or falling in accordance with the severity of the outbreak.[39] Abbeville's town council hired between twelve and sixteen men '*des plus ydoines*' to bury plague victims in the summer of 1458 at wages of 12*s.* per week, whereas the gravediggers employed in Rouen for the same purpose in 1514 were paid at the higher rate of 60*s.* per month, which the *échevins* considered to be '*ung gros et grant proffict*'.[40] Although they received a substantial reward for their work, these people were drawn from the poorer classes and formed a marginal social group. Nonetheless, their role in clearing the streets of bodies and disposing of the remains was one of the key measures taken by magistrates to purify the urban environment.

As well as arranging for the disposal of the dead, urban elites also provided care for the living. Members of religious orders figure prominently among the people whom they employed to tend to plague victims.[41] As secular authorities began to assume greater responsibility in this regard during the second half of the fifteenth century, regular clergy looked to them, rather than to senior members of the ecclesiastical hierarchy, when offering to minister to the sick. When a group of Franciscan monks fleeing conflict in Montreuil came to Amiens in 1478, they pledged their services to a grateful civic council.[42] In return for the provision of pastoral care for plague victims, such bodies supplied members of the religious orders with victuals and money to pay for the upkeep of their buildings. For instance, during the plague of 1459, the rulers of Abbeville gave one *quene* of wine

---

[37]   AMA, BB 4, 91–93v; *La chronique d'Enguerran de Monstrelet*, ed. Louis Douët-d'Arcq (6 vols., Paris, 1857–62), v. 194–8. For the wider context of this revolt, see Neil Murphy, 'Between France, England and Burgundy: Amiens under the Lancastrian Dual Monarchy, 1422–35', *French History*, xxvi (2012), 160–1.

[38]   For the location of plague cemeteries, see *Les ordonnances faictes et publiées à son de trompe par les carrefours de ceste ville de Paris pour éviter le danger de peste 1531*, ed. Achille Chéreau (Paris, 1873), 37; *Registres des délibérations du bureau de la ville de Paris. Tome deuxième, 1527–1539*, ed. Alexandre Tuetey (Paris, 1886), 135, 169; AMA, AA 1, f. 126v.

[39]   For Venice, see J.L. Stevens Crawshaw, 'The Beasts of Burial: Pizzigamorti and Public Health for the Plague in Early Modern Venice', *Social History of Medicine*, xxiv (2011), 570–87. For the appointment and wages of those hired to dispose of the bodies of plague victims at Amiens, see AMA, BB 16, f. 265; BB 17, f. 80; BB 19, ff. 59v, 65v; BB 25, f. 126v; BB 31, f. 77; BB 32, ff. 82, 104v, 150v; BB 34, f. 107.

[40]   Ledieu, *Inventaire sommaire, Abbeville*, 97; AMR, A 10, f. 74.

[41]   John Henderson, *Piety and Charity in Late Medieval Florence* (Chicago and London, 1994), esp. chs. 7 and 8.

[42]   AMA, BB 13, f. 53v.

per week to the sisters of a *béguinage*, '*se disposent à aler viseter, conforter et amonester les malades*'.[43]

One of the key positions created by the burgeoning plague industry was that of the surgeon or barber-surgeon responsible for bleeding the sick, as it was believed that the removal of contaminated blood might arrest the progress of the disease.[44] Some southern towns, such as Saint-Flour, employed surgeons specifically to phlebotomise plague victims from the epidemic of 1414–16 onwards. These regions lay far from the conflicts devastating Normandy, Picardy and the Ile-de-France following Henry V's invasion of France in 1415, where municipal councils were pouring money into the repair of their fortifications. It is interesting to note that Saint-Flour's ruling council struggled to raise the money necessary to care for the sick when fighting between Armagnac and Burgundian factions spread to the Auvergne in the early 1420s.[45] Expenditure had then to be directed towards the costs incurred through conflict, rather than funding preventative measures against plague. By this date many town councils employed surgeons to tend the poor, though they did not always want to assume the unwelcome task of bleeding plague victims. When pestilence hit Amiens in October 1501 the municipal surgeon, Jean Obry, declined to do so. As a result, he was immediately dismissed from his position and replaced with someone who would.[46] During an outbreak of plague at Beauvais in 1520 the master barbers likewise refused to phlebotomise the sick, who were then assigned to the Franciscans for care.[47] Their reluctance is understandable, as the mortality rate among those who performed this operation was high. The barber-surgeon employed at Abbeville in August 1483 died within two weeks of his appointment, and the town council had to double the wages in order to find a successor.[48]

Most surgeons were paid a weekly wage for the duration of an outbreak, which they supplemented by levying an additional charge upon the people whom they bled. These sums were regulated by the authorities and were determined by social status. The rates set at Abbeville in 1458 were: '*riches et puissans de chacun vjs.; des moiens, iiijs.; et des serviteurs et autres mendres personnes, ijs.*' Each phlebotomist was, moreover, warned that '*de ceulx qui sont poures il n'en aura riens, et sy ne les porra refuser à saigner comme les autres*'.[49] As a sanitary measure, barber-surgeons were generally forbidden to practise while they were treating plague victims. At Paris and Rouen, those who opted to bleed the sick were not allowed to open their shops or attend other patients during epidemics.[50] However, they were compensated for any loss of income while they performed this service.[51] Magistrates also made *ad hoc* payments to some surgeons for their help

---

[43]   Ledieu, *Inventaire sommaire, Abbeville*, 98–9.

[44]   Rawcliffe, *Urban Bodies*, ch. 3.

[45]   Marcellin Boudet and Roger Grand, *Epidémies de peste en Haute-Auvergne (XIVe–XVIIIe siècles)* (Paris, 1902), 43–4.

[46]   AMA, BB 19, ff. 59v, 61v, 84.

[47]   Rose, *Inventaire sommaire, Beauvais*, 16.

[48]   Ledieu, *Inventaire sommaire, Abbeville*, 126–7.

[49]   *Ibid.*, 97.

[50]   *Registres de Paris. Tome deuxième*, ed. Tuetey, 169; AMR, A 2, f. 10v.

[51]   During the plague outbreak of 1501–2 the council of Amiens compensated the barber-surgeon, Colart Baude, for his loss of income. He also drew a salary for bleeding plague victims: AMA, BB 19, f. 107.

in treating plague victims, rather than hiring them on a permanent and far costlier basis.[52] While the financial rewards to be gained from this type of activity could be considerable, public-spirited barber-surgeons encountered an additional range of restrictive measures during epidemics. They were not permitted to converse with the general population, and had to wear distinctive clothing and reside in houses marked by a white cross.[53]

Although work of this kind was not without its drawbacks, it could provide a means of climbing the social ladder. After a serious outbreak of plague finally passed, in April 1469, the rulers of Abbeville continued to retain the services of Georges Yot, the surgeon whom they had previously employed as a phlebotomist. This new position came with its own livery, lodgings and an annual pension of 60 *livres*. Yot was made a municipal sergeant four months later, bringing him an additional income of 9 *livres* a year.[54] Service of this kind could, in turn, lead to further advancement. When plague appeared at Amiens, in February 1542, the council was unable to locate its official surgeon, Nicaise Hurtault, who it transpired had left to become master barber to the king, despite the fact he was still claiming his civic pension. The *échevins* declared this to be '*grandement contre les droictz, auctorite et jurisdiction dicelle ville*' and began a case of impeachment against him.[55] Magistrates did not exercise a monopoly over the deployment of phlebotomy during times of plague, though they did attempt to regulate the practice by setting down conditions for resident surgeons to follow, and preventing unqualified outsiders from coming into town to bleed the sick. During the plague year of 1521, for example, the rulers of Amiens redrafted the statutes of the guild of barber-surgeons in order to tackle the '*faultes et abbus quy se commettent chacun jour par gens estrangiers non congnoissans dudit estat*'.[56]

University-trained physicians stood at the social and professional pinnacle of those medical practitioners hired by municipal councils to combat plague.[57] They were responsible for diagnosing cases of pestilence, examining the infected and inspecting the quality of the drugs stocked by apothecaries. Some town councils had employed salaried physicians, along with surgeons, to tend the sick poor and advise on matters of public health from at least the early fifteenth century.[58] Physicians considered themselves to be of superior social standing and intellectual prowess to barber-surgeons, which led to rivalry during outbreaks of plague.[59] A complaint was made to Amiens' civic council on 7 April 1458 by the physicians

---

[52] On 27 Apr. 1484 Amiens' council gave 4 *livres tournois* to Hue de Louvencourt, barber and surgeon, for bleeding plague victims: AMA, BB 14, f. 137v.

[53] See, for example, *Registres de Paris. Tome deuxième*, ed. Tuetey, 168.

[54] Ledieu, *Inventaire sommaire, Abbeville*, 115.

[55] AMA, BB 23, f. 157.

[56] AMA, BB 22, f. 50.

[57] Roger French, 'The "Long Fifteenth Century" of Medical History', in *Medicine from the Black Death to the French Disease*, ed. French, Jon Arrizabalaga, Andrew Cunningham and Luis Garcia-Ballester (Aldershot, 1998), 1–5.

[58] The first mention of an official physician at Amiens comes in 1427, though it concerns an appointment to an existing position which had been unoccupied for some time: AMA, BB 3, f. 62.

[59] Guido Ruggiero, 'The Status of Physicians and Surgeons in Renaissance Venice', *Journal of the History of Medicine and Allied Sciences*, xxvi (1981), 168–84; P.N. Stearns, 'Empirics and Charlatans in Early Modern France: The Genesis of the Classification of the "Other" in Medical Practice', *Journal of Social History*, xix (1986), 583–603.

Jaque Delaquarre and Jehan Lemansier that there were '*plusieurs barbiers, gens estrangierz et autres, qui se merloient et entremetoient de la science et estat de medechine*'.[60] Physicians were highly valued by the authorities, who went to great pains to find the most capable candidates. Like surgeons, however, they were often reluctant to treat plague victims; and magistrates collaborated with other judicial bodies to compel them to act. Since local physicians proved slow to offer their services during the plague outbreak of 1538, the *échevins* of Rouen obtained an order from the city's *parlement* instructing the college of physicians immediately to elect one of their number to assist the community, with the threat of punishment should they refuse.[61] Similarly, when plague struck Paris in late summer 1533, the *parlement* of Paris ordered the Faculty of Medicine of the University to appoint four physicians from its ranks to visit the sick.[62]

The argument advanced by Ann Carmichael and Carlo Cipolla regarding the disparity between the recommendations made by medical experts and the actions taken by civic magistrates in their battle against plague has been overstated.[63] Recent research by Samuel Cohn has demonstrated that physicians and officials in Italian cities could work effectively together to implement quarantine measures based on the shared assumption that plague was spread by person-to-person transmission.[64] The municipal records of northern French towns document similar levels of co-operation between physicians and civic authorities, who collaborated on a range of measures to isolate the sick from the healthy and to minimise contact between people. The expertise provided by physicians in diagnosing plague was crucial in an age when urban populations were increasingly vulnerable to a variety of epidemic diseases. The late fifteenth century, in particular, saw new and devastating diseases, including syphilis, typhus and the sweating sickness, strike European towns, which also succumbed to smallpox, influenza and a wide range of malignant fevers.[65] Urban authorities often faced two or more different epidemics which were raging at the same time. For example, Amiens' council had to respond to outbreaks of both syphilis and plague during the summer of 1503.[66] It was crucial for such bodies to identify each disease quickly and accurately, so that they could intervene in the appropriate manner.[67] Providing reliable information might be difficult, however, as many of these diseases exhibited similar symptoms. In

[60]   AMA, BB 8, f. 113v.
[61]   AMR, A 14, f. 41.
[62]   *Registres de Paris. Tome deuxième*, ed. Tuetey, 169.
[63]   Carmichael, *Plague and the Poor*, 90–107; C.M. Cipolla, *Public Health and the Medical Profession in the Renaissance* (Cambridge, 1976). See also Henderson, 'The Black Death in Florence', 139–41; Brian Pullen, 'Plague and Perceptions of the Poor in Early Modern Italy', in *Epidemics and Ideas*: *Essays on the Historical Perception of Pestilence*, ed. T.O. Ranger and Paul Slack (Cambridge, 1992), 112–13.
[64]   Cohn, *Cultures of Plague*, 252–63; and see the paper by John Henderson in this volume, pp. 175–9.
[65]   J.N. Hays, *The Burdens of Disease*: *Epidemics and Human Response in Western History* (revised edn., New Brunswick, N.J., 2009), 63–71; Roger French and Jon Arrizabalaga, 'Coping with the French Disease: University Practitioners' Strategies and Tactics in the Transition from the Fifteenth to the Sixteenth Century', in *Medicine from the Black Death to the French Disease*, ed. French *et al.*, 48–87; J.A.H. Wylie and L.H. Collier, 'The English Sweating Sickness (*Sudor Anglicus*): A Reappraisal', *Journal of the History of Medicine*, xxxvi (1981), 425–45.
[66]   AMA, BB 20, f. 9v.
[67]   A.G. Carmichael, 'Epidemics and State Medicine in Fifteenth-Century Milan', in *Medicine from the Black Death to the French Disease*, ed. French *et al.*, 221–47.

July 1503, the rulers of Amiens moved an individual initially suspected of suffering from leprosy out of the municipal leper hospital of St. Ladre when it became clear that he had contracted syphilis.[68]

By the fifteenth century the word '*peste*' was generally deployed in the specific context of plague.[69] A precise vocabulary was essential, as the preventative measures adopted in response to plague were more extensive and draconian than those taken against other infectious diseases; and if physicians made a mistake they were quick to correct it. Thus, an epidemic which reached its peak in Amiens and Abbeville during the winter of 1493–4 was at first described as plague in the deliberations of both municipal bodies, though it soon became apparent that it was syphilis, a disease previously unknown to the region. Because of its presumed origins, it came to be called the '*maladye de Naples*' on subsequent occasions.[70] Magistrates wisely insisted on receiving sufficient confirmation before stringent regulations for the containment of plague were put into operation. When an outbreak of suspected plague struck Rouen in December 1537, the city council held three separate meetings (1, 3 and 5 December) in order to validate this diagnosis. The meetings were attended by two physicians in civic employment and another three hired to provide additional opinions on the etiology of the disease. Once all five agreed that plague was indeed present in the city, the authorities immediately set in train the mechanisms customarily taken to manage outbreaks of the disease, which included the unique precaution of closing up the houses of its victims with the residents inside.[71]

Municipal records suggest that several different strains of plague were attacking French towns. Contemporary medical practitioners certainly noted this development. During the early stages of an epidemic in Rouen, in August 1517, the council ordered its physician, Robert Nagerel, to provide appropriate guidance. He reported that '*il y a plusieurs sortes de maladies de peste*', but that the current sickness did not conform to any of them. He advised the council to stay its hand before closing suspect houses, though the *échevins* sought the advice of other experts before reaching a consensus.[72] Many of the measures taken by magistrates to combat plague were initiated in April and continued through to October, which is in keeping with the seasonality now associated with the disease.[73] However, it is also clear that plague could strike at any time of year.[74] Some epidemics began in

---

[68] AMA, BB 20, f. 8v.

[69] S.K. Cohn, Jr., *The Black Death Transformed: Disease and Culture in Early Renaissance Europe* (2002), 135–7. For recent surveys of the wide-ranging debate about the etiology of late medieval and early modern plague, see O.J. Benedictow, *What Disease was Plague? On the Controversy over the Microbiological Identity of Plague Epidemics of the Past* (Leiden, 2010); S.K. Cohn, Jr., 'Epidemiology of the Black Death and Successive Waves of Plague', in *Pestilential Complexities: Understanding Medieval Plague*, ed. Vivian Nutton, *Medical History*, supplement xxvii (2008), 74–100; L.K. Little, 'Plague Historians in Lab Coats', *Past and Present*, ccxiii (2011), 267–90; Susan Scott and C.J. Duncan, *Biology of Plagues: Evidence from Historical Populations* (Cambridge, 2001).

[70] See, for example, AMA, BB 20, f. 8v. Syphilis and leprosy were often confused during this period: French and Arrizabalaga, 'Coping with the French Disease', 248.

[71] AMR, A 14, f. 48.

[72] AMR, A 11, f. 119.

[73] For the seasonal aspects of plague in France, see Cohn, *Black Death Transformed*, 179–81; Carmichael, *Plague and the Poor*, 61–7.

[74] See here Cohn, *Black Death Transformed*, 145–6; and his article below, pp. 202–3.

March and lasted until late summer, while others first occurred in August and persisted through the winter months. Indeed, some of the most devastating outbreaks reached their peak in January and February. In 1508, plague was first diagnosed at Amiens by municipal physicians on 3 November and continued through the winter to reach its height in January 1509, which suggests that it might have been an instance of the more virulent and deadly pneumonic form of the disease.[75]

Contagion and Isolation

Contagion theory gained ground among the ruling elites of northern French towns towards the end of the fifteenth century. In their initial battles against plague, they had been predominately concerned with the elimination of miasmatic air and the ringing of bells at funerals, rather than attempting to separate the sick from the healthy.[76] Although measures for the isolation of potential carriers of plague were adopted in cities such as Milan and Ragusa from the later fourteenth century, the authorities of northern French towns lagged almost a century behind their Mediterranean counterparts where segregation was concerned.[77] Indeed, initially at least, urban administrations took steps which encouraged plague victims to circulate in public. When pestilence struck Abbeville in 1478, the sick were allowed to attend public mass in the centrally-located church of Saint-Sépulchre.[78] Such concessions derived from a belief in the power of the Eucharist to heal the sick and dispel miasmatic air.[79] As a fundamental part of their nascent strategy against plague in the 1450s and 1460s, municipal councils orchestrated general processions to solicit divine intervention. In 1467 the magistrates of Amiens organised a mass procession bearing all the town's relics throughout the streets, which was followed by a sermon exhorting the congregation to avoid sin.[80] There was, however, an official movement away from collective penitence and supplication towards the end of the fifteenth century. Although the Church continued to stress the importance of public demonstrations of faith in the war against plague, town councils tended to avoid promoting measures that directly

---

[75] AMA, BB 21, f. 18v.

[76] See, for example, the actions taken by Tournai's council during the plague outbreak of 1452: La Grange, 'Registres des consaulx, 1431–1476', 186.

[77] Carmichael, 'Plague Legislation', 512; Mirko Grmek, 'Le concept d'infection dans l'antiquité et au Moyen Age, les anciens mésures sociales contre les maladies contagieuses, et la fondation de la première quarantine à Dubrovnik', *RAD Jugoslavenske Akademije Zanosti i Umjetnosti*, ccclxxxiv (1980), 28–32; Bariša Krekić, *Dubrovnik in the Fourteenth and Fifteenth Centuries: A City between East and West* (Norman, Okla., 1972), 99–101; S.S. Stuard, 'A Communal Program of Medical Care: Medieval Ragusa/Dubrovnik', *Journal of the History of Medicine and Allied Sciences*, xxviii (1973), 126–42. Jane Stevens Crawshaw has shown that the public health measures introduced in Milan and Ragusa during the late 14th century inspired the foundation of the world's first permanent plague hospital at Venice in 1423: *Plague Hospitals*, 3, 19.

[78] Ledieu, *Inventaire sommaire, Abbeville*, 124.

[79] Richard Palmer, 'The Church, Leprosy and Plague in Medieval and Early Modern Europe', *Studies in Church History*, xix (1982), 85; Carole Rawcliffe, *Leprosy in Medieval England* (Woodbridge, 2006), 95.

[80] AMA, BB 9, f. 167v.

undermined their attempts to minimise contact between people.[81] Whereas the *pénetencier*, May de Brueil, warned Rouen's magistrates in 1517 that, in order to prevent plague, they should correct '*les vices*' of the inhabitants, especially with regard to the indecent clothing worn by '*plusieurs folles femmes*', the *échevins* themselves were more concerned to separate the infected from the rest of the population.[82]

As John Henderson reminds us, we should not attribute modern definitions to the meaning of terms such as 'contagion' and 'infection' in the later Middle Ages and Renaissance.[83] Yet, although they knew nothing of germ theory, by the late fifteenth century urban authorities did use these words specifically to describe the transmission of plague from person to person. A growing acceptance of ideas about contagion came to exist alongside more traditional theories regarding the role of corrupt air in spreading disease. The attendant concept of 'contingent contagion' also gained widespread currency among urban elites during the early decades of the sixteenth century, with some socio-economic groups being considered especially susceptible to infection, which they then spread by polluting the air and environment. During the plague outbreak of 1534, the Parisian city council observed that those who tended the sick in the Hôtel Dieu '*ne peuvent endurer le gros aer qui y est, et deviennent mallades et meurent commes les autres*'.[84] In this case it was the poor who were believed to have corrupted the air in the hospital, thereby transmitting the disease to others. Surprisingly, despite the longstanding assumption that toxic air was responsible for the spread of plague, there was little emphasis on the lighting of bonfires or any of the other measures taken to dispel miasmas during the fourteenth century.[85] The bulk of the regulations adopted by municipal councils from the late fifteenth century onwards was directed towards limiting contact between the healthy and the sick.

Concern about contagion converged with a drive to improve the morality of urban populations, especially the poor. Many of the measures adopted by magistrates attempted to regulate the behaviour of the lower classes. The appearance of plague in Amiens in 1523 provided the authorities with a welcome pretext for prohibiting an especially notorious dance favoured by the lower classes, which involved young unmarried men and women and was prone to descend into violence.[86] As well as banning dancing, Abbeville's council outlawed gambling

---

[81] For tensions between state and church in this respect, see Biraben, *Les hommes et la peste*, ii. 63–8; Carlo Cipolla, *Faith, Reason and Plague in Seventeenth-Century Tuscany* (New York, 1979), *passim*; Pullen, 'Plague and Perceptions of the Poor', 105–6.

[82] AMR, A 11, f. 3v. For further examples of plague being blamed on the wearing of indecent clothing, see *The Black Death*, ed. Rosemary Horrox (Manchester, 1994), 134–5.

[83] Henderson, 'The Black Death in Florence', 139–41, and below, pp. 175–9; M.D. Grmek, 'Les vicissitudes des notions d'infection, de contagion et de germe dans la médicine antique', *Mémoires de Centre Jean Palerne, V. Texts médicaux: Latins Antiques*, ed. Guy Sabbah (Sainte-Etienne, 1984), 53–70.

[84] *Registres de Paris. Tome deuxième*, ed. Tuetey, 179.

[85] J.M.W. Bean, 'The Black Death: The Crisis and its Social and Economic Consequences', in *The Black Death: The Impact of the Fourteenth-Century Plague*, ed. Daniel Williman (Binghamton, N.Y.,1982), 26.

[86] AMA, BB 23, f. 58. For the prohibition of dances because of the threat of plague, see also AMA, BB 7, f. 134.

when plague struck in 1494.[87] Public gambling was both morally unacceptable in the eyes of urban elites and an encouragement for people to congregate together. There was also an attempt to limit contact between the general populace and members of those social groups which were deemed to be spiritually unclean. Prostitution and sexual promiscuity were regarded as a cause of plague by clergy and physicians alike, and magistrates were keen to remove such a physical and moral threat to the community's health.[88] Prostitutes had long been associated with disease, and increasingly restrictive measures were adopted throughout the fifteenth century to curtail their freedom in plague time.[89] According to contemporary medical thought, sexual activity made people especially vulnerable to infection by raising body heat and opening the pores to miasmatic air. Bathhouses, which were closely connected with prostitution, were either closed down or subjected to tighter regulation during pestilences. Measures of this kind were initially adopted in southern towns, such as Saint-Flour, where one of the very first steps taken by the council in 1402 to combat the spread of plague was to confine all the prostitutes in a house for the duration of the epidemic.[90] It was towards the end of the fifteenth century that northern towns began to direct equally harsh legislation against them. In Abbeville they were not permitted to use public ovens or go outside the walls to gather firewood during plague outbreaks from 1493 onwards.[91]

Municipal councils also sought to exclude people and goods that had come from infected regions. When the rulers of Beauvais learned that plague was endemic in Clermont and Amiens, in August 1514, they prohibited anyone from these areas from entering the town.[92] Notices were attached to the gates informing travellers from suspect places that they were not welcome, while townspeople who sheltered refugees fleeing from pestilence faced punishment.[93] Some town councils took far more aggressive steps to impose a cordon sanitaire. During outbreaks of plague in 1493 and 1519, mercenaries were hired to guard the gates of Amiens against people coming in from the surrounding countryside and to prevent the inhabitants

[87] Ledieu, *Inventaire sommaire, Abbeville*, 151.
[88] Rawcliffe, *Urban Bodies*, ch. 2. See also P.J.P. Goldberg, 'Pigs and Prostitutes: Streetwalking in Comparative Perspective', in *Young Medieval Women*, ed. K.J. Lewis, N.J. Menuge and K.M. Phillips (Stroud, 1999), 172–93.
[89] Much of this legislation predates measures for the containment of prostitutes that followed the appearance of syphilis in the late 15th century: Lotte van de Pol, *The Burgher and the Whore: Prostitution in Early Modern Amsterdam* (Oxford, 2011), 74. Jacques Rossiaud, *Medieval Prostitution*, trans. L.G. Cochrane (Oxford, 1988), 86–9. For attempts to arrest the spread of syphilis, see Anna Foa, 'The New and the Old: The Spread of Syphilis (1494–1530)', in *Sex and Gender in Historical Perspective*, ed. Edward Muir and Guido Ruggiero, trans. M.A. Gallucci (Baltimore, Md., and London, 1990), 26–45; Mary Hewlett, 'The French Connection: Syphilis and Sodomy in Late-Renaissance Lucca', in *Sins of the Flesh: Responding to Sexual Disease in Early Modern Europe*, ed. Kevin Siena (Toronto, 2005), 239–60. Prostitutes were associated with the transmission of other diseases, too: R.M. Karras, *Common Women: Prostitution and Sexuality in Medieval England* (Oxford, 1996), 40, 157; L.L. Otis, *Prostitution in Medieval Society. The History of an Urban Institution in Languedoc* (Chicago, Ill., 1985), 41.
[90] Boudet and Grand, *Epidémies de peste*, 32.
[91] Ledieu, *Inventaire sommaire, Abbeville*, 131. For measures against prostitutes, see also AMA, 12, f. 134.
[92] Rose, *Inventaire sommaire, Beauvais*, 15.
[93] *Registres de Paris. Tome deuxième*, ed. Tuetey, 60.

from escaping elsewhere.[94] Professional soldiers were less likely to have local roots and therefore seemed less prone than residents to subvert the regulations by admitting friends or family from outside the walls. Such concerns reached the very highest levels of society. When plague swept through northern France in August 1510, Louis XII sent orders to the council of Paris from his castle at Blois forbidding anyone from leaving the capital lest they might contract the disease and return to spread it among the citizenry. He claimed to be acting for the protection of his pregnant daughter, Claude of France, wife of the duke of Angoulême, who was then in Paris.[95] The consequences of breaking such embargoes could be serious. In 1457 the municipal council of Tournai ruled that any inhabitant caught travelling to, or selling goods brought from, an infected area would either be imprisoned and fined, or suffer banishment and the confiscation of his possessions.[96]

Fear of contagion made it desirable to set aside a special building in which to house plague victims. When plague was raging through Paris in 1534 and large numbers of people were dying in the Hôtel Dieu, the civic authorities moved to separate the infected from those suffering from '*autres mallades de fiebvres et autres malladies*', as they, too, were rapidly contracting the disease.[97] Perhaps the ultimate manifestation of the drive to isolate the sick from the healthy came with the creation of designated pest houses. Documented in some Italian cities from the mid fifteenth century, the use of *lazaretti* quickly spread into France, with Bourg-en-Bresse, Lyon and Marseilles all founding such establishments in the 1470s.[98] However, it was not until the first half of the sixteenth century that pest houses began to appear in northern French towns. Geography can partly explain the time lag between the north and south of the kingdom, as the demand for institutional segregation was understandably greatest in those regions that lay closest to Italy. The delay was also due to continuing warfare in the north. While the end of the Hundred Years' War had ushered in a period of peace across most of France, the north-east remained a military frontier and the scene of numerous conflicts between 1460 and 1560. It is telling that, when the rulers of Amiens eventually constructed a permanent plague hospital in 1544, they did so within the walls.[99] Had it been built beyond the fortifications, there was every likelihood that it would have been destroyed in one of the numerous conflicts in the region, since buildings lying in the *banlieue* were among the first targeted for demolition, either as a defensive measure by the municipal authorities or by enemy soldiers.

The manner in which urban plague legislation developed in fifteenth- and sixteenth-century France highlights the strikingly regional character of French society. The sharing of information and copying of practices among communities

[94] AMA, BB 16, f. 265; BB 22, f. 13.
[95] As well as organising criers to go through the streets and make this announcement, the council arranged for its sergeants to visit each house under their jurisdiction in order to inform the residents: *Registres de Paris. Tome premier*, ed. Bonnardot, 161–2.
[96] La Grange, 'Registres des consaulx, 1431–1476', 243.
[97] *Registres de Paris. Tome deuxième*, ed. Tuetey, 179. Similar concerns had been voiced in Florence in 1464: see below, p. 179.
[98] Delumeau and Lequin, *Les Malheurs des temps*, 202; Carmichael, *Plague and the Poor*, 108. For these institutions, see Stevens Crawshaw, *Plague Hospitals*, and Daniel Panzac, *Quarantines et lazarets: l'Europe de la peste d'Orient (XVIIe–XX siècles)* (Aix-en-Provence, 1986).
[99] Permanent plague hospitals were still rare even in 17th-century Europe: Cipolla, *Cristofano*, 24.

which were already joined by commercial and political networks led to the adoption of sanitary measures, such as the foundation of pest houses, by clusters of towns at approximately the same time. We can observe this pattern in the north and north-east of the kingdom, where municipal councils began simultaneously to implement regulations designed to combat plague. There was no conscious attempt to follow the model already available in the south of France, and I have found no evidence in urban archives of communication between northern and southern towns during this period. Even Paris, the capital of the kingdom, existed as part of a regional network, and did not develop comprehensive plague legislation in advance of its smaller neighbours. Indeed, the first permanent plague hospital in Paris was not established until 1580.[100]

Prior to the appearance of pest houses in northern French towns, the infected were either confined to their homes or removed to the local hôtel Dieu (general hospital). The implementation of this policy was largely dictated by social and economic factors; the wealthier residents remained in their own homes, while the poor were hospitalised. Although these institutions were frequently run by the clergy under the authority of their local bishop, they relied heavily on the financial support of municipal authorities during times of plague. On 31 August 1511, for example, the *vicaire* of the archbishop of Rouen appealed to the city council for help. Claiming that the Hôtel Dieu had accommodated numerous plague victims over the past four years, and that between sixty and eighty of them were currently being tended there, he made a powerful case for relief.[101] Families which had been confined to their homes could also expect assistance. Once a house had been marked with a white cross, the inhabitants were not permitted to leave for a period of between four to six weeks. This meant that they were reliant on municipal employees to supply them with food and other provisions. At Rouen and Amiens the officers engaged in this potentially risky task were instructed to carry a stick when they went out in public '*affin que on se puist garder d'approcher deulx*'.[102] This compassionate approach contrasts with the much harsher conditions apparent in other French towns. Brutal measures were introduced (if not necessarily enforced) at Troyes, where the sick and all their relatives were to be expelled from the town for a minimum of three months and their houses burned to the ground, while at Châlons-en-Champagne all those who had come in contact with plague victims were also banished.[103]

Although Carlo Cipolla has described the pest house as a 'preview of hell', municipal councils were initially concerned to make such places as healthy and pleasant as possible for their inhabitants.[104] The first pest house established at Amiens in 1520 was a temporary structure erected in the grounds of the Hôtel Dieu. Partly dictated by the need to find a convenient place where the plague

---

[100] Biraben, *Les hommes et la peste*, ii. 173.
[101] AMR, A10, f. 101.
[102] AMA, AA 12, f. 115v. The council of Rouen also ruled that '*lesquelles vergues doibvent estre de telle grandeur et estre tenuz en telle evidence que l'intention de l'ordonnance ne soit défrauldée*': AMR, A 14, f. 48.
[103] Guilbert, 'Châlons-sur-Marne', 1293.
[104] Cipolla, *Cristofano*, 27. For efforts to beautify Renaissance hospitals, see Stevens Crawshaw, *Plague Hospitals*, 45–52, and John Henderson, *The Renaissance Hospital: Healing the Body and Healing the Soul* (New Haven and London, 2006), 70–81.

victims from the hospital could be bled, the decision to locate the pest house here was also informed by the desire to create a salubrious environment in which to tend the sick. Medical literature of the period, including the *Regimen sanitatis* and plague *consilia*, stressed the importance of gardens and agreeable surroundings for the improvement of health.[105] A team composed of *échevins* and physicians inspected the site and declared it to be a *'tres beau lieu pour icelle faire au bout du jardin et pourprins dudit hostel, derriere la chappelle de la Conception respondant sur la riviere'*.[106] The entire exercise was financed out of civic funds, and the council continued to underwrite running costs right through to the end of the epidemic in the spring of 1523.[107] The building was extended during subsequent outbreaks of plague, and by 1540 the council had to purchase an adjoining garden in order to enlarge it.[108] Even so, when plague returned in 1544, the authorities decided to purchase land adjacent to the hospital of St. Roch (the patron saint of those struck by pestilence), in order to construct a more permanent pest house. This was because they planned to accommodate a greater variety and number of people. Prior to 1544, only those who were obviously infected with plague had been removed to the pest house; from then onwards, however, anyone suspected of harbouring the disease, including the friends and relations of victims, was also to be sent there.[109]

Once urban elites started to isolate the sick, they also began to regulate what should be done with their goods.[110] Because it was believed that particles of corrupt air could attach themselves to clothing and thus spread disease,[111] councils sought to prevent the sale of effects that had been removed from the homes of plague victims. During the pestilence of 1467 the officials guarding houses that had been sealed up in Abbeville were under no circumstances *'[à] vende ne expose à vente en la juridition de ladite ville quelques biens meubles demorés de gens qui sont trespasses ou trespasseront de la maladie impédimieuse'*. Those who disobeyed this order were to be imprisoned, banished, stripped of their offices and otherwise *'pugnis à la discretion de messeigneurs prévostz et juréz'*.[112] In spite of attempts by magistrates to prevent this dangerous trade, they were unable to stop it completely. Several people were discovered in Amiens in 1523 selling items from the homes of infected persons, while Rouen's civic council designated two towers along the walls in which to place anyone who contravened similar ordinances.[113] The creation

---

[105] Pedro Gil Sotres, 'The Regimens of Health', in *Western Medical Thought from Antiquity to the Middle Ages*, ed. M.D. Grmek, trans. Anthony Shugaar (Cambridge, Mass., 1998), 291–318, especially 300–14; Rawcliffe, *Urban Bodies*, ch. 3.

[106] AMA, BB 22, f. 30.

[107] *Ibid.*, ff. 37v, 95v.

[108] AMA, BB 23, f. 48v.

[109] AMA, BB 25, ff. 11v, 106, 114.

[110] Similar measures had been employed against infectious diseases in earlier centuries. The clothes of lepers were washed at Chartres from 1208; and, when an unidentified epidemic struck Paris later that century, the prévôt of the city, Etienne Boileau, ruled that the goods, and especially the garments, of the victims were not to be resold: *Cartulaire de la léproserie du Grand-Beaulieu et du prieuré de Notre-Dame de la Bourdinière*, ed. René Merlet and Maurice Jusselin (Chartres, 1909), 72–3, 154, cited in Rawcliffe, *Leprosy in Medieval England*, 276; *Le livre des métiers d'Etienne Boileau*, ed. René de Lespinasse and François Bonnardot (Paris, 1879), 160.

[111] Stevens Crawshaw, *Plague Hospitals*, 28.

[112] Ledieu, *Inventaire sommaire, Abbeville*, 295.

[113] AMA, AA 12, f. 146; AMR, A 9, f. 3.

of special prisons for those caught trading in the goods of the sick served both to punish the offenders and, as potential carriers of the disease, to isolate them from the rest of the population. During the 1530 outbreak of plague in Rouen, the authorities ruled that the contaminated effects (*'biens epydemiez'*) of plague victims should be placed in barrels and brought in a marked boat to a designated place outside the town where they could be washed four or five times in order to be properly cleansed (*'mundiffiez'*).[114] After facing opposition from the prior of the Hôtel Dieu, who argued that this ordinance would endanger the institution's principal farm, the council looked for an alternative spot, far from habitation.[115]

As well as separating themselves from the persons and goods of suspected plague victims, townspeople increasingly sought to keep their distance from the polluted breath of lepers.[116] During the Middle Ages it was customary for the inmates of Amiens' leper hospitals to come into the city at Easter and on All Saints' Day in order to participate in public processions. A growing fear of proximity to the sick led some of the population to request the introduction of measures to restrict, if not entirely prohibit, their customary presence within the walls. Following the devastating plague outbreak of 1457–9, the canons of the cathedral appeared in the council chamber accompanied by a number of *'notables personnes'* to complain that the lepers came dangerously close to their houses as they entered the city, and successfully to petition for an alternative route where there were no dwellings.[117] The severity of the restrictions placed on lepers increased over time; and the plague ordinances issued at Amiens in 1523 explicitly prohibited them from visiting the city at all during Easter.[118] Amiens was not the only place to introduce such draconian measures. When plague hit Paris in 1533, lepers were also excluded. Anyone caught harbouring a leper was to be brought *'devant les juges'*, not only to pay a fine, but for the authorities to proceed *'extraordinairement contre eulx'*.[119] Regulations of this kind had significant financial consequences. Until the late fifteenth century, lepers were permitted to beg in the streets of Amiens. The council gradually clamped down on this activity, however, and by the plague year of 1545 had agreed to pay the two municipal leper hospitals the sum of 40 *livres* every year on the condition that their inmates did not attempt to seek alms there.[120] The place formerly occupied by them in the All Saints' Day procession was henceforward taken by paupers who were also in receipt of official charity. It was hoped that their presence would provoke the pity of the townspeople and encourage them to provide support, thus reducing the

---

[114] AMR, A 10, f. 10; A 13, f. 39.

[115] AMR, A 13, f. 39.

[116] Hammond, 'Contagion, Honour and Urban Life', 104; F.-O. Touati, 'Contagion and Leprosy: Myths, Ideas, and Evolution in Medieval Minds and Societies', in *Contagion: Perspectives from Pre-Modern Societies*, ed. L.I. Conrad and Dominik Wujastyk (Aldershot, 2000), 179–201; Palmer, 'Church, Leprosy, and Plague', 81.

[117] AMA, BB 9, f. 239v. The canons would have been well-versed in Avicenna's ideas about contaminated air and leprosy: Luke Demaitre, *Leprosy in Premodern Medicine: A Malady of the Whole Body* (Baltimore, Md., 2007), 238–9; Rawcliffe, *Leprosy in Medieval England*, 92, 94.

[118] AMA, AA 12, f. 147v. See also S.K. Cohn, Jr., 'Pandemics: Waves of Disease, Waves of Hate from the Plague of Athens to A.I.D.S.', *Historical Research*, lxxxv (2012), 535–55; idem, 'Hate in Times of Pestilence', *Clio's Psyche*, xix (2012), 113–16.

[119] *Registres de Paris. Tome deuxième*, ed. Tuetey, 170.

[120] AMA, BB 25, f. 139.

pressure placed on the municipal budget. We might note, too, that almsgiving was itself believed to be a prophylactic against plague.[121]

Plague became more closely linked with poverty during the late fifteenth century.[122] As well as benefiting from a nutritionally better diet, wealthier families were able to flee the towns for the countryside, where the plague had grown less virulent by this date. In Amiens it was observed that many of the '*bonnes gens d'icelle*', including several members of the civic council, had taken to their heels at the first sign of trouble in 1467.[123] During the epidemic that raged at Beauvais between August and October 1522, a significant proportion of the more affluent residents left, while the authorities estimated that between twenty and twenty-three poor people were dying there each day.[124] At a meeting of Rouen's city council in 1510, one of the *échevins*, Jehan Le Carpentier, declared that plague had been brought to the nearby town of Neufchâtel some years before by a travelling vagrant ('*pelletier*'), resulting in the death of between 1,700 and 1,800 inhabitants.[125] The Amiens plague of 1545 was likewise apparently first discovered in the hospital of St. Julian, where non-native vagrants were housed.[126] Such reports served to justify the increasingly repressive measures taken during this period against the itinerant poor, who were seen by the social elite as the most likely carriers of pestilence.[127] In the plague year of 1509, for example, Abbeville's municipal council ruled that '*nulls belictres en ceste dicte ville ne lez hospitalier d'icellez*' should offer them accommodation.[128] During the outbreak of plague in Paris in 1533, all the sick poor inhabitants of the city were promised food and medical treatment, whereas '*tous vallides vaccabons*' had to remove themselves '*hors la Ville*'.[129]

Such undisguised intolerance towards the vagrant poor sprang from the widespread belief that they were the principal vectors of disease; and ordinances against the plague soon became ordinances against the poor.[130] As Ann Carmichael notes, 'new policies of poor relief, which favoured charity to those at home over hospitality to foreigners, neatly coincided with the elaboration of similar plague policies'.[131] Indeed, the plague ordinance issued at Amiens in July 1514 was almost entirely concerned with regulating and restricting the movement of foreign vagrants in the town. Plague offered an opportunity for magistrates to discipline those whom they regarded as social parasites, and the measures taken against the 'undeserving' poor reflect wider concerns about idleness and vagrancy in the body politic. In the eyes of municipal authorities, plague and poverty were becoming

---

[121] *Ibid.*, f. 169v; Rawcliffe, *Urban Bodies*, ch. 2.

[122] S.K. Cohn, Jr., 'Changing Pathology of Plague', in *Le Interazioni fra Economia e ambiente biologico nell'Europa preindustriale, secc. XIII–XVIII*, ed. Simonetta Cavaciocchi (Florence, 2009), 46–50.

[123] AMA, BB 8, f. 170.

[124] Rose, *Inventaire sommaire, Beauvais*, 16.

[125] AMR, A 10, f. 101.

[126] AMA, BB 24, f. 124.

[127] Carmichael, 'Plague Legislation', 522. For the poor and the plague in the 14th century, see Michel Mollat, *The Poor in the Middle Ages: An Essay in Social History*, trans. Arthur Goldhammer (New Haven and London, 1978), 193–210.

[128] Ledieu, *Inventaire sommaire, Abbeville*, 140.

[129] *Registres de Paris. Tome deuxième*, ed. Tuetey, 167.

[130] AMA, AA 12, f. 115v.

[131] Carmichael, 'Plague Legislation', 523–4.

closely intertwined. At both Rouen and Paris, official positions were created
expressly to deal with the two problems. Debates in the parlement of Paris and
civic council chambers alike depicted them as two sides of the same coin.[132]

Conclusion

Between the mid fifteenth and mid sixteenth century municipal councils in
northern France developed a comprehensive strategy for curtailing the impact of
infectious diseases on their communities.[133] This strategy reflects a growing
acceptance of the ideas about contagion upon which it was grounded. Prior to the
1450s, on the rare occasions when councils did respond to plague, their approach
tended to be reactive. By isolating the sick, cleansing their goods and imposing
sanitary regulations, they now took practical steps to limit the spread and severity
of each epidemic. How effective these measures were is difficult to gauge. Some
outbreaks of plague were less severe than others, though the extent to which this
may have been due to the efficacy of legislation is unclear. Coping with infectious
diseases became a regular part of urban life during this period, as northern French
towns faced outbreaks of plague during every decade from the 1450s to the 1560s,
in addition to the other epidemic diseases, both new and established, with which
they had to contend.

Whereas the ruling elites of the fourteenth and early fifteenth centuries had often
escaped to the country during times of plague, from the later fifteenth century
onwards some *échevins*, at least, stayed to oversee the institutional response to the
problems created by the disease.[134] In doing so, they faced the threat of death
alongside the rest of the population. When plague struck Beauvais in 1520, six
members of the municipal council became ill, three of whom died, while three
échevins also died in Amiens during the plague outbreak of late summer 1519.[135]
By standing firm and rising to the challenges posed by these epidemics, municipal
councils established themselves as the principal agents responsible for urban public
health. Indeed, although health boards were not formally established in northern
French towns until the end of the sixteenth century, by 1560 magistrates had
already accumulated over a century's worth of experience in dealing with
pestilence. These measures also gave them the means to control and regulate more
areas of urban life than ever before, enabling them to demonstrate their power
more forcefully than had previously been possible. We should also remember that,
in northern France, urban authorities were struggling against a backdrop of
intermittent war. Although it may have taken time to put an administrative
infrastructure in place, once it was up and running it continued to function even
during times of intense conflict. By the mid sixteenth century, however, municipal
councils were beginning to call for royal assistance in addressing the growing

---

[132] *Registres de Paris. Tome deuxième*, ed. Tuetey, 168–9; AMR, A 15, f. 60.

[133] For similar measures introduced in English towns and cities during this period, see Rawcliffe, *Urban Bodies*.

[134] When plague broke out in Amiens in August 1433, many of the councillors fled to the countryside, which led to doomed attempts to run the municipal government through an exchange of letters between those who had escaped and those who remained: AMA, BB 4, ff. 40v–41.

[135] Rose, *Inventaire sommaire, Beauvais*, 16; AMA, BB 22, f. 18v.

problems posed by plague and poverty.[136] As a result, the management of epidemics became a national, rather than just a local, concern. This shift towards centralisation was to be checked by the Wars of Religion, though it would re-emerge stronger than ever during the course of the devastating outbreaks of plague that erupted in France in the seventeenth century.

---

[136] See, for example, Amiens' appeals to the crown for financial support in the battle against poverty and disease in 1545: AMA, BB 24, f. 137v.

THE RENAISSANCE INVENTION OF QUARANTINE

Jane Stevens Crawshaw

In 1405, Pietro Filargo (1339–1410) – who was Milan's archbishop, the tutor and ambassador for Giovanni Galeazzo Visconti and future Pope Alexander V – described that city in painful terms. He wrote,

> How can things go well in this most miserable Milan, full of the poor, famished and pestilent who wander through the city showing spots and sores while so great and even adequate provisions are cruelly embezzled? The souls of benefactors are being damned, for no one prays for them any longer, no one gives charity any longer and the souls of those who do not respect the wishes of the dead are also damned. And it is for such great impiety that God, with his three whips of hunger, war and plague, has inflicted Milan with these apocalyptic punishments [*apocalittici castighi*].[1]

In spite of changes in the centralised administration of charity in the early years of the fifteenth century in this Italian city state, it was recognised that more needed to be done. The consequences of inaction, as described by Filargo, were great: eternal damnation for the dead and earthly suffering for the living. In particular, he noted the increased regularity of famine, warfare and plague as natural signs of an impending apocalypse; for Filargo, as for many of his contemporaries, the issues of charitable care and natural disasters were intertwined.[2]

The increased incidence of such natural disasters at the end of the fourteenth and beginning of the fifteenth century was recognised in many parts of Europe. In the sphere of epidemic disease, plague outbreaks were more common than the emphasis on the major episodes in the existing historiography might suggest. In Ragusa (modern day Dubrovnik), for example, plague hit, after the Black Death, in 1363, 1374, 1381, 1400, 1416 and 1438. Just across the Adriatic, in Venice, the senate of the city noted in 1423 that outbreaks of plague were occurring almost annually.[3] The disease was far from occasional and could strike urban communities as often as once every five to ten years.

---

[1] E.S. Welch, *Art and Authority in Renaissance Milan* (1995), 129.

[2] On natural disasters as signs of the apocalypse see L.A. Smoller, 'Of Earthquakes, Hail, Frogs and Geography: Plague and the Inventing of the Apocalypse in the Later Middle Ages', in *Last Things*: *Death and the Apocalypse in the Middle Ages*, ed. C.W. Bynum and Paul Freedman (Philadelphia, Pa., 2000), 156–90.

[3] R.J. Palmer, 'The Control of Plague in Venice and Northern Italy 1348–1600' (Univ. of Kent Ph.D. thesis, 1978), 49–50.

In response to the increased severity and frequency of outbreaks of epidemic disease during the fourteenth century, and in the interests of public health, a number of Italian cities codified legislation.[4] Initially, these ordinances focussed on the cleanliness of the air and consequently hinged upon measures to restrict the presence of animals within cities, to remove open sewers and to clean streets. Regulations concerning the movement of people were also developed. Richard Palmer has shown that, in an Italian context, Pistoia and Lucca prohibited contact and commerce with infected states during the Black Death.[5] In addition, as literary and archival sources indicate, the notion of '*villeggiatura*', escaping to the countryside for health, was well established.[6] It was at the beginning of the fifteenth century, however, that one of the most common and enduring aspects of public health legislation during periods of epidemic disease was codified as a permanent policy. That policy was quarantine, which brought together elements of earlier initiatives for the promotion of cleanliness and charitable effort into a more coherent and complex structure. The basic idea was that the separation of the sick (and eventually of those suspected of having contracted the plague) was essential in order to prevent the spread of the disease. Quarantine measures were imposed upon inhabitants when cities were infected, as well as upon incoming travellers and merchants; they would come to encompass not only individuals but also their clothing, their possessions and their homes. Quarantine could be carried out in the domestic setting, but often separate buildings were set aside or specially constructed to serve communities as plague hospitals and to facilitate the care of patients while they remained in isolation. Care could be necessary for a significant period of time. Quarantine literally meant a period of forty days (it derives from the Italian word *quaranta* meaning forty), but in practice individuals might be sequestered for anything from eight to eighty days, depending on the severity of their symptoms or the extent of their exposure to the disease.[7]

Despite its influence on the formulation of early modern public health measures, the initial development of quarantine has attracted little historiographical attention; it is not even clear when, where and why measures were first introduced. In the absence of such studies, an indication of the date and extent to which quarantine policies were adopted across Europe can be gleaned by charting the spread of plague hospitals. This is an imperfect exercise, since these hospitals were not the only places where quarantine could be implemented; nevertheless, it goes some way to filling a gap in our current understanding of this important public health policy. The first of these hospitals was established on a permanent basis in 1423 in Venice.[8] Plague hospitals were then set up in cities of the Venetian mainland territories: by 1437 for Padua, in 1438 in Brescia and 1473 for Verona, in Salò in 1484 and certainly during the fifteenth century in both Vicenza and Treviso.

---

[4]   For example, Florence in 1324 and Milan in 1330, as described in *ibid.*, 2.

[5]   *Ibid.*, 21–2.

[6]   The best known literary account in a Renaissance Italian context can be found in Giovanni Boccaccio, *The Decameron*, trans. G.H. McWilliam (1995).

[7]   Archivio di Stato Venice [ASV], Sanità 732, f. 149 (13 June 1576) and f. 156v (1 July 1576).

[8]   See the '*atto constitutivo del lazaretto vecchio*' (28 August 1423) which is reprinted in *Venezia e la peste 1348–1797*, ed. Jacqueline Brossollet (Venice, 1980), appendix 7, p. 365. For the *lazaretto nuovo* see the documents reprinted in *Isola del Lazzaretto Nuovo*, ed. Gerolamo Fazzini (Venice, 2004).

Elsewhere on the Italian peninsula, *lazaretti* appeared in Milan in 1448, Naples in 1464 and Genoa in 1467.[9] Beyond Italy, the Ragusan authorities isolated people and goods on two nearby islands in 1377.[10] Quarantine institutions spread in France, where at least one *maison* or *hôpital pour pestiférés* might be found in many cities from the mid fifteenth century.[11] Teresa Huguet-Termes likewise confirms that plague hospitals were established in fifteenth-century Spain, as, for example, in Madrid in 1438.[12] Elsewhere, in the German States, Switzerland and the Low Countries, innovations were made in the sixteenth century. The fifteenth-century establishment of structures will be considered in more detail in this article through a specific focus on Milan, Ragusa and Venice, the three cities which are at the heart of the debate regarding the development of quarantine, both in terms of its date and purpose.

[9] The table constructed by Ann Carmichael presents a useful guideline to the development of these institutions, although it should be cited with care since it is based upon secondary sources and is inaccurate in places. For example, the foundation of the *lazaretto vecchio* in Venice cannot be regarded as a reclassification of an older hospital, and the decision regarding a permanent *lazaretto* in Florence was taken in 1464 not 1463: A.G. Carmichael, 'Plague Legislation in the Italian Renaissance', *Bulletin of the History of Medicine*, lvii (1983), 520. For the Milanese *lazaretto* see Luca Beltrami, 'Il lazzaretto di Milano', *Archivio storico Lombardo*, ix (1882), 403–41. It is also described in A.F. La Cava, *La peste di S Carlo: note storico-mediche sulla pest 1576* (Milan, 1945), which makes extensive use of the account by Fra Paolo Bellintano. The Florentine *lazaretto* was permanent from the 1490s: John Henderson, *The Renaissance Hospital. Healing the Body and Healing the Soul* (New Haven and London, 2006), 91–6. In Naples, the *lazaretto* was founded in 1464 by Archbishop Carafa in an abandoned Benedictine convent with adjacent catacombs which were adopted as a cemetery: Charlotte Nichols, 'Plague and Politics in Early Modern Naples: the Relics of San Gennaro', in *In Sickness and in Health: Disease as Metaphor in Art and Popular Wisdom*, ed. L.S. Dixon (Newark, N.J., 2004), 30.

[10] Although Venice is often credited with the invention of the *lazaretto*, it is likely that the first was established in Ragusa, on a temporary basis, in 1377. These quarantine regulations were extended in 1397. I am grateful to Zlata Blažina Tomić for sharing her work on public health in Dubrovnik with me – particularly the text of the 1397 ordinance. She is currently preparing an English version of her book *Kacamorti i kuga: utemeljenje i razvoj zdravstvene službe u Dubrovniku* (Dubrovnik, 2007). At present, the most useful study of early Ragusan initiatives in English is Bariša Krekić, *Dubrovnik in the Fourteenth and Fifteenth Centuries: a City between East and West* (Norman, Okla., 1972), 99–101. Krekić maintains that the Venetians invented quarantine in 1374 and that Dubrovnik followed suit in 1377 (p. 99), but the precise chronology has not been determined. See also F.W. Carter, *Dubrovnik (Ragusa), A Classic City-State* (1972), 17; and S.M. Stuard, 'A Communal Program of Medical Care: Medieval Ragusa/Dubrovnik', *Journal of the History of Medicine and Allied Sciences*, xxviii (1973), 126–42.

[11] J.-N. Biraben, *Les hommes et la peste en France et dans les pays européens et méditerranéens* (2 vols., Paris, 1975–6), ii. 171–5, describes institutions established in Bourg-en-Bresse in 1472, Lyon in 1474 and Marseilles in 1476. He distinguishes between these institutions and the *lazaret* which developed as a quarantine centre in later centuries. The case of Toulouse, where a *lazaretto* was established in 1514, has been singled out for attention by R.A. Schneider, 'Crown and Capitoulat: Municipal Government in Toulouse 1500–1789', in *Cities and Social Change in Early Modern France*, ed. Philip Benedict (1989), 195–220. See also the survey by L.W.B. Brockliss and Colin Jones, *The Medical World of Early Modern France* (Oxford, 1997), especially 43, 69, 352–3.

[12] For the hospital de San Antón founded in 1438 in Madrid see Teresa Huguet-Termes, 'Madrid Hospitals and Welfare in the Context of the Habsburg Empire', in *Health and Medicine in Habsburg Spain: Agents, Practices, Representations*, ed. eadem, Jon Arrizabalaga and H.J. Cook (2009), 68. For institutions in Seville see K.W. Bowers, 'Balancing Individual and Communal Needs: Plague and Public Health in Early Modern Seville', *Bulletin of the History of Medicine*, lxxxi (2007), 335–58; and Linda Martz, *Poverty and Welfare in Habsburg Spain* (Cambridge, 1983), 89, 117, 152, 155–6, 162.

Milan is well known for its unusual experience of the Black Death of 1348–9, in that the city seems to have been barely touched by that pandemic. It has been suggested that a prohibition on commerce beyond the walls introduced in 1348 may have acted as a form of protection and that its perceived success encouraged further legislation along these lines in later epidemics. The city's most famous plague hospital was founded in 1488 as a large structure which made use of canals to separate the space into zones reserved for different groups; but other types of quarantine had been introduced more than a century earlier. In 1374, for example, the sick were told to leave Milan 'and take to the open country, living either in huts or in the woods until either [they] died or recovered'.[13] By 1399, the civic authorities clearly recognised that the idea of making infected inhabitants live like hermits in nearby woodlands could be improved upon as a public health measure. Plans for future outbreaks included the creation of two plague hospitals, whose express purpose was to separate the sick from the healthy and prevent them from remaining in their own homes. In 1400 (a Jubilee year) the plague hospitals were moved outside the city at the same time that entry was forbidden to the crowds of disease-bearing pilgrims on their way to Rome. The latter were instead directed along obligatory routes through the dominium. As we shall see below, these developments have been regarded as attempts at state building under Visconti rule.

In Ragusa, early, but temporary, innovations in the sphere of public health have been associated with the vital importance of trade for the city. The authorities founded a temporary plague hospital in 1397 on the island of Mljet. In subsequent years quarantine was either carried out in a monastery there or on the nearby islet of Mrkan. Significantly, the 'three main foci of the business life of the small state [were said to be] the port, the caravan route out of town and the quarantine area'.[14] The very first quarantine regulations targeted shipping and trade, ensuring that infected or suspect cargoes and crews were kept safely outside Ragusa for approximately one month a year during the late fourteenth and fifteenth centuries.

Finally, in Venice, Krekić has argued that quarantine was employed on a temporary basis in 1374 (three years before being adopted in Ragusa and in the same year as Milan). In 1400 the Venetian authorities turned the tables on 'the Ragusan policy of denying Venetian shipping access to its ports whilst there was plague in Venice'.[15] The decision was taken to '*respingere*' (which means to reject but also conveys a more forceful sense of driving back the enemy) from all Venetian ports any ships from Ragusa (which might be carrying plague at that time). This directive seems to have been largely political rather than sanitary in purpose, because it was not until 1423 that a prohibition on commerce and a quarantine policy were applied more generally to other plague-infected states. In addition to the commercial and diplomatic implications of this policy, the introduction of quarantine in Venice has been linked to a desire on behalf of the Republic to project an image of solicitude and paternal care to visitors and inhabitants alike.

In studies of the measures taken by individual cities, as summarised above, specific political, economic and charitable concerns have been highlighted by

---

[13]   *The Black Death*, ed. Rosemary Horrox (Manchester, 1994), 199.
[14]   Carter, *Dubrovnik (Ragusa)*, 113.
[15]   Palmer, 'The Control of Plague in Venice', 36.

historians. However, very few attempts have been made to adopt a broader perspective and to explain the widespread introduction of quarantine during the fifteenth century in more general terms. In 1986, Ann Carmichael published, in relation to Florence, her much-quoted conclusion that 'plague did not create the need for controlling the poor and the property-less [but rather] the causal relationship may have been the reverse'.[16] Yet there is little evidence to suggest that changing perceptions of poverty or rising levels of indigence served as a catalyst for the imposition of quarantine in the three cities under consideration here. The other generally applicable explanation has been offered by Richard Palmer, who argues that it was introduced during the fifteenth century because of the changing medical context. He maintains that plague was increasingly understood in terms of contagion, rather than airborne transmission by miasmas, and also emphasises the regularity of urban epidemics, observing that 'the increased frequency of the outbreaks [of plague] caused governments to take action, whilst the disease's attenuated ability to spread rendered it more subject to control'.[17] These factors might account for the adoption of some measures, but they do not fully explain the nature of specific responses. Here, Palmer enlists the example of late medieval reactions to leprosy as a model for current ideas about contagion and for the situation of plague hospitals outside urban centres.

Since so many considerations appear to have made quarantine attractive to urban elites, it is useful to disentangle those which were specific to particular cities (such as the economic priorities apparent in Venice and Ragusa) from others which were much more widely influential. This article will contribute to the ongoing discussion about public health and the state by exploring in greater detail explanations for the form that quarantine took, as well as the reasons for its introduction. First, it will examine Palmer's suggestion that current attitudes to leprosy set the mould for responses to the plague. This presumed connection is worth reconsidering because, since Palmer's thesis appeared, valuable work has been done to revise our assumptions about historical reactions to leprosy, most notably by Carole Rawcliffe in the context of medieval England.[18] Second, some preliminary conclusions will be drawn regarding the Renaissance ideas embedded in the concept of quarantine and the connections that may be made between architecture, civic charity, health and the public good.

Richard Palmer noted that 'the experience of leprosy helped society towards an understanding of the contagiousness of plague and the means of dealing with it'. Carole Rawcliffe has shown that the disease seemed far from mono-causal; it could affect an individual because of sin or as a test of faith.[19] Often, though, explanations were rooted in more general medical theories, such as ideas about unbalanced humours or infected air. Both leprosy and plague were endemic in Europe across the centuries, albeit in different geographical and chronological contexts. It is difficult, therefore, to generalise about a 'standard' or 'common'

---

[16] A.G. Carmichael, *Plague and the Poor in Renaissance Florence* (Cambridge, 1986), 125.

[17] Palmer, 'The control of Plague in Venice', 50.

[18] Carole Rawcliffe, *Leprosy in Medieval England* (Woodbridge, 2006). Other important works on leprosy include F.O. Touati, *Maladie et société au moyen âge* (Paris, 1988); and Luke Demaitre, *Leprosy in Premodern Medicine: A Malady of the Whole Body* (Baltimore, Md., 2007).

[19] Rawcliffe, *Leprosy in Medieval England*, ch. 2 ('The Body and Soul: Ideas about Causation'), 44–103, especially 48–64.

aetiology shared between them, the one thing that can be argued being that they were both understood within society's customary, but wide-ranging, explanative structures.

More work remains to be done on the connections between leprosy and plague in terms of causal explanations but, where they exist, they were applicable to many other diseases as well. The most common of these shared features concerned retribution for sin, but, broadly speaking, there was much less onus on the sinful individual in the context of plague (although certain social groups, as, for example, the Jews, did routinely come in for blame), and pestilence was widely regarded as a form of collective punishment. In terms of transmission, explanations included environmental changes (miasmas), direct contact with people and goods (contagion) and deliberate spread (smears and sabotage).[20] There were also some important differences between the nature of, and therefore assumptions about, the two diseases. In particular, leprosy was a long-term chronic illness, which prompted comparisons with sufferings in purgatory. The plague, in contrast, was characterised by its rapidity and the fact that it could be cured or prove fatal within a comparatively short space of time – hence the introduction of quarantine, which was intended to treat victims, as well as to protect the healthy, and lasted for just over a month.

It has been argued that both leprosy and plague elicited similar responses, crucially with regard to removing first lepers and then the plague sick 'outside the camp', in accordance with the biblical injunction in Leviticus 13. The sites set up for the accommodation of lepers and plague victims have been closely associated, to the extent that leper houses and plague hospitals have been seen by some historians as two generations of the same institution.[21] Plague epidemics were becoming increasingly frequent at a time when leprosy seemed to be on the decline. *Leprosaria* were said to be emptying and were, therefore, available for use as the sites of plague hospitals. This was, indeed, the case in some places, although not, significantly, in Venice, Milan or Ragusa. Yet, even when continuity occurred, the point should not be overemphasised. Monastic and military sites were also requisitioned as plague hospitals, but it does not necessarily follow that plague was understood in the same way as either religious contemplation or military service. In the context of plague, sizeable structures were required which were architecturally suitable for redeployment as hospitals. It was ideal if the sites had been recently abandoned or had just a few inhabitants. Nor is it true that the name *lazaretti* given to plague hospitals, and which came to be adopted more widely, derived from that of the earlier leper hospitals of *San Lazzaro*. The presumed etymological connections between *lazaretti* and *San Lazzaro* constitute a much repeated error in the historiography of the European hospital. The term *lazaretti* actually developed from a corruption of the name of the island on which the first Venetian plague

---

[20] The spread of leprosy was linked with both miasmas and contagion, although Carole Rawcliffe points out that the meaning of the latter term in the past should not be automatically conflated with current definitions – in medieval England 'contagion' could encompass hereditary and congenital transmission: Rawcliffe, *Leprosy in Medieval England*, 90.

[21] Achille Breda, 'Contributo alla storia dei lazaretti (leprosaria) medioevali in Europa', *Atti del reale Istituto Veneto di scienze, lettere ed arti*, lxviii (1908–9), 133–94; G.B. Risse, *Mending Bodies, Saving Souls: a History of Hospitals* (Oxford, 1999), particularly ch. 4 ('Hospitals as Segregation and Confinement Tools: Leprosy and Plague'), 167–229.

hospital was founded (Santa Maria di Nazareth). It is apparent from contemporary records that the hospital became known as the '*nazaretto*' and later '*lazaretto*'.[22] The use of leper hospitals is likely to have been a matter of practical convenience rather than a reflection of some underlying conceptual link between the two diseases.

Although the connections made between leprosy and plague need to be reconsidered, there are useful ways in which the institutions of the leper house and plague hospital can be seen in parallel, not least for nuancing our understanding of what being placed 'outside the camp' meant in practice. Rawcliffe has shown that many leper houses (both rich and poor) admitted the sick on a voluntary basis, that the patients could retain a degree of contact with the outside world and that the sites were often located near city gates rather than far beyond the walls.[23] Still retaining a place within their communities, lepers attended mass and made confession, and thus remained within the body of the church.[24] The issue of burial was more complicated – although it took place in consecrated ground, if not in parish burial sites. Some of these characteristics were also shared by early plague hospitals. Quarantine, during the fifteenth century, was not always compulsory and patients were induced to leave their homes because of the perceived benefits in terms of quality of care and nourishment provided by hospitals. Nor were these institutions necessarily located outside cities. Indeed, they might be found in urban centres well into the sixteenth century. In Verona, for example, it was not until the epidemic of 1575–7 that the authorities decided that communal health was being threatened by the use of urban sites as plague hospitals; and during the 1590s significant investment was made in a plague hospital beyond the city walls.[25] Plague victims also continued to receive communion and to confess. When it comes to the interpretation of these spaces as accommodation for the sick, it is important to recognise that separation was not synonymous with expulsion. In fact, at a time when certain social and religious groups were being expelled from cities, separation should be recognised as an entirely different, and in this case temporary, response which was applied more broadly to the healthy as well.

In a late medieval English context, Rawcliffe has demonstrated that 'official attempts to separate presumed lepers from society tended to occur during periods of crisis, when concerns about epidemic disease, disorder and vagrancy were running high'.[26] In other words, the removal of the sick was not solely motivated by ideas about illness, but was shaped and applied against a wider background of pressing social issues. Such factors not only influenced the treatment of lepers but, as Rawcliffe observes in a characteristically neat turn of phrase, those who appeared either 'physically or morally leprous'. In Renaissance Europe, too, the use of space in response to the problems apparently posed by specific social groups was not limited to a medical context. The development of quarantine in Milan, Ragusa and Venice, therefore, should be understood in terms of more general policies and attitudes towards the urban environment. In so doing, an influential

---

[22] For example, ASV, Provveditori al Sal, b.6 reg. 3, ff. 47v, 72.
[23] Rawcliffe, *Leprosy in Medieval England*, 7.
[24] *Ibid.*, 53.
[25] J.L. Stevens Crawshaw, *Plague Hospitals: Public Health for the City in Early Modern Venice* (Aldershot, 2012), 75.
[26] Rawcliffe, *Leprosy in Medieval England*, 253.

genre of writing – the tract on the ideal Renaissance city – can be helpful. In such works, emphasis was placed on the creation of a well-ordered cityscape as a means of promoting a well-ordered society; the relationship between people and place was significant and intricate, and fostered a deep-rooted belief in the notion of 'safe space'. What follows is a preliminary study of such tracts in order to link Renaissance urban planning with state efforts in the sphere of public health.

In the Italian Renaissance city, policy was based on the association between the *urbs* and the *polis*, the city and its people. Studies of the relationship between specific parts of buildings or cities likewise drew upon the proportions and functions of the human body. The contemporary relevance of such anthropomorphic imagery also relied upon the analogy made between man as the microcosm and his habitat or environment as the macrocosm. This series of correspondences fed into a more general connection between the characteristics of places and those of people. Works on ideal cities, therefore, were essentially about ideal societies, however implicit or explicit authors chose to make this point. One of the most famous examples of such writing is by Antonio Averlino, known as 'Filarete' (c.1400–1469), who described his ideal city as a body.[27] In his tract, Filarete explored the close relationship between the nature of place and people. The foundation stone of his ideal city was to be buried along with a bronze book recording the notable things of the age, a jar of wheat and glass jars of water, wine, milk, oil and honey. He explained that this was to be done so that the city would be full of the things which give life to man. He elaborated further on the importance of each of the substances and its role in strengthening the physical foundations. Water was clean, pure and useful to all people, just as every inhabitant should be. Being composed of distilled blood, milk ranked as one of the best substances for giving nutriment. Drawing on humoral theory, Filarete urged that sanguine men should purge themselves of excess blood, becoming 'white', or charitable, rather than 'red'. Oil was said to be equally beneficial, coming from a plant dedicated to Pallas Athena, the goddess of wisdom, with branches that signified victory and peace. Finally, honey was chosen because it was sweet, useful and made by animals that were attentive, obedient and good. Each bee carried out the tasks assigned to it and obeyed every command, just as the model citizen should; not surprisingly, bees and hives offered a plethora of similes for the well governed state.[28]

The exercise of state power not only influenced theories about the architectural form of the ideal city, but also prompted official intervention in the management of the environment both within and beyond the walls. Elements of the built fabric of a city are often considered apart from their immediate location, in the same way that a city is often separated from its rural surroundings in historical studies. It was clear to Renaissance rulers that the effective use of the natural landscape could complement the beauty, safety and health of the urban setting. In Milan, for example, the association between the beauty of the city and its outskirts was

---

[27]   What follows derives from Antonio di Pietro Averlino ('Filarete'), 'Sforzinda', in *La città ideale nel Rinascimento*, ed. G.C. Sciolla (Turin, 1975), 70–84.

[28]   For the political image of the bee and the hive see W.J. Farrell, 'The Role of Mandeville's Bee Analogy in "The Grumbling Hive"', *Studies in English Literature 1500–1900*, xxv (3) (1985), especially 511–13; and Bee Wilson, *The Hive: the Story of the Honeybee and Us* (2004), ch. 3 ('Politics'), 106–40.

recognised by an admiring observer during the late thirteenth century. Friar Bonvesin de la Riva reported that,

This city has a circular form, and such a marvellous roundness is the sign of its perfection. A trench of surprising beauty and breadth surrounds this city and contains, not a swamp or a putrid pool, but living water from fountains stocked with fish and crayfish.[29]

These assets could be developed in the interests of defence, trade, health and aesthetics, and became the focus of political intervention during the Renaissance, partly because of the way in which notions of public and private ownership and interest were blurred. The use (or abuse) of a city's environment by its inhabitants could clearly have communal implications; the heightened concerns regarding sanitary nuisances and the management of shared resources in times of epidemic disease offer a case in point. Those seeking to establish or to secure their hold over political structures, therefore, did well to consider initiatives which appeared to promote the public good. In 1457, Francesco Sforza added the development of the Milanese river network to his list of the public works that were intended to 'establish his political legitimacy'.[30]

Both the built and natural environments could be used to provide appropriate sites for potentially dangerous groups or activities. In Venice, for example, by the thirteenth century, certain trades had been banned from the city for health reasons and relocated to lagoon islands.[31] This policy was extended to others during the following centuries.[32] Works on ideal cities also identified safe spaces within the walls, particularly for hospitals and the care of the sick. Leon Battista Alberti's treatise on this theme, for example, suggests that those with contagious diseases ought to be given separate quarters, the creation of which was encouraged by growing demands for appropriate care, as well as concerns about the infectious nature of the sick and especially of their breath. During the fifteenth century, there was a well-documented specialisation of charitable and medical foundations, which has been widely studied by historians and closely linked to the important civic functions which these institutions served. Their purpose was both to protect the populace and to make visible the care for different social groups provided in the name of the public good.

This civic purpose of hospitals on the Italian peninsula is comprehensively illustrated in John Henderson's monograph of 2006, in which he establishes Florence as the home of 'the Renaissance Hospital'. He cites a number of contemporary descriptions of Florence's hospitals as, *inter alia*, 'beautiful and capacious ... adapted and organised to receive any sick or healthy person who is wretched and needs to be received for whatever reason', although, at this point, the

---

[29] Patrick Boucheron, 'Water and Power in Milan, c.1200–1500', *Urban History*, xxviii (2001), 180–93.

[30] *Ibid.*, 191.

[31] In 1271, for example, the *conciatori di pelli* were sent to the Giudecca: Nicolo Spada, 'Leggi veneziane sulle industrie chimiche a tutela della salute pubblica dal secolo XIII al XVIII', *Archivio veneto*, 5th series, vii (1930), 126–56.

[32] In 1413, for instance, dyeing was banned within the city. For the growing use of these islands and civic hygiene measures see, for example, *Venezia e la peste 1348–1797*, ed. Brossollet, 118.

care was not extended to the plague sick.[33] The same encomium goes on specifically to note this fact, for, at the time of writing, early Renaissance Florence lacked a *lazaretto*. In 1479, though, when the decision was taken to set up a permanent plague hospital, it too was said to be 'couched in terms of Christian charity to show the world that the city's door of charity was as open as in other parts of the world'. The investment was further justified 'on the grounds that "the greater the danger to those who look after the sick and the more these people are abandoned by everybody, the greater the merit in the eyes of God to whomever receives them and provides for their needs"'. Such sentiments underscore the significance of specialised structures in the context of Renaissance civic governance, not least as a means of demonstrating centralised, charitable endeavours.[34]

This same goal was pursued in each of the three cities at the forefront of the development of quarantine. In Milan, Gian Galeazzo Visconti (1378–1402) famously attempted to centralise authority within the duchy, not least through the control of charitable institutions. Giangaleazzo purchased the title of duke from the Holy Roman emperor in 1395. Jane Black has argued that his investiture did not dramatically alter the nature of Visconti rule in practical terms, but that the title was intended to shape perceptions of the coup of 1385, in which Giangaleazzo had ousted his uncle Barnabò, and to unite a previously divided state.[35] This strategy provides an important context in which to consider public health issues, since Giangaleazzo's policies were concerned with the expansion of the state, as well as his attempts to make its structures more visible. Significant innovations were also made, in relation to quarantine, during the period of the Ambrosiana Republic between 1447 and 1450. Temporary *lazaretti* were located in a castle at Cusago, which the Visconti had used for recreation and pleasure; within Milan, the ducal castle of Porta Giovia assumed a similar role, 'as signorial power was transformed into a symbol of civic charity'.[36] The Republic's authorities, therefore, also recognised the importance of controlling charitable and welfare institutions as a means of demonstrating political power and forging links between the populace and the communal government.

Ragusa was a small city-state and independent republic which, during the fifteenth century, accommodated a population of approximately 3,000 people within its walls.[37] Even at its peak in the sixteenth century, the population was only approximately 9,000. Irena Benyovsky Latin's work in particular has drawn attention to the striking number of hospitals established in Renaissance Ragusa, especially given the size of the population, although they are less well documented in the historiography than they should be because many archival sources were destroyed in an earthquake and fire in 1667.[38] The best known of them was the *Hospedal del comun*, founded in 1347. It would eventually become a hospital for

---

[33]   Henderson, *The Renaissance Hospital*, 70.
[34]   *Ibid.*, 94. See also Henderson's article, below, p. 183.
[35]   Jane Black, *Absolutism in Renaissance Milan: Plenitude of Power under the Visconti and the Sforza, 1329–1535* (Oxford, 2010), 68–72.
[36]   *Ibid.*, 135.
[37]   Stuard, 'A Communal Program of Medical Care', 138.
[38]   I.B. Latin, 'Dubrovnik Renaissance Hospitals: Between Lay and Religious', unpublished seminar paper delivered to the Renaissance Society of America, Venice, 8 April 2010.

the care of the sick poor, but its first function was to accommodate foreign merchants and their goods in a location conveniently close to the port. Most of the city's medieval hospitals were small and run by private benefactors, but, during the late fourteenth and early fifteenth centuries, foundations increased in number, grew more specialized and, crucially, became an important element in negotiations between church and state for the control of systems of charity and welfare. They were brought under the remit of the Republic and managed in the name of the public good.

As is well known from Brian Pullan's work, Venetian hospitals did not develop along the same lines as those of many other cities in Europe into larger, more specialised institutions.[39] Only the Pietà (the city's orphanage and foundling hospital) fits that bill before the sixteenth century. By contrast, most hospitals continued to serve particular neighbourhoods or guilds. The city was also very late to establish a central body to administer its hospitals. The introduction in 1423 of a quarantine hospital, which was both centralised and state-funded, was, therefore, the exception rather than the rule. A number of attempts have been made to identify the inspiration for this institution. In his study of Doge Francesco Foscari (1373–1457), Denis Romano gives the credit for this innovation to Foscari himself, and cites it as an illustration of the Doge's paternal care for the wider community. The plague hospital was classified as a 'pious institution' and made part of the charitable networks of the city.[40] Testators were encouraged to donate money to it alongside local institutions. The hospital featured prominently in attempts to weave centralised, civic initiatives into the fabric of neighbourhood charity. In all three cities, quarantine structures were used in various ways to make the authority and influence of Renaissance governments more visible in the early fifteenth century.

It should be acknowledged that these three cities were not operating in isolation from one another, or from communities elsewhere. In particular, this is true of Ragusa and Venice, not least because of the so-called 'Venetian period' in Ragusan history between 1205 and 1358; indeed it is clear that Venetian influence endured beyond the mid fifteenth century. The Ragusan constitution was said to have been virtually copied from that of Venice and remained almost unchanged after the end of Venetian sovereignty.[41] Ragusa had neither a school of medicine nor a guild or fraternity of surgeons, and consequently until the fourteenth century Ragusans travelled to Venice to recruit medical men.[42] There were institutional borrowings too: in 1432, the Ragusan authorities established a foundling hospital, or *Ospedale della Misericordia*, modelled on the Venetian Pietà with one of the famous revolving *ruote*.[43] In terms of influence from elsewhere, Siena and its celebrated hospital of *Santa Maria della Scala* were explicitly cited as examples for the reform of Milan's hospitals by Gian Galeazzo in 1399.[44] San Bernardino of Siena's successful preaching and subsequent request to the Venetian authorities for

---

[39] Brian Pullan, *Rich and Poor in Renaissance Venice: the Social Institutions of a Catholic State, to 1620* (Oxford, 1971).

[40] Palmer, 'The Control of Plague in Venice', 185.

[41] Carter, *Dubrovnik (Ragusa)*, 116.

[42] Stuard, 'A Communal Program of Medical Care', 128.

[43] Latin, 'Dubrovnik Renaissance Hospitals', 3. The Ragusan system for the administration of charitable institutions was also modelled on that of the Venetian Procurators: *ibid.*, 4.

[44] Welch, *Art and Authority*, 128.

the city to develop designated institutions for quarantine were together said to have inspired the foundation of the Venetian system.[45] Given his powers of persuasion, it is worth considering the sentiments expressed by San Bernardino regarding responses to epidemic disease and illness in general. Preaching during the 1420s, he asked his congregation:

> Do you want to survive corporal death, epidemics or pain in the side or the illnesses which beset you day after day? And you, woman, do you want to be free of pestilence, do you want to be healed of the disease that you have? Yes? Now go, run to charity, and I promise you that if you take the medicine which I will teach you, you will be cured of every ill.[46]

San Bernardino's emphasis on the importance of charity in response to epidemics brings us full circle to Filargo's complaint about 'miserable Milan' with which this article started. The introduction of civic institutions was not only intended to provide care for the sick but also to prevent outbreaks of epidemics and natural disasters by engaging with the all-important issue of charity. Quarantine was one policy of the late fourteenth and early fifteenth centuries which promoted a centralised response to a natural disaster and which could be made in the name of the public good. It also reflected the broader concerns of Renaissance governments – particularly the reshaping of urban space in the interests of aesthetics, health and welfare. Emphasising the significance of these attitudes in the formulation of responses to plague does not preclude the historical connection previously made with reactions to leprosy, but it does argue against the perceived exceptionalism of medical responses, and suggests that it is sensible to consider assumptions about each of the two diseases in their wider social contexts. One of the benefits of continuing to recognise a link with leprosy is that it reminds us how well-established many of these concepts actually were. However, there was something distinctive about Renaissance ideas, which was expressed most clearly in the tracts about ideal cities: namely the close association between good governance, ordered city space and ordered societies, which often promoted intervention by civic authorities in both built and natural environments.

The specific contexts of Ragusa, Milan and Venice meant that the chronology and form of innovations did differ, but in each case the Renaissance, civic solutions to the kind of problems Filargo was bemoaning and about which San Bernardino was preaching became, initially, spatial and subsequently architectural or institutional. Quarantine – through its regulation of movement and control of space – evolved into a structure for providing, distributing and demonstrating charity and for facilitating the practice of medicine. It was developed as a result of the contemporary association between charity and natural disasters. It allowed Renaissance governments to devise collective responses and to make civic charity more prominent. Unlike many charitable and medical institutions which bridged the public and private divide, quarantine initiatives and hospitals were public. They

---

[45] This is discussed in Iris Origo, *The World of San Bernardino* (1963), 32–3.
[46] San Bernardino of Siena, cited in Palmer, 'The Control of Plague in Venice', 86. See *idem*, 'The Church, Leprosy and Plague in Early Modern Europe', *Studies in Church History*, xix (1982), 79–99, especially 89.

served to make the connection between the creation of safe space and good governance overt, strengthening a sense of authority within Renaissance states, as well as providing protection against disease and the potential damage that an outbreak of pestilence could cause to a state's reputation in both the political and economic spheres.

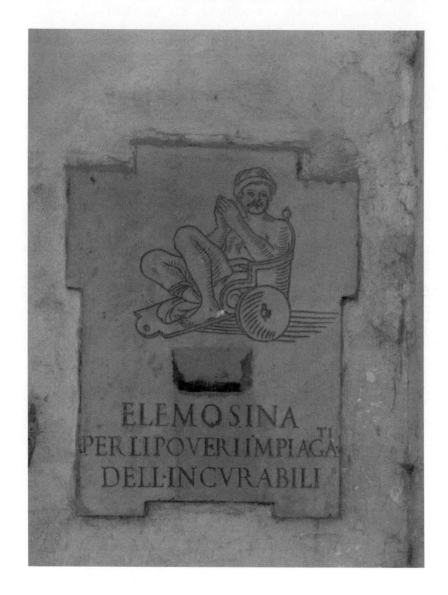

Plate 1: Plaque on the Incurabili Hospital of S. Giacomo, Rome.
Photograph: John Henderson.

COPING WITH EPIDEMICS IN RENAISSANCE ITALY: PLAGUE AND THE GREAT POX

John Henderson

This article will examine and compare the way that society coped with two of the major epidemics to affect Renaissance Italy: plague and the Great Pox. Even though these diseases impacted on Italy as severely as they did on the rest of Europe, different countries devised different solutions to the same problems. Discussing the strategies that Italy adopted in the long fifteenth century is valuable not just to those who work on Italian Renaissance history, but also to historians of countries such as England which developed very different measures. Indeed, in the sixteenth century, in the case of plague, the privy council and statesmen such as William Cecil, Lord Burghley, looked to continental and particularly Italian plague measures as a reflection of their 'civility', which made them worthy of imitation.[1]

The main elements which constituted this 'civility' will be the subject of the first part of this article, which will examine society's reactions to plague in Renaissance Italy through the prism of how contemporaries understood the nature of the disease. One of the more traditional themes of historical studies of Italian plague is the idea that at the time there was a marked division in beliefs between doctors and health boards about how disease was spread, with the former supporting the idea of infected air, or miasma, and the latter espousing contagionist views. This story is complicated still further from the late fifteenth century by the emergence of the Great Pox. It has been suggested that, particularly under the influence of Girolamo Fracastoro, this epidemic led to the 'true' understanding of contagion, as the Pox was seen to have been spread by human contact. Indeed, Fracastoro has even been hailed as the first bacteriologist.[2] More recent scholarship has recognised that the situation was actually much more complex.[3] This can be

---

[1] For a discussion of foreign influences on English plague provisions, see Paul Slack, *The Impact of Plague in Tudor and Stuart England* (1985), 203, 207–19.

[2] Col. Fielding H. Garrison, writing in 1910, cited approvingly in Wilmer Cave Wright's 'Introduction' to her edition and translation of Girolamo Fracastoro, *De contagione et contagiosis morbis et eorum curatione libri tres* (New York, 1930), p. xxxi. The editor of Fracastoro's 1533 prose work on the French Disease, Francesco Pellegrini, attributed to him the discovery of germ theory: *Trattato inedito in prosa di Gerolamo Fracastoro sulla sifilide* (Verona, 1939), 197.

[3] Vivian Nutton, 'The Reception of Fracastoro's Theory of Contagion. The Seeds that Fell Among Thorns?', *Osiris*, 2nd series, vi (1990), 196–234; reprinted in Nutton, *From Democedes to Harvey: Studies in the History of Medicine* (1988), 15–34; Jon Arrizabalaga, John Henderson and Roger

seen from two short passages which reflect the reactions of the Italian authorities, first to plague and secondly to the Great Pox, and also their understanding of both diseases. First, a law of the Florentine government of 21 August 1476 promulgated during an epidemic of plague:

> The Magnificent and Excellent Lords, Lord Priors of Liberty and Standard-Bearer of Justice of the Florentine people desiring to maintain health in the city from any *contagion* of plague and in order to achieve this effect every possible human remedy is to be taken … so that plague, through *contagion*, does not offend the city …[4]

Second, a decree of the Venetian Health Board, or *Sanità*, in 1523, responding to the problem of the '*mal franciosati*', those sick from the French Disease:

> Some of these persons in their bodily weakness languish in the streets and the doorways of churches and public places both at San Marco and at the Rialto to beg for a living; and some, being inured to their profession of begging, have no wish to seek a cure, and loiter in these same places, giving forth a terrible stench and *infecting* their neighbours and those with whom they live. This [abuse] gives rise to the most vociferous complaints … especially as we are told that the stench may breed *infection* and disease, to the universal damage of this our city.[5]

Given what has been said above about the historiographical tradition, what is intriguing here is that the Florentine authorities used the term 'contagion' in relation to plague, while the Venetians referred to 'infection' when discussing the transmission of the French Disease, which they evidently believed to be spread by stench.[6] This already serves to underline the slipperiness of contemporary use of these terms and the inherent problems in setting up an artificial opposition between miasmatic and contagionist ideas.

One of the main reasons that this paradigm has remained so popular in traditional Italian historiography is the continued influence of Alfonso Corradi, the physician turned medical historian who was writing in the second half of the nineteenth century. His influence stems from his fundamental collection of sources,

   French, *The Great Pox. The French Disease in Renaissance Europe* (New Haven and London, 1997), ch. 1. Most recently on Fracastoro, see *Girolamo Fracastoro. Fra medicina, filosofia e scienze della natura*, ed. Alessandro Pastore and Enrico Peruzzi (Florence, 2006).

[4]   Archivio di Stato di Firenze [henceforth ASF], Provvisione Registri [henceforth Provv. Reg.], 167, f. 75v; cf. Andrea Corsini, *La 'moria' del 1464 in Toscana e l'istituzione dei primi lazaretti in Firenze ed in Pisa* (Florence, 1911), 44 (my italics).

[5]   *Venice. A Documentary History, 1450–1630*, ed. David Chambers and Brian Pullan (Oxford, 1992), 308–9 (my italics).

[6]   Francois-Olivier Touati makes the same point in relation to leprosy: 'Contagion and Leprosy: Myth, Ideas and Evolution in Medieval Minds and Societies', in *Contagion: Perspectives from Pre-Modern Societies*, ed. L.I. Conrad and Dominik Wujastyk (Aldershot, 2000), 179–201. See also, F.-O. Touati, 'Historiciser la notion de contagion: L'exemple de la lèpre dans les societés médiévales', in *Air, miasmes et contagion: Les épidemiés dans l'antiquité et au moyen âge*, ed. Sylvie Bazin-Tacchella, Danielle Quéruel and Évelyne Samama (Langres, 2001), 157–86.

the *Annali delle epidemie in Italia*, published between 1865 and 1895, at a time when debates were most heated between contagionists and miasmists in relation to the nature and causes of disease.[7] Indeed, given the number of times Corradi published passages including the word 'contagion', one could be forgiven for concluding that a sub-text of his *Annali* was to further the cause of the contagionists.[8] These references to 'contagion' have provided persuasive evidence for those more recent historians who have wished to document the presumed contrast between the health boards' belief in contagion and doctors' belief in the spread of disease by infected air. In the second half of the twentieth century it was Carlo Cipolla's series of ground-breaking studies of Tuscany in the seventeenth century which proved the most influential on plague historiography; and in his work we find the continued suggestion of a gulf between lay and medical understanding of the nature and methods of transmission of plague.[9] The implication is that the men who ran governments and the members of the health boards were more 'rational' and showed greater common-sense in their approach to plague control, which was based on empirical observation and belief in contagion. This has been portrayed as more 'scientific' when compared with the more theoretical stance of the physician, whose vision was seen as befogged by belief in miasma and corrupt air.

In fact, once one begins to examine the evidence, and in particular to analyse contemporary use of language, belief in this gulf becomes clearly unsustainable. To stress the obvious, health boards specifically appointed well-known physicians to determine the nature of epidemics and to give them advice based on their diagnosis about the best course of action to follow. This happened from the time of the Black Death, when Italian governments had asked physicians to anatomise publicly the bodies of plague victims, had commissioned plague treatises, and increasingly asked Colleges of Physicians for their expertise and the provision of specialist advice.[10] Samuel Cohn in his recent work has shown that there was a growing emphasis by the medical profession in Italy on the value of observation and experience. The corollary of this pragmatism was that physicians for at least a century following the Black Death felt a new confidence in their ability to heal plague victims, though their confidence in time began to fade once it became all too obvious that plague had come to stay.[11]

[7]   Giorgio Cosmacini, *Storia della medicina e della sanità in Italia dalla peste europea alla prima guerra mondiale, 1348–1918* (Rome and Bari, 1989), 349, 358–64.

[8]   See Claudio Pogliano, 'L'utopia igienista (1870–1920)', in *Malattia e medicina. Storia d'Italia. Annali, VII*, ed. Franco Della Peruta (Turin, 1984), 589–631.

[9]   Two of the best known are C.M. Cipolla, *Public Health and the Medical Profession in the Renaissance* (Cambridge, 1976), and *Cristofano and the Plague. A Study in the History of Public Health in the Age of Galileo* (1973). More recently, see A.G. Carmichael, *Plague and the Poor in Renaissance Florence* (Cambridge, 1986), and 'Contagion Theory and Contagion Practice in Fifteenth-Century Milan', *Renaissance Quarterly*, xliv (1991), 213–56.

[10]   For Florence, see John Henderson, 'The Black Death in Florence: Medical and Communal Responses', in *Death in Towns. Urban Responses to the Dying and the Dead, 100–1600*, ed. Steven Bassett (Leicester, 1992), 136–47.

[11]   S.K. Cohn, Jr., *Cultures of Plague. Medical Thinking at the End of the Renaissance* (Oxford, 2010), 10–16.

To examine further this shared use of language and its practical implications, I shall investigate developing public health measures formulated to cope with plague, which I shall then compare with reactions to the Great Pox, prefacing my discussion by briefly summarising contemporary medical theory regarding the causes and spread of plague.

Government measures were based on a shared belief that plague derived from the atmosphere, being formed by poisonous vapours spread from place to place by wind. An epidemic was seen to have been created in a variety of ways from primary, sometimes extra-terrestrial, causes (divine wrath, conjunction of planets) to volcanic eruptions and earthquakes which released poisonous vapours from beneath the earth's surface. The more proximate secondary cause of corrupt vapour or 'poison' often appeared to be the generation of corrupt matter from a series of sources, the most common of which was stagnant water in bogs. Another was the effluence generated by humans living in close proximity; from well before the Black Death Italian communes had passed a series of measures to clean up the environment through the effective disposal of human waste and the banning of butchery of animals in city centres. Indeed, by the mid sixteenth century the importance of this approach was underlined by the revival of Neo-Hippocratic ideas about the link between airs, waters and places and the health of an individual and a city.[12] These ideas had an important impact on Italian public health policies, leading, for example, to the commissioning of detailed surveys of urban and rural landscapes in order to determine the link between corrupt air and environmental conditions.[13]

Despite their best efforts, the continuing level of stench convinced contemporaries that bad smells must be the cause of plague. It was, then, from the recognition of the necessity of preventing the spread of corrupt air that all the well-known provisions taken by Italian governments during periods of plague ultimately derived.[14] It is important to stress this point because it helps us to understand the role of air and its relationship to ideas about putrefaction and smell in the theory of disease and disease transmission in Renaissance Italy. In the case of plague, which was deemed to have been spread through breath or the transmission of vapours which had impregnated the clothes worn by the sick, this led to the burning of cloth or its lengthy exposure to the air as a preventative measure. The idea that at the time there was any clear-cut distinction between 'contagion' and 'infection', or, indeed, that the term 'contagion' had any one single meaning in this period, is too simple-minded, as has been amply demonstrated in the work of more recent

---

[12]   On Tuscany, see C.M. Cipolla, *Miasmas and Disease. Public Health and Environment in the Pre-Industrial Age* (New Haven and London, 1992); and, more generally, Andrew Wear, 'Making Sense of Health and the Environment in Early Modern England', in *Health and Healing in Early Modern England*, ed. Wear (1998), 119–47, and Mary Dobson, *Contours of Death and Disease in Early Modern England* (Cambridge, 1997).

[13]   Cipolla, *Miasmas and Disease*; John Henderson, 'Public Health, Pollution and the Problem of Waste Disposal in Early Modern Tuscany', in *Le interazioni fra economia e ambiente biologico nell'Europa preindustriale, secc. XIII–XVIII*, ed. Simonetta Cavaciocchi (Florence, 2010), 373–82.

[14]   For the most detailed discussion of medical theory of plague at the time of the Black Death, see Jon Arrizabalaga, 'Facing the Black Death: Perceptions and Reactions of University Medical Practitioners', in *Practical Medicine from Salerno to the Black Death*, ed. Luis Garcia-Ballester, Roger French, Jon Arrizabalaga and Andrew Cunningham (Cambridge, 1994), 237–88.

historians, such as Vivian Nutton, Jon Arrizabalaga and Samuel Cohn.[15] This was as true of medical men as of the health officials who organised the administrative measures taken during plague epidemics.

Public Health and Plague

In the period I am surveying, from roughly the mid fourteenth to the mid sixteenth century, Italian states evolved a system to deal with plague which grew gradually more sophisticated as it was realised that the disease was not just a temporary phenomenon. I shall look at developments in north-central Italy, and especially Florence, which was one of the major cities of Europe and whose experience of the Black Death remains one of the best known through the description by Giovanni Boccaccio in the 'Introduction' to *The Decameron*. The city, like many others, suffered from outbreaks of plague at regular ten- to fifteen-year intervals during these two centuries, which varied in severity, but effectively prevented it from returning to its pre-Black Death population of about 100,000.[16]

Boccaccio's celebrated account of the plague begins by mentioning the measures taken by the commune, even if the purpose of this passage was to emphasise that they were largely ineffective:

And in that pestilence no wisdom nor provision was of any use, such as the cleansing of the streets of much refuse by officials appointed for that purpose, and the prohibition of any sick persons from entering the city and many counsels [of the doctors] given for the preservation of health ...[17]

Boccaccio conflates a series of strategies here. First, he speaks of 'officials appointed for that purpose'. In common with some other northern and central Italian states, city governments instituted *ad hoc* magistracies specifically to supervise the necessary measures to deal with the emergency.[18] The second element to which Boccaccio alludes is the role of the Florentine magistracy in 'cleansing of the streets of much refuse'. This clearly was based on existing sanitary practice; and the reason for such activity in March 1348 at the outset of the Black Death was, in the words of contemporary legislation, 'to avoid the corruption and infection of the air', which stemmed from the 'putrefaction and corruption of things and bodies'.[19] Talk of putrefaction of bodies leads to one of the gravest

---

[15] Nutton, *From Democedes to Harvey*, 15–34; Arrizabalaga, 'Facing the Black Death', 237–88; and Cohn, *Cultures of Plague*.

[16] On plague in medieval Florence, see Carmichael, *Plague and the Poor*, and Henderson, 'The Black Death in Florence'.

[17] Giovanni Boccaccio, *Decameron*, ed. Vittore Branca (Florence, 1976), 9–10.

[18] For Venice, see Mario Brunetti, 'Venezia durante la peste del 1348', *L'Ateneo Veneto*, xxxii (1) (1909), 5–42, 289–311; and, more recently, *Venezia e la peste, 1348–1797* (Venice, 1979); for Siena, W.M. Bowsky, 'The Impact of the Black Death upon Sienese Government and Society', *Speculum*, xxxix (1964), 1–34; and for Orvieto, Élisabeth Carpentier, *Une ville devant la peste. Orvieto e la peste noire de 1348* (Paris, 1962).

[19] ASF, Provv. Reg. 35, f. 133v.

problems associated with the Black Death: the burial of tens of thousands of corpses. A contemporary Florentine chronicler, Marco di Coppo Stefani, points to another element of government policy which became a standard feature of strategies adopted during plague:

> At every church they dug deep pits down to the water level; and thus those who were poor who died during the night were bundled up quickly and thrown into the pit, they then took some earth and shovelled it down on top of them; and later others were placed on top of them and then another layer of earth, just as one makes *lasagne* with layers of pasta and cheese.[20]

The preoccupation with rapid burial was to avoid the stench and toxic vapours which would spread the pestilence and corrupt the humours of the survivors. Fear of corruption of the air was also behind measures to deal with cloth, which was believed to absorb and retain within itself the diseased air. This led famously to the restriction of the import of cloth into Italian cities and to the quarantining and disinfection of clothes which were deemed to have come into contact with plague victims. The obsession with cloth is clearly reflected in the 'Ordinances' passed by the Tuscan city of Pistoia at the time of the Black Death in spring to summer 1348:

> The foresaid wise men provided and ordered that no person whether citizen, inhabitant of the district or county of the city of Pistoia or foreigner shall dare or presume in any way to bring ... to the city of Pistoia, its district or county, any used cloth, either linen or woollen, for use as clothing for men or women on penalty of £200.[21]

Policies adopted during the Black Death sowed the seeds of the strategies which developed in northern and central Italy over the following 150 years. In Florence, as in other cities, existing sanitary legislation for cleansing the streets and the disinfection of cloth was combined with social measures for the welfare and containment of the sick poor.

The structures put into place during emergencies caused by epidemics in Florence, as elsewhere in Italy, combined public and semi-private initiatives. Public health boards emerged from the magistracies traditionally appointed to deal with specific problems, such as warfare or famine. Over the next two centuries these magistracies were established on a more permanent basis, although there was some variation from city to city, depending on need and the type of government in operation. Milan, ruled over by the authoritarian regimes of the Visconti and then the Sforza, had from the first imposed more draconian measures, reputedly bricking up alive the first victims of the Black Death.[22] The city established a

---

[20] *Cronica Fiorentina di Marchionne di Coppo Stefani*, ed. Niccolò Rodolico (Città di Castello, 1903), in *Rerum Italicarum Scriptores*, new series, xxx (1), 230–1: rubric 634.

[21] 'Gli ordinamenti sanitari del Comune di Pistoia contro la Pestilenza del 1348', ed. Andrea Chiappelli, *Archivio Storico Italiano*, 4th series, xx (1887), 8–22.

[22] On plague in Milan, see Giuliana Albini, *Guerra, fame, peste. Crisi di mortalità e sistema sanitaria nella Lombardia tardomedioevale* (Bologna, 1982); Carmichael, 'Contagion Theory and Contagion Practice'.

permanent health board in 1448,[23] followed in 1486 by republican Venice, which was particularly vulnerable to plague through its geographical position and its role as a centre for trade between the west and east Mediterranean. Florence appointed temporary magistracies during plague epidemics from the Black Death onwards, as in 1448 when the role of the *Otto di Guardia e Balìa* was defined as being 'to preserve the health of the people and to prevent plague and to avoid [the spread of] contagion'.[24] In other words, the city-states of northern and central Italy adopted similar administrative structures, whether a regime was princely or republican, though it is a mistake to assume that they all immediately became permanent. For example, despite what is generally believed, Florence did not establish a permanent health board until well into the sixteenth century; and, in the event, plague did not return to the city for a hundred years after 1530.[25]

Health boards eventually came to co-ordinate the overall control of plague measures within the city, including the inspection and disinfection of infected houses or those suspected of harbouring plague, the provision of medical treatment, the transport of the sick, the isolation of those who had come into contact with them and the burial of the dead. Also, in time, health passes were introduced for goods from infected places and *cordons sanitaires* were set up, as a result of which frontiers were closed with neighbouring states infected with plague and trade was stopped with the rest of the peninsula.[26] One of the reasons that plague boards became more permanent was not just to direct responses during epidemics, but also to provide conduits of communication with other cities and countries in order to learn about the spread and progress of an epidemic.[27]

If the overall control of plague measures was a public responsibility, in many cities much of the actual work in dealing with the sick and dead was undertaken by semi-private organisations. In Florence until the late fifteenth century those sick from plague were removed to the main medical hospital of Santa Maria Nuova, an independent institution which served the poor of the city.[28] Here they would have been provided with clean beds and treated with an appropriate diet, as well as the wonder drug of theriac, which was believed to be a panacea against even the most severe diseases.[29] Then, from the 1490s, the actual transport of the sick or those who had died from plague became the responsibility of a private fraternity of laymen called the 'Misericordia', whose members undertook this arduous work in a spirit of Christian charity.[30] This intermeshing of public and private initiatives remained characteristic of Italian systems designed to cope with epidemic and

---

[23] On dates for the establishment of health boards, see A.G. Carmichael, 'Plague Legislation in the Italian Renaissance', *Bulletin of the History of Medicine*, lvii (1983), table 5, p. 521.

[24] ASF, Provv. Reg. 139, f. 125.

[25] Carmichael, 'Plague Legislation', table 5, p. 521; cf. Cipolla, *Public Health and the Medical Profession*, 13–14, for the assertion that the Florentine health board was made permanent in 1527.

[26] Carmichael, 'Plague Legislation', table 1, p. 513.

[27] For a fuller discussion of this topic, see Cipolla, *Public Health and the Medical Profession*.

[28] On the role of this hospital, see John Henderson, *The Renaissance Hospital. Healing the Body and Healing the Soul* (New Haven and London, 2006).

[29] *Ibid.*, 307.

[30] See John Henderson, 'Plague in Renaissance Florence: Medical Theory and Government Response', in *Maladies et société (XII–XVIIIe siècles)*, ed. Neithard Bulst and Robert Delort (Paris, 1989), 165–86.

endemic disease throughout the post-Reformation period, compared with many countries in northern Europe where the state became increasingly central to policies concerned with the poor and sick.[31]

The gradual emergence of public health boards has been seen as a significant achievement of Italian plague controls, but the one for which Italy became most renowned was the pest-house or *lazaretto*. Between 1423 and 1462 some eleven different cities in northern-central Italy passed legislation to establish isolation hospitals. While initially, as in the case of Florence, many were based in existing hospitals,[32] in time the vast majority of cities established new and permanent *lazaretti*. One of the largest was in Milan; it was built in 1488 and consisted of a vast square courtyard measuring some 368 by 370 metres. At the centre of the courtyard was a chapel open on all sides so that the sick could see the celebration of the Host, designed to cure the plague through the strength of God's spiritual medicine. It was surrounded by a moat to keep out the public and enclosed a structure of 280 small rooms. During the 1630 epidemic it came to accommodate over 16,000 sick people, many of whom were housed in temporary huts.[33] Venice, on the other hand, was the first to initiate another aspect of plague control, through the foundation of a second *lazaretto* as a quarantine station for contacts and those who had recovered from the epidemic. Both were established on islands in the Lagoon, in 1423 and 1471 respectively. At the time of one of the worst epidemics to hit Venice, in 1575, they proved insufficient and the city requisitioned a veritable armada of 3,000 boats which were moored off the island and catered for between 8,000 and 10,000 people.[34]

It would be easy to extrapolate from the examples of Venetian and Milanese responses over the whole of Italy, but in fact the development of isolation hospitals varied considerably according to the geographical location and resources of individual states. The example of Florence shows that governments could be reluctant to devote the necessary funds to establish one of these extremely expensive institutions. It was only in 1464 – over a century after the Black Death – that the government recognised the necessity of providing a separate isolation facility for the sick rather than placing them in the general medical hospital of Santa Maria Nuova, because it was observed that 'others who are sick from other diseases become infected with the contagion of those with plague and therefore those die who should not have died'.[35] In the event, little was done in 1464 because the *morbo* disappeared; and it was only in 1479 that an isolation hospital was begun, in response to another attack of plague, though it did not open until 1494. Despite the good intentions voiced at the time of foundation, intriguingly its capacity was minimal; it had beds for only twenty-six patients, hardly sufficient to house plague victims in an epidemic when hundreds of people might be infected

---

[31]   As in England: Slack, *Impact of Plague*.
[32]   Carmichael, 'Plague Legislation', table 4, p. 520.
[33]   R.J. Palmer, 'The Control of Plague in Venice and Northern Italy, 1348–1600' (Univ. of Kent Ph.D. thesis, 1978), 36.
[34]   On Venice, see Palmer, 'The Control of Plague in Venice', 195–6; the article by Jane Stevens Crawshaw in this volume, pp. 162–4; and her *Plague Hospitals: Public Health for the City in Early Modern Venice* (Aldershot, 2012).
[35]   ASF, Provv. Reg. 155, f. 58; Corsini, *La 'moria' del 1464*, p. 34 (12 June 1464).

each day! It is tempting to see these moves as part of a strategy designed to make the Florentine republic seem both philanthropic and proactive to the outside world during epidemics which were not in fact very severe. Legislators in the mid fifteenth century couched their enactments in terms of Christian charity towards those sick of plague. They claimed that their 'door of charity is as open as in other parts of the world' to all, for 'the greater the danger to those who look after the sick plague victims ... the greater the merit in the eyes of God to whomsoever receives them and provides for their needs'.[36] In this context, reflecting again the cross-over between medical texts and government pronouncements, it is significant that some plague tracts describe charity as another important plank in their preventative policies, for it helped to convince God of man's repentance in the face of His wrath and was thus seen as spiritual medicine against infection.[37]

These were brave sentiments indeed. Attitudes had changed by the 1520s when plague returned to Florence in a much more virulent form.[38] The Florentine administration was forced to construct a veritable shanty town of huts of wood and straw outside the city walls, where those who had been in contact with somebody who had died of plague were housed and fed free of charge on a daily basis. The impetus at this time had changed from Christian charity to concern about the disorders that might arise; gallows were erected as a deterrent to those who broke the law and stole from empty houses or deliberately spread the plague. It was the poor who now became the butt of the government's policy; and, while efforts were made to present a charitable façade, behind it were the sentiments voiced by Niccolò Machiavelli in 1527: 'The clean and beautiful neighbourhoods which are usually full of rich and noble citizens, now are stinking and ugly, full of the poor whose fearful clamours make it difficult to walk through the streets.'[39]

A range of plague controls was developed in Renaissance Italy for the prevention of the spread of the disease, from the isolation and quarantine of people and cloth to the rapid burial of corpses to prevent corrupt fumes from infecting the air. Underwriting these measures lay a shared understanding on the part of magistrates and their medical advisors of the nature of plague and its methods of transmission through infected air. Added to this pragmatic approach were the mixed motives of Christian charity and fear, which increasingly came to underpin official policies towards the poor and sick and led to their increased marginalisation.[40]

The rest of this article will examine how far this shared interpretation of the nature of plague and its methods of transmission informed the reactions of medical and non-medical men to the second great epidemic of this period, the Great Pox,

---

[36] ASF, Provv. Reg. 155, f. 58; Corsini, *La 'moria' del 1464*, p. 34 (12 June).

[37] For charity as a prophylactic, see, for example, BL, Add. 27582, f. 71; Anon., *Here Begynneth A Litill Boke Necessarye & Behouefull agenst the Pestilence* (1485), f. 3v; Richard Palmer, 'The Church, Leprosy and Plague in Medieval and Early Modern Europe', *Studies in Church History*, xix (1982), 79–99, on pp. 86, 89. I am grateful to Carole Rawcliffe for this information.

[38] On plague in the 1520s, see Henderson, 'Plague in Renaissance Florence'.

[39] Niccolò Macchiavelli, 'Descrizione della peste di Firenze dell'anno 1527', in *Opere di Niccolò Machiavelli cittadino fiorentino* (7 vols., Florence, 1813), v. 36.

[40] See Brian Pullan, 'Plague and Perceptions of the Poor in Early Modern Italy', in *Epidemics and Ideas*, ed. Terence Ranger and Paul Slack (Cambridge, 1992), 101–23.

and, furthermore, whether this 'new disease' led to the evolution of new public health strategies.

The Great Pox: Initial Reactions

The epidemic of the French Disease, the *Mal de Naples*, the Great Pox, or the Sickness of St. Job, exploded in Italy in the mid 1490s and from thence spread like wildfire throughout the rest of Europe.[41] The majority of contemporaries described this sickness as an unprecedented phenomenon associated specifically with the invasion by the French army and more generally with the discovery of the New World. One of the fullest accounts of the appearance of the disease is to be found in Francesco Guicciardini's *History of Italy*:

> This disease which was either altogether new or at least unknown up to this time in our hemisphere ... was for many years especially so horrible that it deserves to be mentioned as one of the gravest calamities. For it showed itself either in the form of the most ugly boils, which often became incurable ulcers, or very intense pains in the joints and nerves all over the body. And since the physicians were not experienced in dealing with such a disease, they applied remedies which were not appropriate, but often harmful, frequently inflaming the infection ... This disease killed many men and women of all ages, many became terribly deformed and were rendered useless, suffering from almost continuous torments; indeed, most of those who appeared to have been cured, relapsed in a short space of time into the same miserable state ...[42]

Guicciardini begins by defining the main characteristics of the Great Pox: namely that it was perceived to have been a new disease, notable for intense pains and then boils which became ulcerated; and that a period of respite would be followed by the onset of deformity and eventually death. These symptoms were repeated by most chroniclers throughout Italy from the mid 1490s onwards, many of whom added their own theories of causation and transmission. Neither were medical men initially united in their understanding of the nature of the disease, a fact which led to public disputations in a number of north Italian cities. Some leading academics believed that it was possible to identify the Pox from among those diseases described by the classical authorities whose texts formed the basis of the medical curriculum. The dispute in Ferrara in 1497, for example, involved three main contenders: Niccolò Leoniceno, who believed that it was an epidemic 'disease of the summer' to be found among the Hippocratic works; Sebastiano Dall'Aquila, who thought it was '*elephantiasis*' (or leprosy) as described by Galen; and Coradino Gilino, who maintained that it was the 'Holy Fire', identified by the

---

[41]   The most detailed study of the Great Pox in Italy is Arrizabalaga, Henderson and French, *The Great Pox*.

[42]   Francesco Guicciardini, *Storia d'Italia, I*, ed. Silvana Seidel Menchi (Turin, 1971), 233.

celebrated Muslim scholar Avicenna.[43] The dispute was important because the Great Pox was seen as a threat to medical authority. The fear was that, if it was indeed a new disease, its novelty might call into question the authority of the medical Canon, which was largely derived from the works of Hippocrates, Galen and Avicenna, and in turn challenge the authority of the faculties of medicine within their respective universities.

While disputes were taking place within medical faculties about the nature, novelty and even the name of the Great Pox, contemporary chroniclers had little doubt that it was new, even if there were many contradictory views about how exactly the *morbo* was spread and the degree of its infectiveness. Two Bolognese chroniclers recording events in the mid 1490s, at the time of the public disputations in Ferrara and Bologna, provided very different explanations of transmission: one said quite bluntly that 'the majority of people get this sickness through coitus'; while the second, Friano degli Ubaldini, argued that 'the said sickness is caught ... through eating and through drinking and through carnal intercourse'.[44] Fear of the disease spreading through corrupt air remained powerful. In 1504 in Florence, for example, the canons of the cathedral, anxious lest they might catch from communicants 'French boils and the French Disease', requested a new cupboard so that they might keep separate the 'chasubles, chalices and liturgical vestments' used in public. This precaution suggests they believed that, in common with the miasmas of plague, the vapours of disease might be absorbed within the cloth.[45] Twenty years later, although many contemporaries had by then made the connection between sexual activity and *Morbus Gallicus*, it was still not regarded as the exclusive method of transmission. As in Bologna, so in Venice, different views were recorded in the same city. Marin Sanudo, for instance, wrote in his *Diario*: 'And this sickness begins first in the area of the genitals; and in coitus it is contagious, otherwise not.'[46] However, in the same period, the health board complained of the 'terrible stench' which was generated by beggars with the French Disease, who it was feared might infect those living in the area.[47]

A recognition that it was possible to advance a multiplicity of ideas about transmission explains the lack of any common programme which could be dignified with the term 'government policy' in Italy during the first decade or so after the onset of this new disease. The problem for the authorities was that, unlike plague, it did not kill off its victims rapidly. Instead, those afflicted by the disease, and especially those reduced to poverty, remained to clutter up the streets and to molest passers-by. This lamentable state of affairs was confirmed by the papal physician, Gaspar Torella, writing in c.1500:

[43] Arrizabalaga, Henderson and French, *The Great Pox*, ch. 4.
[44] Cited in Alfonso Corradi, 'Nuovi documenti per la storia delle malattie veneree in Italia dalla fine del Quattrocento alla metà del cinquento', *Annali universali di medicina e chirurgia*, cclxix (1884): 'Cronica Bianchina', 344; Friano degli Ubaldini, 'Cronaca dalla creazione del mondo fino all'anno di N.S. 1513', in Corradi, 'Nuovi documenti', 345.
[45] Cited in Francesco Puccinotti, *Storia della medicina* (3 vols., Livorno, 1850–70), ii (2), 505.
[46] Marin Sanudo, *I Diarii*, ed. Rinaldo Fulin *et al.* (58 vols., Venice, 1879–1902), xxxiii. 233–4.
[47] *Venice. A Documentary History*, ed. Chambers and Pullan, 308–9.

Neither the Pope nor the Emperor and not even kings and other princes or lords have done anything to combat this disease; it would certainly be simple in the cities to elect ancient matrons to seek out these sick people (including prostitutes) and with the authority of the secular arm to separate them from those who are not sick, placing them in a house or hospital so that they are treated by physicians.[48]

Despite his position at the papal court, it took another fifteen years for any of Torella's suggestions to be put into effect in Rome, during which period the number of *mal franciosati* (those sick from the French Disease) multiplied. However, moves were on foot in other parts of Italy based on the two mainstays of medieval poor relief, the confraternity and the hospital. Although it is often difficult to distinguish private from public initiatives, the specialist hospitals for incurables, the 'Incurabili', which treated those sick from the Great Pox, were usually set up by independent confraternities of lay men and women, who received the blessing and financial backing of local governments.[49] A closer look at the identity of those who promoted and ran these institutions reveals that many were from the ruling classes. In Venice a group of noble ladies from some of the city's leading families, including the Gabrieli, Giustiniani and Grimani, were from the start deeply involved in hospital life. Their support was reflected in a very public ceremony at Easter 1524 on the steps of the newly-founded Incurabili hospital, where a group of patricians 'with great humility washed the feet of the poor who were sick from the French Disease'.[50]

The same link between high status families and these hospitals can be found in other Italian cities. In Bologna, for example, the name of the ruler, Count Battista Bentivoglio, was among the list of members of the Company of St. Job which ran the Incurabili hospital.[51] In Florence the first prior and councillors of the hospital of SS. Trinita included representatives from prominent families, such as the Albizzi, Benci and Macinghi.[52] In Naples the patrician Maria Lorenzo Longo was involved closely in the foundation of the hospital of S. Maria del Popolo. Subsequently, the city kept a close eye on the running of this institution, for its statutes were subject to civic approval, as was the nomination of its governors.[53] Many of the brotherhoods which established the Incurabili hospitals were linked through a

[48]   Cited in Arrizabalaga, Henderson and French, *The Great Pox*, 34.
[49]   On Incurabili hospitals, see Cassiano Carpanetto da Langasco, *Gli ospedali degli incurabili* (Genoa, 1938); Anita Malamani, 'Notizie sul mal francese e gli ospedali degli incurabili in età moderna', *Critica storica*, xv (1978), 193–216; and, above all, Arrizabalaga, Henderson and French, *The Great Pox*, chs. 2, 7, 8.
[50]   Marin Sanudo, *I Diarii*, xxxvi. cols. 102–3 (24 Mar. 1524). On the Incurabili in Venice, see Andrea Nordio, 'L'Ospedale degli Incurabili nell'assistenza veneziana del '500', *Studi veneziani*, new series, xxxii (1966), 165–84.
[51]   Arrizabalaga, Henderson and French, *The Great Pox*, 319, n. 37.
[52]   ASF, Ospedale degli Incurabili 1, f. 1.
[53]   Giuliana Vitale, 'Ricerche sulla vita religiosa e caritativa a Napoli tra medioevo ed età moderna', *Archivio storico per le province napolitane*, lxxxvi-vii (1970), 228.

federation of 'Companies of Divine Love'.[54] These initiatives owed much to what has been labelled by Brian Pullan as the 'new philanthropy' of the sixteenth century. Under the influence of the Catholic reform movement, charitable institutions came to extend their redemptive arms to include those marginalized by society, especially indigents reduced to extreme misery through a sickness which disfigured their bodies and induced disgust in those whom they encountered.[55] This development casts a fascinating light upon the religious inspiration which led to the foundation, maintenance and staffing of the Incurabili hospitals. It also underscores another important aspect of the treatment of the *mal franciosati*, that is the spiritual role of the hospital and its mission for the moral reform of even diseased beggars, a motivation which is often easy to forget when reading traditional histories of public health.

It is precisely these two elements – growing intolerance and hospitalisation – which came to characterise the reactions of many of the major Italian cities: discrimination towards the diseased poor as they came to fill the streets with their lamentations, and the foundation of substantial new hospitals to provide treatment for these unfortunates.

The Great Pox: Incurabili Hospitals[56]

The Incurabili hospitals arose out of a series of initiatives; and, just as sometimes it is difficult to distinguish public from private inspiration, so it is not always easy to disentangle the complex interaction of charity and disgust. The way in which these very different responses were presented depends on the type of source one reads. A bland and reassuring account emerges from the chronicle of Friano degli Ubaldini:

> The [existing] hospitals did not want to receive or give shelter to anyone who had such a sickness for which reason a large number of poor people, both men and women, did not have anywhere to go. [Therefore] certain good men from Bologna began a hospital for such a sickness and began to put beds and other furnishings in the hospital of San Lorenzo dei Guarini and it was called the hospital of St. Job, which was given many alms and it was full of the said poor people, men and women, and they were looked after well.[57]

Compare this with Pope Leo X's Bull of 1515, *Salvatoris nostri*, in which the sick were described as not simply a nuisance to themselves, but also a threat to public order:

---

[54] On Companies of Divine Love, see Langasco, *Gli ospedali degli incurabili*, and Pio Paschini, 'Le Compagnie del Divino Amore e la beneficenza pubblica nei primi decenni del Cinquecento', in *Tre ricerche sulla storia della chiesa nel cinquecento* (Rome, 1945).

[55] Brian Pullan, 'Support and Redeem: Charity and Poor Relief in Italian Cities from the Fourteenth to the Seventeenth Century', *Continuity and Change*, iii (1988), 177–208.

[56] For the most detailed overview of Incurabili hospitals in Italy, see Arrizabalaga, Henderson and French, *The Great Pox*, chs.7 and 8.

[57] Cited in Corradi, 'Nuovi documenti', 345–6.

For a number of years large numbers of sick poor have come together in Rome, all infected with incurable diseases. [They have come] in such great numbers that they cannot find shelter in the hospitals of the city for their incurable sicknesses, [which] give annoyance to the sight and sense of smell, so that they are obliged to beg for their living through Rome, dragging themselves along on little carts.[58]

Both passages emphasize that existing general hospitals did not want to treat victims of this incurable disease, just as they had come to reject those with plague. Building on their experience of plague, some cities opted to house pox sufferers in separate institutions; within thirty-five years of the appearance of the Great Pox (1497–1530) eleven substantial Incurabili hospitals had been established in Italy. It is, however, indicative of the relationship between contemporary perceptions of the nature of different diseases that all these institutions were established *within* city walls. Indeed, instead of founding a completely separate hospital, some places set aside a ward of an existing one to treat those suffering from the Great Pox, as was the case at the Ospedale Maggiore in Milan. This was in direct contrast, as has been seen, to the *lazaretti* which either had been, or were in the process of being, set up at much the same time *outside* city walls in order to avoid the spread of plague to the general population. Such was notably the case in Milan, which had established one of the largest *lazaretti* in Italy.[59]

Thus, even though contemporaries may have believed that the French Disease could be caught through infected air, this was seen as far from the only method of transmission, and therefore represented a much lesser threat to public health than the miasmas of plague. In this sense, then, *Mal Francese* seemed to be more of a social and less of a medical problem than plague, which explains the very different strategies of Italian cities in dealing with these two major new epidemic diseases.

The first Incurabili hospital was founded in Genoa by the original Company of Divine Love. The two people associated most closely with this initiative were a pious notary called Ettore Vernazza and an even more pious lay woman called Caterina Fieschi.[60] She must have been a formidable character indeed. She was already the first female director of the city's main hospital, the Pammatone, and, according to her biographer, was reputed to have been so devout and penitential that she 'never shunned any patient with any type of horrible sickness even though they stank' and never avoided any filth, even though it led her to vomit.[61] By behaving in this way she was clearly modelling herself on earlier generations of women who cared for lepers, or those like Elizabeth of Hungary or Catherine of Siena who tended to the sick in less specialised medieval hospitals.

---

[58]   *Salvatoris Nostri Domini Jesu Christi*, in *Bullarium Romanum* [henceforth *Bull. Rom.*] *a B. Leone Magno usque ad S.D.N. Innocentum X, Vol. I*, ed. A.M. Cherubini (Lyon, 1655), 15 Aug. 1515.

[59]   One of the major hospitals in the city, the Brolo, was designated for the treatment of the '*brossolosi*' in response to the worsening of the epidemic: *Storia di Milano*, ed. Giovanni Treccani degli Alfieri (16 vols., Milan, 1958), xi. 624–5.

[60]   See Paschini, 'Le Compagnie del Divino Amore', 11–32.

[61]   Cattaneo Marabotto and Ettore Vernazza, *Vita mirabile e dottrina celeste di Santa Caterina Fiesca Adorna di Genova* (Padua, 1743), 31–2.

The influence of the Company of Divine Love gradually spread south, leading to the establishment of Florentine, Roman and Neapolitan hospitals. Indeed, one of the main reasons for their success was their association with the Catholic reform movement. Well-known people who supported these initiatives included leading reformers such as Gaetano Thiene and Filippo Neri, founders of the Oratorians.[62] The new religious orders of the Counter-Reformation, not least of which were the Jesuits and the Cappucins, also came to be linked closely to this network of confraternities and hospitals, followed by the new nursing orders, such as the Ministri degli Infermi (Ministers of the Sick) founded by Camillo de' Lellis at the Incurabili hospital of S. Giacomo in Rome.[63] They not only became members of the Divine Love companies, but also often served in the Incurabili hospitals, relishing the chance they provided to help the sick, and in particular the real outcasts of society.

The close link between these and other charitable ventures inspired by the Catholic reform movement can make it more difficult to penetrate behind the hagiographical accounts of incurabili hospital foundations.[64] The traditional view of charity in early sixteenth-century Italy in general, and reactions to those sick from the Great Pox in particular, tended to present a cosy picture of Christ's compassion and to ignore the authorities' increasingly intolerant attitude to the poor. The wretched in this period came to suffer from a new moralistic intolerance towards those who did not apparently make a proper and honest contribution to society. It is, however, over-simplistic to envisage a binary opposition between religious charity and secular intolerance. As I have suggested, states provided support for initiatives which were designed to care for and treat the *mal franciosati*, while the religious confraternities and orders which ran the hospitals for the incurable fulfilled a useful supporting role for city governments in coping with the problems generated by this new epidemic. The intermeshing of the secular and sacred can be seen clearly in the Bull of 1515 cited above, in which the pope promoted the establishment of the hospital of San Giacomo in Rome and in which the sentiments expressed were as intolerant as those of any other ruler [Plate 1].

The inter-dependence of public and private initiatives in dealing with the Great Pox, together with a shared perception of the problems caused by the sick, was reflected in the way that the policies of those who established and ran the Incurabili hospitals mirrored the public health concerns of the state. In 1500, when the administrators of the Genoese hospital sought approval for their regulations, they asked for a subsidy to help them in their work on behalf of 'many who are ill, labouring with incurable diseases, crushed by extreme poverty and misery and lying on the ground [and who] are to be found in almost all parts of the city'. The hospital appointed 'inquisitors' to search the city for these unfortunate victims of

[62]   Pietro Tacchi Venturi, *Storia della Compagnia di Gesù in Italia* (4 vols., Rome, 1930), i (1), chs. 18–19; J.W. O'Malley, *The First Jesuits* (Cambridge, Mass., and London, 1993), ch. 5; *I Frati Cappuccini. Documenti e testimonianze del primo secolo*, ed. Costanzo Cargnoni (3 vols., Perugia, 1991), iii (2), 341–6; Piero Sannazzaro, *Storia dell'Ordine Camilliano, 1550–1699* (Turin, 1986).

[63]   See Sanzio Cicatelli, *Vita del P. Camillo de Lellis*, ed. Piero Sannazzaro (Rome, 1980).

[64]   See, for example, the works cited above in Venturi, *Storia della Compagnia di Gesù*; *I Frati Cappuccini*, ed. Cargnoni; and Cicatelli, *Vita*.

the Pox and to provide them with treatment.[65] In Rome Leo X gave the Incurabili hospital power to elect syndics to search the streets for those 'afflicted by any illness [and] begging throughout the city', and to take the incurably sick to San Giacomo and those who seemed curable to general hospitals, such as Santo Spirito in Sassia.[66] The statutes suggest that the syndics even had the power to hospitalise incurables against their own will, although this policy would have soon fallen into disuse, as the demand for free treatment outstripped supply.

The link between Incurabili hospitals and state authorities was clearly of mutual benefit. The hospitals gained privileges and financial backing, while governments obtained institutions with pro-active policies to deal with what rapidly came to be perceived as a growing social problem. In Ferrara the ruling family represented by Ercole d'Este granted a licence to the members of the newly constituted Company of St. Job to solicit alms throughout his duchy for the establishment of an Incurabili hospital in Ferrara.[67] In Florence more direct subsidies were provided. The foundation of the Spedale di S. Trinita was backed by Cardinal Archbishop Giulio de'Medici, under the influence of his uncle, Pope Leo X. Both church and state gave substantial sums in 1520, the archbishop alone presenting 200 florins and the communal treasury 330 florins. The ruling Medici family continued their support. In 1534 Duke Alessandro provided the hospital with a guaranteed annual income from indirect taxes; and in 1560 the Grand Duchess Elenora of Toledo gave a generous donation, plus an annual income.[68] Although these sums reflect commitment to the enterprise, when compared with the annual income of two merchant banking firms in the same period, such as the Capponi (*fl.*2,600) and Gondi (*fl.*4,500), they seem substantial but not enormous.[69]

All this cash was necessary to pay for the ever-increasing number of people who were treated by the Incurabili hospitals during the sixteenth century, and whose presence also reflects the demographic growth of many Italian cities. Venice's population, for example, increased by about 50 per cent to 175,000 between 1509 and 1563, while its hospital's capacity grew from eighty to 450 patients between 1524 and 1567.[70] Naples expanded even more dramatically – from 150,000 in 1500 to 210,000 by 1550 – helping to explain why the Incurabili hospital already had 600 patients by 1535.[71] Rome also grew, more than doubling in size from 45,000 to 110,000 over the course of the sixteenth century. The city's major period of demographic growth was in the second half of the century, reflected again in the

[65] Langasco, *Gli ospedali degli incurabili*, doct. 2, pp. 205–6.
[66] *Salvatoris Nostri*, in *Bull. Rom.*, i. 568.
[67] Arrizabalaga, Henderson and French, *The Great Pox*, 152.
[68] *Ibid.*, 161, 321, n. 77.
[69] R.A. Goldthwaite, *The Economy of Renaissance Florence* (Baltimore, Md., 2009), 59.
[70] *Venice*, ed. Chambers and Pullan, 106; R.J. Palmer, 'L'assistenza medica nella Venezia cinquecentesca', in *Nel Regno dei poveri. Arte e storia dei grandi ospedali veneziani in età moderna, 1474–1797*, ed. Bernard Aikema and Dulcia Meijers (Venice, 1989), 39; Brian Pullan, *Rich and Poor in Renaissance Venice: The Social Institutions of a Catholic State to 1620* (Oxford, 1971), 375. Most recently, see L.J. McGough, *Gender, Sexuality and Syphilis in Early Modern Venice. The Disease that Came to Stay* (Basingstoke, 2011).
[71] Vitale, 'Ricerche sulla vita religiosa', 227–8.

increase in the numbers of patients at San Giacomo from about 200 in the late 1520s to over 2,200 in 1581.[72]

Growth in demand led to the physical expansion of these hospitals in the same period. Some were constructed on a very considerable scale, were important buildings in their own right and were designed by leading architects. In Venice two distinguished architects, Jacopo Sansovino and Antonio da Ponte, were employed between 1566 and 1600 to rebuild and to expand the Incurabili hospital. Their new creation boasted one of the first elliptical churches in Italy, which stood within the main courtyard.[73] The same period saw the extension of the Florentine Incurabili hospital through the efforts of the well-known local architect, Giovanni Battista Pieratti.[74] The potential scale of the operation of these institutions can be appreciated from the size of the new male ward of San Giacomo in Rome, which, when opened in 1600, measured 100 metres long and ten metres wide, and provided accommodation for almost 300 beds.[75] The association of celebrated architects with these institutions led them to be included in the itinerary of gentlemen on their grand tour and to be described in contemporary guidebooks, as in the passage on San Giacomo by Gregory Martin in *Roma sancta* (1581). He noted that 'upon St James day in Julie, when al the citie visiteth this Hospital, there are set forth in lively purtraicts Job with his sores upon the dunghill, his wife holding her nose for niceness not abiding her husbands stinche, his three frenddes weeping and lamenting his case'.[76]

The scale of investment in these hospitals clearly reflected society's belief in the efficacy of the role of such institutions in dealing with the epidemic of the French Disease. It also suggests, given the growing demand for admission, that the poorer members of society believed in the benefits of treatment. Confidence in the efficacy of the Incurabili hospitals derived from two main factors, one traditional and the other new. The former was the long history of care offered by medieval hospitals. In many major cities in southern Europe these institutions were imposing in size and scope, and provided free services for the poor, who entered voluntarily, knowing that they would receive the most up-to-date treatment from leading physicians, surgeons and apothecaries, combined with the cure of the soul through spiritual medicine. The search for novel remedies is apparent from the second factor, the use of the new wonder drug of guaiacum. It was imported from the Indies – where the Pox is thought to have originated – and was a hard wood which was used to induce sweat in order to eradicate the effects of the contagion, thus

---

[72] For the population of Rome, see C.M. Cipolla, *Before the Industrial Revolution. European Society and Economy, 1000–1700* (1976), 281; and, for a discussion of the number of patients at San Giacomo, see Arrizabalaga, Henderson and French, *The Great Pox*, ch. 8.

[73] Deborah Howard, *Jacopo Sansovino, Architecture and Patronage in Renaissance Venice* (New Haven and London, 1987); Bernard Aikema and Dulcia Meijers, 'Gli Incurabili. Chiesa e Ospedale del Santissimo Salvatore', in *Nel Regno dei poveri*, ed. Aikema and Meijers, 132–4.

[74] Walter and Elizabeth Paatz, *Die Kirchen von Florenz* (6 vols., Frankfurt-am-Main, 1940–55), v. 394.

[75] On the hospital of San Giacomo, see Arrizabalaga, Henderson and French, *The Great Pox*, ch. 8; Alessandra Cavaterra, 'L'ospedalità a Roma nell'età moderna: il caso di San Giacomo (1585–1605)', *Sanità, scienza e storia*, i (1986), 87–123.

[76] Gregory Martin, 'The Charitie of Rome', in *Roma Sancta*, ed. G.B. Parks (Rome, 1969), 187.

cleansing the body from pestilential matter and promoting resistance to putrefaction.[77]

Holy Wood, as guaiacum was known, quickly became fashionable and was adopted all over Europe during the 1520s. Its reputedly miraculous effects were trumpeted by practitioners and patients alike. The Spanish priest Francisco Delicado, for example, was so enthusiastic about Holy Wood that in 1529 he published a treatise on its many benefits because, as Pope Clement VII said in his preface:

> Our beloved son Francisco Delicado ... suffered for a while in the Arch-hospital of San Giacomo Apostolo, of our noble city, the greatest pains and almost incurable sickness as a result of the Morbo Gallico, and through the gracious intervention of God and the Apostles, with the amazement of everybody, has recovered his original health.[78]

Belief in the curative effect of this expensive drug encouraged individuals and states to subsidise the Incurabili hospitals, which could thus afford to provide treatment with Holy Wood free to thousands of people each year. In the process they helped society to cope with the nuisance posed by the *mal franciosati*, their work also being facilitated by a general perception that, by the mid sixteenth century, if not earlier, the Great Pox had modified its nature and those infected with the disease now posed less of a threat. When Girolamo Fracastoro wrote his famous treatise *De contagione et contagiosis morbi* in the mid 1540s he observed that 'though the contagion is still flourishing today, it seems to have changed its character since those earliest periods of its appearance'.[79] Fracastoro did not explain this change, but Francesco Guicciardini did suggest a number of possible reasons, including successful treatment: 'because of astrological influence, or through the long experience of doctors, or the appropriate remedies to treat the sickness, or it had found itself able to transform into other types of diseases different from the original'.[80] The changing nature of the Great Pox meant that it had become more of a social than a medical problem; the disease and its victims could be more easily contained than those suffering from plague.

Conclusion

We return, then, to the questions raised at the beginning of this article: the extent to which the strategies devised by Italian society to deal with the Great Pox built on those initially developed to combat plague, and the relationship between these strategies and contemporary medical theory. We have seen that institutional responses to these two epidemics had much in common. Both the *lazaretto* and the

---

[77] Robert S. Munger, 'Guaiacum, The Holy Wood from the New World', *Journal of the History of Medicine and Allied Sciences*, iv (1) (1949), 196–229.
[78] Francisco Delicado, *La Lozana Andaluza* (Milan, 1970), 294.
[79] Fracastoro, *De contagione*, ed. Wright, 139, 155–7.
[80] Guicciardini, *Storia d'Italia, I*, 233.

Incurabili were based on the model of large-scale Italian medieval medical hospitals and both aimed to provide free what was believed at the time to have been the best of treatments, theriac for plague and guaiacum for the Pox. These hospitals should also be seen in the wider context of society's strategies for coping with the poor sick. Institutions offered a useful means of hiding the problems of poverty and sickness behind tasteful façades.

There were, though, some significant differences in attitudes towards, and policies for, the containment of these two epidemics, stemming from the way that each disease was perceived. In each case the intention was to isolate patients for the protection of society, but those with plague were housed in extra-mural isolation hospitals, while those with Pox were treated in institutions within the city. Furthermore, the distinctive characteristics of each of these diseases led to separate outcomes, with most who entered the *lazaretti* dying from plague, while the majority of Pox sufferers were released alive into the community.

These differences in turn reflect divergent medical opinions about the two diseases. Plague was perceived to have been so infectious that the sick apparently spread the miasmatic vapours through their infected breath. Although this assumption may also have held good in the early stages of the Pox, it was not long before the principal agent of transmission was seen to be physical contact. But even here, the distinction between transmission through touch and through the air was far from absolute, as is reflected in Fracastoro's subtle division of 'contagion' into three types: transmission by direct contact, such as by sexual intercourse; indirect contact through fomites; and at a distance through infected air.[81] The demarcation between the first and third types would seem to justify historians' idea of a contemporary contrast between physicians' miasmatic concept of plague compared with governments' contagionist views. However, this distinction clearly breaks down when we consider Fracastoro's second type of contagion, indirect contact through fomites. His idea combined the concept of 'seedlets of contagion' (as an infective agent) with that of '*fomes*' or fomites, a term applied to any medium in which the seeds could be stored. He suggested that the '*seminaria contagionis*' could be absorbed by an individual through inhalation, but that the 'seeds' could also enter another medium, such as cloth, within which they could be stored for a long time until they were passed on to another person.[82] The belief that plague was spread through infected air, whether carried by cloth or on the breath of an individual, had, as we have seen, been around since at least the time of the Black Death. However, infected air was not just the vehicle of transmission; it was also identified as the disease itself. Although Fracastoro wrote that these 'seeds' were external to the human body, he believed that they could be reactivated within an individual by an unhealthy regime.[83]

This particular aspect of Fracastoro's contagion theory also had important implications for social policies in the sixteenth century, particularly when combined with the contemporary revival of Neo-Hippocratic ideas about the close association between health, sickness and the environment. It came to form a crucial

---

[81] Fracastoro, *De contagione*, ed. Wright, 7, and 3–21, 135.
[82] *Ibid.*, 13–14; cf. Nutton, 'The Reception of Fracastoro's Theory of Contagion', 200–4.
[83] Fracastoro, *De contagione*, ed. Wright, 7, and 3–21.

John Henderson

element in the growing belief by doctors and governments alike that there was a causal link between diet, poverty and disease.[84] Thus, dealing with the *mal franciosati* now fell more within the realms of poor relief than of public health strategies, an important element in the increasing discrimination against the poorer members of society, as sixteenth-century populations began to rise and more centralised states moved to establish greater distinctions between the worthy and unworthy poor. The French Disease played a major role in the growth of discrimination because, unlike those who caught the plague, Pox sufferers continued to clutter up the streets of cities and importune their social betters. Furthermore, as we have seen from both the official reactions of health boards and individual writers, such as Machiavelli, there was a very real fear that the poor might infect their superiors, with potentially fatal consequences.

[84] On England, see Andrew Wear, *Knowledge and Practice in English Medicine, 1550–1680* (Cambridge, 2000); and, for a further discussion of Italy, see Henderson, 'Public Health, Pollution and the Problem of Waste Disposal', 373–82.

THE HISTORIAN AND THE LABORATORY:
THE BLACK DEATH DISEASE

Samuel K. Cohn, Jr.

The Black Death, along with subsequent strikes of plague into the early modern period, has been the spark of academic debates over the past century or more. Before the 1990s discussion concentrated on the disease's consequences, first the demographic ones, then the plague's effects on economy, society, and religion: did the great destruction of population have a silver lining, leading to higher standards of living, especially for the lower tiers of the population?[1] Did it lead to a more rational distribution of resources and a better organization of commercial society, as David Herlihy, Richard Goldthwaite and others have argued for Italy and especially Tuscany?[2] Was it the trigger of the tidal changes in Renaissance and early modern culture? Did the deaths of so great a proportion of clerical populations across Europe serve to promote the importance of literature written in the vernacular? Did this demographic catastrophe among the clergy encourage a new dependence on the laity for religious solace and confraternity, while at the same time provoking challenges to religious authority and hierarchy? Was the Black Death at the origins of the Reformation?[3]

None of these questions has been resolved; much depends on when and where in Europe, as well as the Middle East, such changes are, or their absence is, being observed. Many subsequent changes in culture and economy can be seen rising before 1348, and afterwards factors other than the Black Death or its demographic consequences contributed to these broad transformations in civilization. But, despite the liveliness of these debates and their importance for understanding European history, they have been largely pushed aside over the past decade. Another question has hogged the limelight of Black Death studies and of historic plague: what was the disease? This question has enlisted a new group of researchers, a wide interdisciplinary collaboration among geneticists, pathologists, microbiologists, archaeologists, osteoarchaeologists, mathematicians, statisticians, physical anthropologists, specialists in ancient DNA, and more. Surprisingly missing from the numerous co-authors of these articles has been the historian.

---

[1] For England, see especially Christopher Dyer, *Everyday Life in Medieval England* (2001); and *idem*, *Making a Living in the Middle Ages: The People of Britain 850–1520* (New Haven, Conn., 2002).

[2] See David Herlihy, *Medieval and Renaissance Pistoia: The Social History of an Italian Town, 1200–1430* (New Haven, Conn., 1967); and, most recently, R.A. Goldthwaite, *The Economy of Renaissance Florence* (Baltimore, Md., 2009).

[3] On these questions, see David Herlihy and S.K. Cohn, Jr., *The Black Death and the Transformation of the West* (Cambridge, Mass., 1997).

As early as 1998 a team of paleomicrobiologists at Marseilles examined plague pits in Provence of the sixteenth to eighteenth century and claimed to have extracted the ancient DNA of *Yersinia pestis* from the dental pulp of plague victims.[4] Despite criticisms of their methods and charges that their laboratories were contaminated, this équipe persevered, employed new tools for isolating and amplifying ancient DNA, and extended its investigation to Black Death plague pits. Two years later, its members claimed to have ended 'the controversy: Medieval Black Death was plague'. By this, they meant that the pathogen of the Black Death was *Yersinia pestis*, and, in the spirit of Robert Koch's late-nineteenth-century reductionism, this was sufficient to claim that the 'disease' of the Black Death or 'Second Pandemic' was the same as that of the 'Third Pandemic' – the sub-tropical, rodent illness that had slowly arrived at Hong Kong in 1894 and then circumnavigated coastal areas by steam vessels across much of the globe during the early twentieth century. Yet, unlike the Black Death and successive bouts of that disease, the 'Third Pandemic' hardly penetrated the old haunts of the historic plagues in temperate Europe.[5] Over the next decade, investigations of plague pits extended geographically to Germany, northern Italy, Denmark, England, and other areas of France, as well as back in time to the Justinianic plague from the mid sixth to mid eighth century. The results were mixed; in fact, most of these researchers came up with negative findings.[6]

At the end of 2010 and in 2011, however, several studies appeared, which, the scientific community seems to have judged, have given closure to the question of the Black Death's pathogen. From new investigations of plague pits, especially that of East Smithfield, London, new techniques of ancient DNA analysis, the detection of antigens and 'protein signatures', and the construction of phylogenetic evolutionary trees of the pathogen's origins and mutations, these interdisciplinary teams have confirmed that the pathogen was a variant of *Yersinia pestis*.[7] But have these articles really ended debate about the nature of the 'disease', as their titles and certain proclamations within them may suggest? One of them begins boldly:

---

[4]   Didier Raoult, *et al.*, 'Detection of 400-year-old *Yersinia pestis* DNA in Human Dental Pulp: An Approach to the Diagnosis of Ancient Septicemia', *Proceedings of the National Academy of Sciences of the USA* [hereafter *PNAS*], xcv (1998), 12637–40.

[5]   Didier Raoult, *et al.*, 'Molecular Identification by "Suicide PCR" of *Yersinia pestis* as the Agent of Medieval Black Death', *PNAS*, xcvii (2000), 12800–3.

[6]   On these discussions and developments, see, for instance, S.K. Cohn, Jr., *The Black Death Transformed: Disease and Culture in Early Renaissance Europe* (2002), 248–50; and, for more recent developments, see J.L. Bolton in this collection, above pp. 17–26; and L.K. Little, 'Plague Historians in Lab Coats', *Past and Present*, ccxiii (2011), 267–90. For negative results, see, for instance, M.B. Prentice, Tom Gilbert and Alan Cooper, 'Was the Black Death caused by *Yersinia pestis*?', *The Lancet Infectious Diseases*, iv (2) (2004), 72; M.T.P. Gilbert, *et al.*, 'Response to Drancourt and Raoult', *Microbiology*, cl (2004), 264–5; M.T.P. Gilbert, *et al.*, 'Absence of *Yersinia pestis*-Specific DNA in Human Teeth from Five European Excavations of Putative Plague Victims', *ibid.*, 341–54; C.M. Pusch, *et al.*, 'Yersinial F1 Antigen and the cause of Black Death', *The Lancet Infectious Diseases*, iv (8) (2004), 484–5.

[7]   Stephanie Haensch *et al.*, 'Distinct Clones of *Yersinia pestis* Caused the Black Death', *PLoS Pathogens*, vi (2010), 1–8; and Giovanna Morelli, *et al.*, '*Yersinia pestis* Genome Sequencing Identifies Patterns of Global Phylogenetic Diversity', *Nature Genetics*, xlii (2010), 1140–3; V.J. Schuenemann, *et al.*, 'Targeted Enrichment of Ancient Pathogens Yielding the pPCP1 Plasmid of *Yersinia pestis* from Victims of the Black Death', *PNAS*, cviii (38) (2011), E746–52 ; and K.I. Bos, *et al.*, 'A Draft Genome of *Yersinia pestis* from Victims of the Black Death', *Nature*, cccclxxviii (2011), 506–10.

'We demonstrate unambiguously that *Y. pestis* spread over Europe during the second pandemic … [i.e. 1347 to the mid eighteenth century] … Our results thus resolve a long-standing debate about the aetiology of the Black Death.' However, the detail embedded in these technical articles adds a new wrinkle to the question of the Black Death's agent and to its consequence for understanding the disease: 'Our aDNA results identified two previously unknown but related clades of *Y. pestis* associated with distinct medieval mass graves … [that] may no longer exist.'[8]

The most recent of these contributions – one from the summer of 2011 that examines new samples from the London plague pit at East Smithfield, clearly dated to 1348–50 – highlights the findings of the first équipe but is more cautious. The authors of the Smithfield study also discovered 'a *Y. pestis* variant that has not previously been reported', and confirmed that 'no extant *Y. pestis* strain possesses the same genetic profile as our ancient organism'.[9] Unlike the first group, they further acknowledge that the genetic ancestry of the plague cannot as yet explain the vast differences in the disease's transmission, seasonality, and other aspects of its epidemiology between the late medieval and early modern 'Second Pandemic' and that of the 'Third' at the end of the nineteenth century:

[O]ur data suggest that few changes in known virulence-associated genes have accrued in the organism's 660 years of evolution as a human pathogen, further suggesting that its perceived increased virulence in history may not be due to novel fixed point mutations detectable via the analytical approach described here. At our current resolution, we posit that molecular changes in pathogens are but one component of a constellation of factors contributing to changing infectious disease prevalence and severity, where genetics of the host population, climate, vector dynamics, social conditions and synergistic interactions with concurrent diseases should be foremost in discussions of population susceptibility to infectious disease and host-pathogen relationships with reference to *Y. pestis* infections.[10]

In short, the recent scientific literature has now recognized more clearly than was the case a decade earlier that ancient DNA and the construction of phylogenetic charts from laboratory samples may not be enough to resolve the problem of the extreme differences in plague from the Black Death to the present: isolation of the pathogen alone cannot resolve what was the Black Death disease. The door appears open again to the historian and his or her analysis of contemporary sources to aid in the understanding of historic plague. First, we shall examine the discoveries of the plague pathogen between the end of the nineteenth century and the First World War, which highlight aspects of the 'Third Pandemic', the protean character of *Yersinia pestis*, and the vital differences between it and the late medieval-early modern plagues that directly impinged on medicine and politics at the turn of the century in India. We will then outline the major differences between these two periods of plague.

[8] Haensch, *et al.*, 'Distinct Clones of *Yersinia pestis*', 2.
[9] Schuenemann, *et al.*, 'Targeted Enrichment of Ancient Pathogens'; and Bos, *et al.*, 'A Draft Genome of *Yersinia pestis*'.
[10] Bos, *et al.*, 'A Draft Genome of *Yersinia pestis*'.

The Discoveries of Yersinia pestis

Two accounts of the discovery of late nineteenth- to early twentieth-century plague stand side by side, a French and a British one. The French story has dominated introductions to plague in scientific text books and numerous articles over the past century. It was one of David and Goliath, in which the essential events happened fast. The first and principal actor was the Swiss-born Alexandre Yersin, attached to the Institut de Pasteur in Paris and the understudy of Émile Roux. When the plague reached Hong Kong, Yersin, in the spirit of the contemporary microbe-hunters, rushed there to discover the pathogen. He was late. Already the German-Japanese contingent linked to Koch, under the direction of the Japanese bacteriologist Shibasaburo Kitasato, who had studied in Berlin, had occupied the major plague hospital in Hong Kong. Yersin's access to the hospital and its supply of plague corpses was blocked. Nonetheless, with one assistant he constructed a straw hut outside the hospital and bribed orderlies to hand bodies over to him. The assistant quickly calculated the odds and left Yersin, stealing his money and equipment. Yet against these odds, Yersin cultured the plague bacillus at the same time as Kitasato. At first, credit was given equally to both, with the pathogen being christened 'Bacterium pestis', then 'Pasteurella pestis'. By 1954, however, Kitasato's identification was recognized as mistaken, and, thereafter, the pathogen has been called *Yersinia pestis*.[11] The next act of this drama came in 1898, when it centred on another scientist from Pasteur's organization, Paul Louis Simond, who hypothesized that plague transmission depended on a flea biting an infected rat and then transmitting the bacillus by biting a human. Finally, a third act focuses on the Jewish Russian, W.H. Haffkline, who contemporaries believed had discovered an effective serum against plague.[12] They were mistaken: still today no effective vaccination exists.[13]

Another story of plague's discovery plays out a more protracted history; its centre is India, and its scientists are mostly British. By this account, the importance of Yersin's discovery, at least initially, appears less decisive in leading to an understanding of the disease's basic characteristics of transmission, its prevention, or its remedies. It was not the expected scenario of a discovery of a pathogen leading swiftly to a disease's control and treatment, and to the manufacturing of an effective serum or vaccination. Yersin may have speculated that rats were involved, but this was only one hypothesis among many: he also thought that larger mammals, such as pigs and water buffaloes, were as important, if not more so.[14] Further, he conjectured that the plague might have an insect vector but pinned it on

---

[11] On this nomenclature, see, among others, Thomas Butler, *Plague and Other Yersinia Infections* (New York, 1983), 25.

[12] Myron Echenberg, *Black Death, White Medicine: Bubonic Plague and the Politics of Public Health in Colonial Senegal, 1914–1945* (Portsmouth, N.H., 2002), 69, 105.

[13] See Bei Li *et al.*, 'Humoral and Cellular Immune Responses to *Yersinia pestis* Infection in Long-Term Recovered Plague Patients', *Clinical and Vaccine Immunology*, CVI, xix (2) (2012), 228–34, who state that 'an effective vaccine against both bubonic and pneumonic plagues is urgently needed...' (p. 228).

[14] Larger mammals can become infected with *Yersinia pestis* and can transmit the disease to humans, as has happened occasionally in Uzbekistan, when humans have eaten diseased camel meat, but neither this carrier nor mode of transmission have ever produced an epidemic of plague.

the house fly, not the flea, and he thought that the bacillus lived in the ground and was transmitted by exposure to dirt.

The significance of Act II can also be called into question. First, Simond was not the first to suggest fleas as the vector. Two years earlier the Japanese bacteriologist Masanori Ogata had advanced that hypothesis, and the following year the German Bombay Plague Commission found plague bacilli in fleas but refused to attribute to them a major role in plague transmission. More importantly, after Simond's 1898 publication in *Annales de l'Institut Pasteur*, leading authorities in plague research, such as Sir Patrick Manson and entomologist and editor of the *Journal of Hygiene*, G.F.H. Nutall, who published the Indian Plague Commission Reports, rejected his speculations and experimental proof. It took many more experiments with guinea pigs in separate cages, mainly published in Nutall's journal, before the medical world became convinced, twelve years later, upon the publication of Glen Liston's experiments.[15] Furthermore, it was not until the eve of the First World War that medical scientists understood the mechanisms by which the flea transmitted the bacillus from the rat into the bloodstream of the human: namely, that in most cases the proventriculus of the flea became blocked, forcing the flea to regurgitate its blood meal contaminated with the bacillus into the human, and that these events occurred in only 13 per cent of bites by infected fleas. Again, British plague scientists, working in India, were its discoverers.[16]

Moreover, despite recognition by hospital workers at the end of the nineteenth century that plague was failing to manifest the lightning speed and person-to-person transmission characteristic of the Black Death and its recurrent strikes, colonial governments and medical establishments held fast to their historical identification of their current plague as the Black Death disease. As a result, they imposed strict quarantine and isolation policies, including the wholesale disinfection of property, even the burning of natives' homes. These practices went against locals' understanding of how their plague was transmitted and gave rise to the worst riots against doctors, the British army and regional administrators in the history of disease in colonial India, cholera included. Major riots exploded in Calcutta, Bombay, Puna, and Kampur between 1898 and 1900. But by 1901 these disturbances had ended, and the reason seems to rest with the British: they now realised that their bubonic plague was not behaving like the Black Death; after many reports from Indian and foreign hospital workers, they concluded that 'the safest place during plague was the plague ward of hospitals'.[17] In contrast to the Black Death and its successive strikes, hardly any nurses or others caring for plague patients caught the disease. Primary and secondary cases of pneumonic plague were rare and plague in this form also spread ineffectively, except, as happened in Manchuria in 1911 and 1922, when forty or more inexperienced tabagan trappers were crammed into 12ft. x 15ft., poorly-ventilated underground bunkers.[18] Even then, the worst manifestations of pneumonic plague known since

---

[15] David Arnold, *Colonizing the Body: State Medicine and Epidemic Disease in Nineteenth-Century India* (Berkeley, Calif., 1993), 210.

[16] A.W. Bacot and C.J. Martin, 'Observations on the Mechanism of the Transmission of Plague by Fleas', *Journal of Hygiene* [hereafter *JH*], *Plague Supplement III* (1914), 432–4.

[17] W.B. Bannerman, 'The Spread of Plague in India', *JH*, vi (1906), 179–211, quotation on p. 180.

[18] Wu Lien-Teh (G.L. Tuck), 'First Report of the North Manchurian Plague Prevention Service', *JH*, xiii (1913–14), 237–90; *idem, A Treatise on Pneumonic Plague* (Geneva, 1926); 'Historical

Yersin's discovery did not spread in any way comparable to historic plague, or even to the plague's spread in bubonic form in India or China. In Manchuria during these two exceptional plagues less than 0.4 per cent of the population were afflicted,[19] despite the fact that the percentage was higher along certain railway corridors,[20] and the small town of Fujiadian (population 8,000) lost a third of its inhabitants.[21] After 1905, efforts by plague researchers to substantiate or understand their findings through the prism of historic bubonic plague disappear almost completely from leading medical journals. As early as 1901 the renowned bacteriologist Robert Koch defined bubonic plague in a way that bears little resemblance to the experience of late medieval and early modern Europe: 'plague is a disease of rats in which men occasionally participate'.[22] That definition has now changed slightly, but in a direction that distances it still further from the late medieval experience: *Yersinia pestis* is primarily a rodent pathogen, to which humans are only 'accidental hosts'.[23]

The Character and Epidemiology of the Black Death Disease

So what is the epidemiological picture of the Black Death and its successive waves until the early nineteenth century, drawn not only from chronicles and other literary sources, but from records that can be analyzed quantitatively, such as numerous last wills and testaments, tax surveys and censuses, burial records and necrologies of religious establishments, as well as of confraternities of the laity? In rare places such as Milan, the researcher can turn to necrologies, or death books, of the mid fifteenth and early sixteenth century, in which physicians diagnosed plague deaths by recording the number and positions of buboes, the appearance of other skin disorders, headaches, muscle pains, vomiting, fevers, and the days, even hours, from the onset of illness to death. From this ensemble of records we find that the rates of mortality differed massively between the 'Second' and 'Third' Pandemics. As many as 95 per cent of cases and deaths attributed to *Yersinia pestis* have occurred in the Indian subcontinent since Yersin cultured the pathogen in 1894. Yet, even here, the disease in no year approached being India's major killer.

Aspects', in Wu Lien-Teh, J.W.H. Chun, Robert Pollitzer and C.Y. Wu, *Plague: A Manual for Medical and Public Health Workers* (Shanghai Station, 1936), 1–55; and Wu Lien-Teh, *Plague Fighter: The Autobiography of a Modern Chinese Physician* (Cambridge, 1959).

[19] Wu Lien-Teh, 'First Report of the North Manchurian Plague Prevention Service'. The history of heavy-handed policies of strict quarantine and the burning of natives' belongings and homes persisted longer in other colonies, as was the case in Senegal, where such assumptions and policies continued until that colony's last major outbreak of bubonic plague in 1944; see Echenberg, *Black Death, White Medicine*, 242. On pneumonic plague's ineffective transmission, see Raymond Gani and Steve Leach, 'Epidemiologic Determinants for Modelling Pneumonic Plague Outbreaks', *Emerging Infectious Diseases*, x (4) (2004), 608–14.

[20] W.C. Summers, *The Great Manchurian Plague of 1910–1911: The Geopolitics of an Epidemic Disease* (New Haven, Conn., 2012), 19.

[21] Mark Gamsa, 'The Epidemic of Pneumonic Plague in Manchuria, 1910–1911', *Past and Present*, cxc (2006), 154.

[22] Cited in 'Digest of Recent Observations on the Epidemiology of Plague', *JH*, vii (1907), 694–723, on p. 696.

[23] See Michael Begon, Colin Townsend and John Harper, *Ecology: From Individual to Ecosystems* (Oxford, 2006), 352.

Even at the plague's zenith, nine or ten other diseases killed greater numbers in the subcontinent. In large cities, the highest plague mortality occurred in Bombay in 1903, when plague felled 2.7 per cent of the population.

Compare these statistics to mortality during the Black Death, as estimated from tax records, or seen on the micro-level from monastic necrologies. In four late spring and summer months, Florence may have lost three-quarters of its residents.[24] Such remarkably high figures occur not only in 1348–9 but also later, when state censuses and church surveys (*'stato dell'anime'*) provide more precision. Milan, for instance, lost at least half its urban population during the plague of 1630–1,[25] and Genoa and Naples upwards of two-thirds during mainland Italy's last major plague of 1656–7.[26] To be sure, certain country villages lost greater proportions of their populations than cities in Indian plagues of the early twentieth century. Losses in the Punjab may have reached as high as one third of the population. In fact, the patterns of epidemic *Yersinia pestis* during the 'Third Pandemic' differed from those of person-to-person diseases, and especially of measles, which rely on high population densities in large compact conurbations. As the statistician Major Greenwood discovered early in the twentieth century, plague manifests an inverse relationship between per capita case numbers and the population size of communities.[27] The Black Death disease, however, never showed such patterns, even if certain villages could have high mortalities.[28] By the early modern period, plague appears to have become generally a disease predominantly of cities and towns in various regions and countries of Europe.[29]

Second, the speed of transmission, its diffusion, and levels of contagion show marked differences between the two periods of plague pandemic. Because 'the Third' has been tied to rodents (usually rats when the disease reaches epidemic proportions), it is a slow-moving disease. Early in the twentieth century, its speed was measured overland in places such as New Orleans and in South Africa and found to travel only 6.5 to 15 kilometres per annum.[30] By contrast, the Black Death could cover such distances almost in a day. Even by the slowest estimates, 1.5 to 2 kilometres a day, historic plague would have sped fifty times more quickly than

---

[24] See S.K. Cohn, Jr., 'Epidemiology of the Black Death and Successive Waves of Plague', in *Pestilential Complexities: Understanding the Medieval Plague*, ed. Vivian Nutton, *Medical History*, supplement xxvii (2008), 82.

[25] See the estimates in *Processo agli untori: Milano 1630: cronaca e atti giuriziari in edizione integrale*, ed. Giuseppe Farinelli and Ermanno Paccagnini (Milan, 1988), 139–42.

[26] C.M. Cipolla, *Public Health and the Medical Profession in the Renaissance* (Cambridge, 1976), 57.

[27] Major Greenwood, 'Statistical Investigation of Plague in the Punjab. Third Report', in *JH, Plague Supplement I* (1911), 62–156; and *idem, Epidemics and Crowd-Diseases: An Introduction to the Study of Epidemiology* (1935).

[28] See, for instance, the calculations of George Christakos, *et al.*, *Interdisciplinary Public Health Reasoning and Epidemic Modelling: the Case of Black Death* (Berlin, 2005), 148; and for Florentine Tuscany, David Herlihy and Christiane Klapisch-Zuber, *Les Toscans et leurs familles: une étude du 'catasto' florentin de 1427* (Paris, 1978), 166–7, 177–81. For examples of certain villages in France and England with extraordinarily high mortality rates during the Black Death, see Cohn, 'Epidemiology of the Black Death', 82.

[29] See for instance, Paul Slack, *The Impact of Plague in Tudor and Stuart England* (Oxford, 1985), 63, 93, 110. Yet, during certain plague waves, such as that of 1629 to 1633 in the north of Italy, rural villages were stricken as badly as the large cities, but certainly not worse; see Guido Alfani, *Il Grand Tour dei Cavalieri dell'Apocalisse: L'Italia del 'lungo Cinquecento' (1494–1629)* (Venice, 2010).

[30] L. Fabian Hirst, *The Conquest of Plague: A Study of the Evolution of Epidemiology* (Oxford, 1953), 304.

modern plague, despite the latter having the benefit of the railway and motorized transport. By collecting extensive data from across Europe and employing sophisticated stochastic and mapping tools, George Christakos and his co-researchers have gone further. The Black Death sped between 1.5 to 6 kilometres per day, depending on place and season, but, more astonishing, it covered an area per unit time ('power of time') that was two orders of magnitude greater than that witnessed by the most widespread and devastating plague of the twentieth century – that of India between 1897 and 1907.[31] Had their calculations of the time-space propagation been compared with other twentieth-century outbreaks, as in Brazil or even China, the differences would have been greater still.

The reasons for these differences depended on the mechanisms of transmission. Even scientists who hold fast to the conviction that these historic plagues were *Yersinia pestis* are now coming to the conclusion that the medieval-early-modern plagues differed fundamentally from the modern ones in one important respect: the medieval and early modern plagues could not have been a rat or rodent disease. Not only do the statistics of diffusion defy any such assumption, the archaeology, especially in northern Europe, gives no signs of any substantial rat populations in the late Middle Ages to support even the lowest levels of twentieth-century plague diffusion.[32]

In addition, physicians and chroniclers marvelled at the Black Death's lightning transmission, reporting that mere speech was enough to pass it directly from one person to the next. Before 1348, the word '*contagium*' rarely appeared outside medical texts, and, when it did, it referred either to the spread of heresy or rebellion. Afterwards, merchant chroniclers and other lay writers used the word to describe the transmission of one disease in particular – plague – and by it they meant primarily person-to-person transmission by breath, touch and occasionally sight, or through contact with infected goods, especially cloth. Early on during the late fourteenth and fifteenth century, physicians and chroniclers distinguished their plague from other infectious diseases, such as *pondi*, *dondi*, or smallpox, which seemed to manifest similar symptoms. Chronicles such as 'the Brut' in England, reporting an epidemic of 1369, the nobleman-chronicler 'pseudo-Minerbetti', describing one of 1390 in Tuscany, and the Florentine merchant Giovanni Morelli, recording plagues in the early fifteenth century, used epidemiological evidence to distinguish plague from other diseases. They all stressed its capacity to spread and kill swiftly, more so than any other disease they knew, and, as a result, commonly named their new disease 'the contagion' – *morbo contagioso, contagioso male, voracissimo contaggio*.[33]

The seasonality of plagues is another epidemiological trait that separates the 'Second' from the 'Third Pandemic'. As plague commissioners in India discovered early in the twentieth century, plague seasons recurred with great consistency, depending on climatic conditions, principally temperature and humidity. By correlating temperature and plague incidence, they suspected an insect vector – the

---

[31]   Christakos, *et al.*, *Interdisciplinary Public Health*, 205–7, 223, 230.
[32]   See, most recently, A.K. Hufthammer and Lars Wolløe, 'Rats Cannot have been Intermediate Hosts for *Yersinia pestis* during Medieval Plague Epidemics in Northern Europe', *Journal of Archaeological Science*, xl (2013), 1752–9; and earlier, Gunnar Karlsson, 'Plague Without Rats: the Case of Fifteenth-Century Iceland', *Journal of Medieval History*, xxii (1996), 263–84.
[33]   Cohn, 'Epidemiology of the Black Death', 81.

rat flea – given the close match between the cycle of flea fertility and plague cases. By contrast, medieval and early modern bubonic plague could occur in any season, as is apparent from the spread of the Black Death in France and England, and even in places such as Bergen, Norway, where it endured into the winter months. Nor was the Black Death's first strike exceptional in this regard. As Karl-Erik Frandsen has recently shown, plague broke out during the severe winter of 1708–9 and again in 1710–11, with the Baltic Sea frozen over, blocking trade to harbours such as that at Danzig.[34] Moreover, unlike the plague of 1348–9, which the pope's physician, Guy de Chauliac, described as pneumonic during the winter months, the greater detail for the early-eighteenth-century Baltic plagues makes clear that these winter outbreaks were bubonic, with the tell-tale skin disorders of buboes in lymph nodes, along with other carbuncles and pustules, despite the frigid conditions.[35] Primary pneumonic plague, whether of the medieval or modern sort, kills so quickly that such skin disorders have no time to develop.[36]

Yet, despite medieval and early modern plague's capacity to flare up at any season, outbreaks of the 'Second Pandemic' had their seasonal patterns, which do not conform to those of modern bubonic plague. In Mediterranean places, where documents such as last wills and testaments, burial records, and necrologies survive in significant numbers, plague normally peaked in June or July, that is, during the hottest and driest periods of the year, when flea populations are at their lowest ebb, even lower than in January. When *Yersinia pestis* has erupted in these regions in the twentieth century, June and July have been the least likely months to encounter plague cases. Instead, the season begins after the rains and cooler temperatures of early autumn and peaks in October or November – exactly when late fourteenth and fifteenth century plagues in the Mediterranean had disappeared. Curiously, in the cooler north, in places such as Douai and the cities of northern Germany, the late medieval plague season differed from that of the south; deaths peaked in their cooler autumn, when in fact temperatures there would not have been optimal for the flea vector.[37]

The patterns of the 'Second' and 'Third' Pandemics differed in other respects. Especially during the fourteenth and for most of the fifteenth century, plague rarely recurred in successive years and never for seven years or more, as was the case with plague in twentieth-century Brazil or Thailand, or persisted more or less

---

[34] Karl-Erik Frandsen, *The Last Plague in the Baltic Region 1709–1713* (Copenhagen, 2010), 25, 78, 80, 143–4.

[35] Examples of earlier outbreaks of plague in bubonic form during extremely cold months can also be cited. For instance, a Genoese chronicler reports the outbreak of plague around Christmas 1493, when an extraordinary cold snap had hit Genoa, freezing the port and blocking the entrance of ships. Nonetheless, during these frigid conditions, without precedent in Genoa, according to the chronicler, he confirms that 'true plague' erupted, 'in which the ulcer first appears'; Bartholomaeus Senaregae, *De rebus Genuensibus commentaria ab anno MCDLXXXVIII usque ad annum MDXIV*, ed. Emilio Pandiani, *Rerum Italicarum Scriptores* [hereafter *RIS*], xxiv (8) (Bologna, 1932), 80.

[36] Frandsen, *The Last Plague in the Baltic Region*, 44, 152, 153, 193. In fact, Frandsen is convinced that these diseases were modern bubonic plague, despite the unfavourable climatic patterns, principally because of the supposed similarities of the signs – the buboes and black spots (p. 153). Nor is he surprised by the positions of these buboes and carbuncles in multiple numbers across the plague victims' bodies, as well as in extraordinary places not seen with modern plague – in the vagina and navel (p. 44), the anus (p. 163), and the corners of the eyes (p. 193).

[37] For this evidence, taken from a quantitative analysis of a variety of records but primarily from last wills and testaments, see Cohn, *The Black Death Transformed*, 178–86.

continuously over a twenty-year period, as in cities and villages in the Bombay Presidency and Punjab from 1896 to the 1920s. Instead, during the first hundred years following the Black Death, plagues recurred roughly once every seven to ten years, with few repeat hits in successive years. For instance, in Siena plague struck in 1348, 1363, 1374, 1383, 1390, 1400, 1411, 1417, 1420, 1433 and 1436–7.[38] By contrast, human plague cycles of the late nineteenth and twentieth century have depended on the time it takes for rat or other rodent populations to become mostly immune to the pathogen and thus to contain it within their own populations. Another difference was the relationship between grain harvests and plague. Plague severity during the twentieth century has corresponded with bumper crops and times of plenty, when the health and population numbers of rats and their fleas have been boosted along with those of humans. By contrast, late medieval and early modern plagues coincided consistently with periods of dearth, even famine, as the demographic historian Henri Dubois has shown over the fifteenth century,[39] and more recently Frandsen has demonstrated for the Baltic region in the early eighteenth century. These plagues not only created periods of dearth, they came on the heels of food shortages and famine, when population resistance was low.[40]

Finally, a fourth pattern distinguishes the 'Second' from the 'Third Pandemic'. For most of the twentieth century, scientists had concluded that humans possess little or no natural immunity to *Yersinia pestis*.[41] Recently, however, they have revised these claims but only slightly: researchers have found in a study of Chinese plague patients (n = 65), that the antibody of *Yersinia pestis* has survived in 69.5 per cent of the patients ten years after infection.[42] But 'the immune mechanism against *Y. pestis* is extremely complex',[43] and 'specific memory T cell responses to *Y. pestis* proteins F1 and LcrV could not be detected in plague patients four to six years post infection'.[44] Furthermore, the experience since Yersin's discovery has been that acquired immunity has been short-lived, offering no protection against second attacks of plague; and no evidence thus far has charted populations adapting to the disease either by declining rates of mortality or morbidity, even in regions, such as the Punjab, that have been hardest hit by plague, or by changes in the age structure of plague victims. Unlike infectious diseases such as measles,

---

[38] See the careful recording of plague outbreaks in Siena and other places in Tuscany in the contemporary chronicle, *Cronaca senese di Donato di Neri e di suo figlio Neri in Cronache senesi*, ed. Alessandro Lisini and Fabil Iacometti, *RIS*, xv (6) (Bologna, 1936), i. 599–600, 654, 698, 737, 760, 768, 788, 794, 847, 849–50.

[39] Henri Dubois, 'La dépression: XVIe et XVe siècles', in Jacques Dupâquier, *et al.*, *Histoire de la population française* (4 vols., Paris, 1988), i. 327.

[40] Frandsen, *The Last Plague in the Baltic Region*, 22, 27, 46–7, 65.

[41] Robert Pollitzer, *Plague* (Geneva, 1954), 133, concluded: 'No convincing evidence is available to show that a natural immunity to insect-borne plague exists in man.' And for pneumonic plague: 'there can be little doubt that instances of natural resistance to pneumonic plague infection exist; [but] these are of such rare occurrence as to be of no practical importance' (p. 511). Also, see Pollitzer, 'Immunology', in Lien-Teh, Chun, Pollitzer, and Wu, *Plague: A Manual*, 92–138, esp. p. 114. More recent textbooks have followed Pollitzer's conclusions: for instance, the most used of the manuals for tropical diseases, *Manson's Tropical Diseases*, ed. P.E.C. Manson-Bahr and D.R. Bell (19th edn., 1987), 591, states that '[t]here is no known natural immunity to plague. Acquired immunity is short-lived and there is no protection against second attacks.'

[42] Li, *et al.*, 'Humoral and Cellular Immune Responses to *Yersinia pestis*'.

[43] *Ibid.*, 228.

[44] *Ibid.*, 223.

rubella and mumps, *Yersinia pestis* has shown no tendency to become a childhood disease. Children may have succumbed more readily to plague than adults in places such as on Indian reservations in the western United States, but their vulnerability results from their greater exposure to plague-infected rodents and fleas rather than from any physiological change in the overall population arising from greater exposure to the bacillus.[45]

Compare these twentieth-century patterns to those of the fourteenth and fifteenth century. Contemporaries, such as the pope's physician, Raymundo Chalmelli de Vinario, writing after four bouts of plague in 1383, boasted that rates of mortality and morbidity had declined sharply since the Black Death:

> In 1348, two thirds of the population were afflicted, and almost all died; in 1361, half the population contracted the disease, and very few survived; in 1371, only one tenth were sick, and many survived; while in 1382, only one twentieth of the population became sick, and almost all of these survived.[46]

While Chalmelli's assessment may have been exaggerated, last wills and testaments, burial records, and monastic and confraternal necrologies point in the same downward direction, charting a rapid adaptation between Black Death's pathogen and human hosts over the plague's first hundred years.[47] Furthermore, along with a steady decline in mortality, chroniclers across Europe from 1361 onwards described their plagues as ones of children. The contemporary chronicler of Pisa, Ranieri di Sardo, went further. By the third plague, in 1374, he recorded that 80 per cent of the plague deaths in his city were among those aged twelve or younger (precisely the number of years since plague had last hit Pisa).[48] A surviving parish register of Siena supports Ranieri's estimates. From the second plague in 1363 to the third in 1374, the proportion of plague deaths among children rose from a third to over half (136 of 233), and by the fourth, in 1383, children had become a staggering 88 per cent of the victims (230 of 260).[49]

---

[45] In India mortality rates occasioned by *Yersinia pestis* fail to show any pattern of adaptation: first they increased for a decade or more, then jumped randomly from year to year before declining in the 1920s, because rats (not humans) were acquiring immunity to the bacillus. (For these trends, see Cohn, *The Black Death Transformed*, 190–1.) Similar patterns of mortality and cases of infection can also be seen in Brazil, Thailand, Vietnam and other subtropical regions later in the century, even after the introduction of DDT, the use of effective antibiotics, and the adoption of modern sanitary measures. See the tables in Pollitzer, *Plague*, 22–27, 56–9.

[46] Cited in Hans Zinsser, *Rats, Lice and History* (New York, 1935), 89.

[47] For evidence of decline in other European cities, see Cohn, *The Black Death Transformed*, 192–203; and for further discussion of these records and trends, *idem*, 'Epidemiology of the Black Death', 86.

[48] *Cronaca di Pisa di Ranieri Sardo*, ed. Ottavio Banti, Fonti per la Storia d'Italia, xcix (Rome, 1963), 186.

[49] For 1348, the records are fragmentary and do not distinguish the burials according to age. Afterwards, the proportion fell to 67 out of 151 and 62 out of 182, in 1390 and 1400, respectively, lower than in 1383 but still higher than in the supposed children's plague of 1363; analyzed from *I necrologi di San Domenico in Camporegio (epoca cateriniana)*, ed. M.-H. Laurent, *Fontes vitae S. Catherinae senensis historici*, xx (Siena, 1937). In the late-fifteenth and sixteenth centuries, with increased spacing between plague outbreaks, the age of victims drifted upwards. For evidence of child mortality in medieval English plagues, see above, p. 54.

Signs and Symptoms Compared

Before interdisciplinary teams of microbiologists, archaeologists, and geneticists had turned to the analysis of ancient DNA, why had most historians and nearly all scientists assumed that the 'Second Pandemic' was the same disease as the 'Third'? The connection turned almost exclusively on the supposedly undeniable similarity of signs and symptoms between the two pandemics. In Ann Carmichael's words, 'Boccaccio leaves no doubt that bubonic *Y. pestis* ravaged Florence in 1348 ... If the bubo predominated as a sign, we could still be reasonably comfortable after five centuries that there was not much error in the ascription of a death to plague'.[50] Among medical authorities, Carmichael certainly has not been alone in adopting such a retrospective clinical analysis. After cautioning historians that signs and symptoms of diseases can be extremely malleable over time, and maintaining that, as a means of identifying diseases in the past, epidemiological evidence might prove more reliable, the double Nobel Prize winner and immunologist Sir MacFarlane Burnet appears to have forgotten his lessons when he came to plague.[51] Like Carmichael, he turned to Boccaccio's signs: they are 'enough to make it easy to recognize the disease ... we can be sure that the two greatest European pestilences, the plague of Justinian's reign (A.D. 542) and the Black Death of 1348, were both the result of the spread of the plague bacillus'.[52]

Were the signs of the two pandemics really so identical? Neither Burnet nor Carmichael mentions that Boccaccio goes on to describe other skin disorders seen with the Black Death: the larger swellings 'big as an apple and others the size of an egg' in the armpits and the groin, spread beyond the principal lymph nodes across plague-ridden bodies, along with black or blue spots (*macchie nere o livide*) on arms, thighs, and in other places, 'sometimes large and few in number, at other times tiny and closely spaced'. [53] These may have been purpuric and ecchymotic skin lesions caused by septic shock, and as such could accord with infection by *Yersinia pestis*. However, other physicians and chroniclers, such as Michele da Piazza describing plague in Sicily in 1347, Geoffrey le Baker on plague in England in 1348–9, and Giovanni Morelli recording plagues in late-fourteenth- and early-fifteenth-century Florence, note the frequent appearance of little pustules, sometimes brown, sometimes red, but mostly black, that covered entire bodies. These were a normal clinical feature of the 'Second Pandemic' from 1347 to the plague that swept across Malta, Corfu and other Greek Islands and into southern Italy (Naja) in 1814–15.[54] They could appear alone, covering infected bodies from head to toe, or along with larger buboes. These pustules were not incidental or unimportant signs of plague. In the Milanese death books, physicians of the city's

---

[50] A.G. Carmichael, *Plague and the Poor in Renaissance Florence* (Cambridge, 1986), 26, 79.
[51] Sir Frank MacFarlane Burnet, *Natural History of Infectious Disease* (3rd edn., Cambridge, 1962), 296.
[52] *Ibid.*, 323. The fourth edn., of 1972, updated by D.O. White, left this remark intact on p. 225.
[53] Giovanni Boccaccio, *Decameron*, ed. Vittore Branca (Milan, 1976), 10.
[54] S.K. Cohn, Jr., *Cultures of Plague: Medical Thinking at the End of the Renaissance* (Oxford, 2010), 61–5; *idem*, 'Epidemiology of the Black Death', 89; Frandsen, *The Last Plague in the Baltic Region*, 152, 161, 163, 493; and Vitangelo Morea, *Storia della peste di Noja* (Naples, 1817), 23, 103, 151, 181, 219, 263, 301, 438–9.

health board recorded them as afflicting over a third of the victims of six plagues from 1452 to 1524. Chroniclers such as Geoffrey le Baker in the fourteenth century and Giovanni Morelli in the fifteenth, as well as Paolo Bellintani, the Capuchin governor of *lazaretti* in Milan, Brescia and Marseilles in the late sixteenth, regarded them as the most deadly signs of plague. The afflicted might survive the larger glandular boils, but the lentil-like bumps led to certain death. The Milanese death books give credence to these judgments, even though precise rates of lethality cannot be calculated from them: those with the black spots tended to die slightly more rapidly than those with buboes alone.[55]

As Robert Pollitzer, J.W.H. Chun and other plague doctors of the early twentieth century observed: 'Plague is a disease of so protean a character that it would be misleading to generalize the results of observations in one or a few areas, however suggestive they appear to be.'[56] Indeed, Chun and other researchers, such as Atilio Macchiavello and N.H. Choksy, have observed 'dark pustules' (sometimes called 'plague smallpox') in plague epidemics of the twentieth century, as in Chile in 1903. But, by contrast with the 'Second Pandemic', they were never common, even as incidents of 'atypical plague'. More importantly, in the rare instances when they have appeared in the twentieth century, instead of being plague's most deadly signs, they signalled the very opposite: 'the pustules have been of low toxicity and their prognosis [has been] generally benign'.[57]

Finally, the six epidemics covered by the Milanese *Libri di morti* bring to bear 6,993 plague cases, in which the signs and symptoms, numbers and bodily positions of buboes and carbuncles, and whether pustules covered infected bodies, have been described in detail. The analysis of this evidence differs radically from clinical statistics compiled for plague epidemics in the Bombay Presidency in 1898, for various Indian hospitals from 1898 to 1909, and for plagues in two parts of China during the early twentieth century, comprising together over 15,000 cases. The Milanese patients displayed almost twice the proportion of multiple swellings (buboes and carbuncles) apparent in late-nineteenth- and twentieth-century cases. Even more striking is the percentage of buboes and carbuncles recorded during the Milanese plagues that strayed from the principal lymph nodes – under arms, in the groin, and in the cervical region, behind the ears and on the neck. While in as few as 2 per cent of the cases from China and 5 per cent from India buboes formed outside these lymph nodes, nearly a quarter of the larger swellings appeared elsewhere on victims' bodies during the Renaissance Milanese plagues. Many of them, moreover, formed in places where few, if any, buboes have been found in cases of modern plague – in the anus and vagina, on penises, noses, faces, foreheads, and even eyelids.[58] Evidence from other descriptions of plague during the 'Second Pandemic', as in Frandsen's recent survey of plague in numerous villages, regions, and cities during the last epidemics in the Baltic from 1709 to

[55]   Cohn, *Cultures of Plague*, 64.
[56]   Robert Pollitzer, 'A Review of Recent Literature on Plague', *Bulletin of the World Health Organization*, xxiii (1960), 361.
[57]   Atilio Macchiavello, 'Plague', in *Clinical Tropical Medicine*, ed. R.B.H. Gradwohl, Luiz Benitez Soto and Oscar Felsenfeld (1951), 444–76, esp. 460. Also, see N.H. Chosky, 'The Various Types of Plague and their Clinical Manifestations', *American Journal of the Medical Sciences*, cxxxviii (1909), 357; and J.W.H. Chun, 'Clinical Features', in Lien-Teh, *et al.*, *Plague: A Manual*, 322.
[58]   For these comparisons, see Cohn, *Cultures of Plague*, ch. 2, 'Signs and Symptoms'.

1712, shows that the Milanese cases were not atypical: here too buboes formed in vaginas, anuses, navels and the corners of eyes;[59] and similar patterns were observed at Naja during its plague of 1815.[60] Without photographs or illustrations to confirm these accounts, and allowing for changes in cultures of observation and terminology, it is possible that eye-witnesses describing the 'Second' and 'Third' Pandemics might have been seeing more or less the same cutaneous realities, despite their radically different reports. My point, however, is that these descriptions made across the two epochs of plague, separated by as many as 664 years, are not incontestably the same, and hardly make a retrospective diagnosis based on signs and symptoms as 'easy' today as prominent doctors and scientists of the twentieth century have assumed.

Conclusions

Let us return to the recent breakthroughs in the ancient DNA of the Black Death. Scientists now concur that the agent belonged to the *Yersinia* family of pathogens and was thus a bacterium, which, given the speed and spread over territory of the Black Death, is surprising. Such a rapid dissemination would be more likely with viruses. The genetic researchers have, however, also discovered that this agent was a variant of *Yersinia pestis* yet to be found at any place or time during the 'Third Pandemic' from 1894 to the present.

The significance of this second finding has yet to be fully digested by researchers into the Black Death and its successive strikes during the 'Second Pandemic'. Thus far, historians and scientists in their reasoning have returned to assumptions about the nature of the disease that have characterized investigations since at least 1913 and became particularly prevalent in the 1970s.[61] To explain the striking differences in the epidemiology of the two pandemics, some now question whether rats may have been necessary for the transmission of the late medieval and early modern plagues, that men and women of those epochs may not have been so blind as to have overlooked the supposed billions of rodents littering streets and lanes. Yet, at the same time, several of these researchers continue to assume that an insect vector was necessary to transmit the Black Death disease.[62] The weight has fallen mainly on the promiscuous *pulex irritans*. Often called the human flea, it also feeds on a number of mammals – rats, cats, dogs – and here lies its advantage. However, it is a flea with one of the lowest vector co-efficiencies in the transmission of *Yersinia pestis* to any mammal, especially from human to human. After speculating on the possibility of *P. irritans* transmitting the much more

[59] Frandsen, *The Last Plague in the Baltic Region*; see note 36 above.
[60] Morea, *Storia della peste di Noja*, 151, 188.
[61] See especially the work of J.-N. Biraben, *Les hommes et la peste en France et dans les pays européens et méditerranéens* (2 vols., Paris, 1975–6). Such speculations, however, reach further back. The earliest I have found is C.J. Martin in 1913: see note 63, below. They were also advanced by Ricordo Jorge, *Les anciennes épiémies de peste en Europe comparées aux épidémies mordernes* (Lisbon, 1932); and Ernst Rodenwaldt, *Pest in Venedig, 1575–1577: Ein Beitrag zur Frage der Infektkette bei den Pestepidemien West-Europas* (Heidelberg, 1953), 366–77.
[62] See Huffthammer and Walløe, 'Rats cannot have been Intermediate Hosts for *Yersinia pestis*', which seriously questions the presence of rats at times of historic plague but insists on an insect vector.

extensive plagues of the 'Second Pandemic', C.J. Martin in 1913 raised doubts: 'the direct transmission of the disease from man to man cannot, at the present time, be of frequent occurrence ... because in human cases the average degree of septicaemia before death is so much less than in rats that the chance of a flea imbibing even a single bacillus is small'.[63] Later, Graham Twigg added that 'man is a biological dead end' as far as plague goes.[64] In other words, unlike typhus, Lyme disease and various other insect-borne diseases, the bacterial concentrations in the much larger human are too low in the case of *Yersinia pestis* to infect a second human by a flea, much less by a tick or a louse that may have imbibed the infected blood from another human.

At present the evidence of *P. irritans* as the vector spreading plague is circumstantial.[65] Even where such evidence seems convincing, as with the household clustering of plague cases in Iranian villages in the 1960s, the disease has never reached epidemic proportions beyond small hamlets or villages, despite the lack of effective medical intervention (as in Iran) until the plague had run its course. The argument in favour of plague's spread by *P. irritans* or by another ectoparasite, such as lice (as has been recently proposed to explain the much quicker and wider dissemination of the 'Second Pandemic'),[66] faces further problems, especially in warmer Mediterranean zones. As noted above, here the disease was 'a summer contagion',[67] which regularly occurred during the warmest periods of the year, when (as Renaissance artists illustrate) people were wearing the least amount of clothing. Further, as chroniclers and story-tellers in Florence and Siena have revealed, even those among the upper echelons of the labouring classes went regularly to the baths.[68] Had *Pulex irritans* or lice been the vector,

---

[63] C.J. Martin, 'Insect Porters of Bacterial Infections: Lecture II: The Transmission of Plague by Fleas', *British Medical Journal* (11 Jan. 1913), i. 59–68, at p. 63.

[64] Graham Twigg, *The Black Death: A Biological Appraisal* (1984), 170.

[65] Most recently, see Anne Laudisoit, *et al.*, 'Plague and the Human Flea, Tanzania', *Emerging Infectious Diseases*, xiii (5) (2007), 687–93, who find a correlation between villages with higher frequencies of plague cases and a greater presence of the *P. irritans*, but admit that 'the vectoral status of *P. irritans* is still under discussion', and that, given the correlative nature of their results, other underlying factors may be at work: that the presence of this flea may only be 'a biologic indicator of the conditions that are conducive for the occurrence of plague in a village' (pp. 691–2). (I thank Professor J.L. Bolton for bringing this article to my attention.) But here, in contrast to the earlier evidence assembled by F.M. Laforce, *et al.*, 'Clinical and Epidemiological Observations on an Outbreak of Plague in Nepal', *Bulletin of the World Health Organization*, xlv (1971), 693–706, the authors of the Tanzania study do not produce circumstantial evidence that plague spread from person to person.

[66] See, for instance, Saravanan Ayyadurai *et al.*, 'Body Lice, *Yersinia pestis*, and Black Death', *Emerging Infectious Diseases*, xvi (5) (2010), 892–3. Their argument in favour of lice as a possible plague vector is based only on experiments in the laboratory with rabbits.

[67] Aeneas Silvius Piccolomini (Pope Pius II), *I Commentarii*, ed. Luigi Totaro (Milan, 1984), 1615.

[68] See, for instance, Giovanni Sabadino degli Arienti, 'The Tale of the Friar and Priest', in Lauro Martines, *An Italian Renaissance Sextet: Six Tales in Historical Context*, trans. Murtha Baca (New York, 1994), 71–92; or the expectation that Catherine of Siena as a young girl would visit the baths with her family. It is important to note that, well before the Black Death, there was a growing assumption that civilised people did not have vermin, as is apparent from a remark by the French physician, Henri de Mondeville (*d.* by 1330), who taught medicine at Montpellier. He recorded a remedy for destroying lice, adding that both the poor and members of religious orders were infested because of their phlegmatic and melancholic diets, '*similiter homines ferales qui de cultu sui corporis modicum currant*' [my italics]: Luke Demaitre, *Doctor Bernard de Gordon: Professor and Practitioner* (Toronto, 1980), 27–8. I am grateful to Carole Rawcliffe for this reference.

then the disease should have flared up most often during the cooler months of the year. Such speculations also assume that medieval people, even across social classes, were universally and consistently filthy, no matter where they lived or from what class they came.[69] Yet medical advice manuals and governmental legislation, spurred on by the devastation of medieval plagues, reveal that health authorities and the public were becoming increasingly aware of the connections between filth, uncovered latrines, the dumping of excrement and plague. Systems for collecting garbage and street cleaning, and even controls to keep individuals' houses in hygienic order, became more frequent by the sixteenth century; yet these plagues could return with vicious force, especially in Italy where such laws and controls were the most advanced.[70] In addition, even during the worst famines of Europe in 1848 or in Russia from 1921 to 1923, diseases such as typhus, with lice as vectors of person-to-person transmission, have never spread to an extent or at a speed comparable to the plagues of late medieval and early modern Europe.[71]

If we do not need the rats to transmit all variants of *Yersinia pestis*, why must we assume that an insect vector was necessary for the spread of the Black Death variant of this pathogen? The ancestor of this family, *Yersinia pseudotuberculosis*, which geneticists argue gave birth to the new strain of *Yersinia*, perhaps as late as on the eve of the Black Death, and which continues to survive today, does not rely on rodent hosts or the inefficient mechanism of a flea or any other insect for its transmission. Although its spread is still not completely understood, it reaches humans by the faecal-oral route, through contaminated food and water. Its symptoms, moreover, differ from those of *Yersinia pestis* and are similar to another strain within the *Yersinia* family – *Y. enterocolitica*. In historical times, these strains have lacked *Yersinia pestis*'s virulence; rarely have they killed their hosts

---

[69] Although plague, at least in places such as northern Italy, had become primarily a disease of the poor by 1400, chroniclers and diarists continued to record the names of aristocrats, cardinals, bishops, doctors, and other notables who died of plague, despite their ability to change clothing frequently, and their cleaner and more sophisticated lifestyles. Plague deaths reached the peaks of society, as in the case of Cardinal Ascanio Sforza, brother of the duke of Milan, and a prominent papal diplomat in 1485, and Giovanni Mocenigo, doge of Venice in 1505; *I diarii di Girolamo Priuli, 1494–1512*, ed. Arturo Segre and Roberto Cessi, *RIS*, xxiv (3) (4 vols., Città di Castello, 1912–41), iii. 377; and *Diario Ferrarese di Bernardino Zambotti, 1409–1502*, ed. Giuseppe Pardi, *RIS*, xxiv (7) (2 vols., Bologna, 1934–7), i. 170–1. See also the diary of the church official and notary, Johannis Burckardi, *Liber Notarum ab anni MDCCCCLXXXIII usque ad anno MDVI*, ed. Enrico Celani, *RIS*, xxxii (1) (2 vols., Città di Castello, 1910), for the names of many other notables felled by plague in Rome from 1485 to 1506, especially papal officials and courtiers.

[70] For these laws and medical awareness, see Cohn, *Cultures of Plague*, esp. ch. 8. Nor was Italy exceptional. As E.L. Sabine showed in the 1930s ('Butchering in Mediaeval London', *Speculum*, viii (1933), 335–53; and *idem*, 'Latrines and Cesspools of Mediaeval London', *ibid.*, ix (1934), 303–21), and Carole Rawcliffe has argued more systematically since ('Sources for the Study of Public Health', in *Understanding Medieval Primary Sources*, ed. Joel Rosenthal (London and New York, 2012), 177–95), the Black Death and successive plagues of the late Middle Ages encouraged the English to pay greater attention to public hygiene and private cleanliness.

[71] On the limited spread of typhus across Europe, see Paul Weindling, *Epidemics and Genocide in Eastern Europe 1890–1945* (Oxford, 2000), 14, 424–7, and appendix. Even when lice were so numerous that victims' bodies were encrusted with them, giving the impression of being covered in black fur, this disease did not spread as many had feared; and certainly not in a manner akin to the Black Death.

and they have never been responsible for epidemics.[72] By the fifteenth century, however, historic plague bears some resemblance to these *Yersinia* strains: vomiting and diarrhoea (and not vomiting of blood as observed during the Black Death and the earliest plagues of the fourteenth century) had become a consistent symptom of the plague observed in physicians' manuals and diagnoses of plague. Could the earlier variety of the ancestor *Yersinia* suddenly have developed pathogenic factors such as plasmids or, on the level of protein biosynthesis, abilities to form a capsule or to release endotoxin, thus suddenly transforming the benign *pseudotuberculosis* into a new and vicious pathogen, but without diminishing its ability to spread efficiently from person to person?

The question of virulence would now be relevant (and not, as scholars previously explained, because a more virulent strain of *Yersinia pestis* would somehow have enabled the Black Death to spread much more quickly and widely than the bubonic plagues of the 'Third Pandemic'). *Yersinia pestis* today is toxic enough – it is certainly one of the most toxic bacteria known to man. Given the mortality rates suggested by physicians in early modern plagues, especially during the later stages of an epidemic,[73] the modern bacillus may actually be more toxic than that of the pathogen of historic plague. Consequently, instead of reflecting its relative virulence, the reason for *Yersinia pestis*'s much lower rates of mortality compared to those of medieval and early modern plague rests on its much less efficient mechanisms of transmission. Only after killing off their rodent hosts must the hungry flea vectors seek out a much less desirable host – humans – for their blood meals, and because of the far greater body mass of humans compared to rats, much lower concentrations of the bacterium make the continuation of the chain of transmission highly unlikely. Already well before the genetic revolution and the availability of techniques for extracting ancient DNA, C.J. Martin speculated in 1913 that possible genetic changes in the pathogen would account for differences between Black Death and the plague he then confronted in India. He reasoned that 'a variation of the plague bacillus' would have had to have been 'in the direction of greater infectivity with perhaps diminished toxicity'.[74]

As Vivian Nutton asked in 2008, does knowing the causal agent of Black Death help to solve the problem of the vast differences in the character of plague between the 'Second' and 'Third' Pandemics?[75] If the agent is established as *Yersinia pestis*, how and why did the epidemiology of the 'Third' differ so radically from the 'Second' and probably also the 'First Pandemic' of the sixth to eighth century? If we accept the most recent conclusions that the agent of Black Death was a strain of *Yersinia pestis*, one in fact that has been unknown in modern times, we might also need to begin with new questions that acknowledge that a pathogen is not a

---

[72] Mark Achtman, *et al.*, '*Yersinia pestis*, the Cause of Plague, is a Recent Emerged Clone of *Yersinia pseudotuberculosis*', *PNAS*, xcvi (21) (1999), 14043–8; Julian Parkhill *et al.*, 'Genome Sequence of *Yersinia pestis*, the Causative Agent of Plague', *Nature*, ccccxiii (2001), 523–7; and Maria Fredriksson-Ahomaa, 'Epidemiology of Human *Yersinia pseudotuberculosis* Infection', *Archiv für Lebensmittelhygiene*, lx (2) (2009), 82–7.

[73] For numerous descriptions in sixteenth-century Italian sources of the decline in the virulence of plague during the last weeks or even months of an epidemic, see Cohn, *Cultures of Plague*.

[74] Martin, 'The Transmission of Plague by Fleas', 59.

[75] Vivian Nutton, 'Introduction', in *Pestilential Complexities*, ed. Nutton, 1–16, concludes: 'Indeed, one might argue that the identification of the agent of the Black Death with *Yersinia pestis* adds very little to what the historian could gain from the sources themselves' (p. 12).

'disease' (as the scientific community came to realise, Robert Koch included, around 1900).[76] Factors other than the pathogen – changes in climate, environment, and in the physiology of the hosts, and more – also play their part in changing relationships between pathogens and hosts, and thereby in the creation of new diseases and epidemics. As regards Black Death and the 'Third Pandemic', when and by what criteria does 'a strain' of a pathogen come to be reckoned as the causal agent of another 'disease', which has to be classified differently from that caused by a related pathogen of the same genetic family, as is currently recognized in the case of *Yersinia pestis* and its older relative, *Yersinia pseudotuberculosis*?[77] Even if scientists thought that the pathogens of the 'Second' and 'Third' Pandemics were identical (and now they do not), should we then return to the strict reductionism of Koch circa 1890, that a pathogen is the equivalent of the disease it in part causes, that it is the only pertinent defining feature? The extraordinary differences in the mechanisms of transmission, seasonality, speed of travel and diffusion between historic plague and the present *Yersinia pestis* certainly call into question any such equivalence.

---

[76] Christoph Gradmann, 'Robert Koch and the Invention of the Carrier State: Tropical Medicine, Veterinary Infections and Epidemiology around 1900', *Studies in History and Philosophy of Biological and Biomedical Sciences*, xli (3) (2010), 232–40; and *idem, Laboratory Disease: Robert Koch's Medical Bacteriology*, trans. Elborg Forster (Baltimore, Md., 2009). See also C.E. Rosenberg, 'Epilogue: Airs, Waters, Places. A Status Report', *Bulletin of the History of Medicine*, lxxxvi (4) (2012), 661–70.

[77] See note 72 above.

INDEX

Index

CONTENTS OF PREVIOUS VOLUMES

I

Concepts and Patterns of Service in the Later Middle Ages
ed. Anne Curry and Elizabeth Matthew (2000)

II

Revolution and Consumption in Late Medieval England
ed. Michael Hicks (2001)

III
Authority and Subversion
ed. Linda Clark (2003)

IV
Political Culture in Late-Medieval Britain
ed. Linda Clark and Christine Carpenter (2004)

Benjamin Thompson	Prelates and Politics from Winchelsey to Warham
Miri Rubin	Religious Symbols and Political Culture in Fifteenth-Century England
Caroline M. Barron	The Political Culture of Medieval London
Christopher Dyer	The Political Life of the Fifteenth-Century English Village
John Watts	The Pressure of the Public on Later Medieval Politics
Jenny Wormald	National Pride, Decentralised Nation: The Political Culture of Fifteenth-Century Scotland

V
Of Mice and Men: Image, Belief and Regulation in Late Medieval England
ed. Linda Clark (2005)

Jon Denton	Image, Identity and Gentility: The Woodford Experience
S.A. Mileson	The Importance of Parks in Fifteenth-Century Society
Alasdair Hawkyard	Sir John Fastolf's 'Gret Mansion by me late edified': Caister Castle, Norfolk
Jenni Nuttall	'*Vostre Humble Matatyas*': Culture, Politics and the Percys
Clive Burgess	A Repertory for Reinforcement: Configuring Civic Catholicism in Fifteenth-Century Bristol
Anne F. Sutton	Caxton, the Cult of St. Winifred, and Shrewsbury
Thomas S. Freeman	'*Ut Verus Christi Sequester*': John Blacman and the Cult of Henry VI
P.R. Cavill	The Problem of Labour and the Parliament of 1495
Colin Richmond	Mickey Mouse in Disneyland: How Did the Fifteenth Century Get That Way?

VI
Identity and Insurgency in the Late Middle Ages
ed. Linda Clark (2006)

Anthony Goodman	The British Isles Imagined
Andrea Ruddick	Ethnic Identity and Political Language in the King of England's Dominions: a Fourteenth-Century Perspective
Katie Stevenson	'Thai War Callit Knychtis and Bere the Name and the Honour of that Hye Ordre': Scottish Knighthood in the Fifteenth Century
Jackson Armstrong	Violence and Peacemaking in the English Marches towards Scotland, c.1425–1440
Matthew Tompkins	'Let's Kill all the Lawyers': Did Fifteenth-Century Peasants Employ Lawyers when they Conveyed Customary Land?

Simon Payling	Identifiable Motives for Election to Parliament in the Reign of Henry VI: The Operation of Public and Private Factors
David Grummitt	Deconstructing Cade's Rebellion: Discourse and Politics in the Mid Fifteenth Century
Jacquelyn Fernholz and Jenni Nuttall	Lydgate's Poem to Thomas Chaucer: A Reassessment of its Diplomatic and Literary Contexts
Maureen Jurkowski	Lollardy in Coventry and the Revolt of 1431
Carole Hill	Julian and her Sisters: Female Piety in Late Medieval Norwich

VII
Conflicts, Consequences and the Crown in the Late Middle Ages
ed. Linda Clark (2007)

Christine Carpenter	War, Government and Governance in England in the Later Middle Ages
Anne Curry	After Agincourt, What Next? Henry V and the Campaign of 1416
James Ross	Essex County Society and the French War in the Fifteenth Century
Michael Brown	French Alliance or English Peace? Scotland and the Last Phase of the Hundred Years War, 1415–53
J.L. Bolton	How Sir Thomas Rempston Paid His Ransom: or, The Mistakes of an Italian Bank
Catherine Nall	Perceptions of Financial Mismanagement and the English Diagnosis of Defeat
Hannes Kleineke	'Þe Kynges Cite': Exeter in the Wars of the Roses
Lucy Brown	Continuity and Change in the Parliamentary Justifications of the Fifteenth-Century Usurpations
Peter Fleming	Identity and Belonging: Irish and Welsh in Fifteenth-Century Bristol
Anthony Goodman	The Impact of Warfare on the Scottish Marches, c.1481–c.1513
G.M. Draper	Writing English, French and Latin in the Fifteenth Century: a Regional Perspective

VIII
Rule, Redemption and Representations in Late Medieval England and France
ed. Linda Clark (2008)

Carole Rawcliffe	Dives Redeemed? The Guild Almshouses of Later Medieval England
Kathleen Daly	War, History and Memory in the Dauphiné in the Fifteenth Century: Two Accounts of the Battle of Anthon (1430)

IX
English and Continental Perspectives
ed. Linda Clark (2010)

X
Parliament, Personalities and Power:
Papers Presented to Linda Clark
ed. Hannes Kleineke (2011)

XI
Concerns and Preoccupations
ed. Linda Clark (2012)

Printed and bound by CPI Group (UK) Ltd, Croydon, CR0 4YY

28/10/2024

14581363-0001